And a Seed was Planted

Volume I
Theoretical views and shifting perspectives

And a Seed was Planted

Volume I.
Theoretical views and shifting perspectives

Edited by
Hanneke van Bruggen
Sarah Kantartzis
Nick Pollard

Forewords by
Sridhar Venkatapuram
and
Elizabeth Townsend

w&b

MMXX

Published by Whiting & Birch Ltd,
London SE23 3HZ

ISBN 9781861776044 (this volume)
Set ISBN 9781861776242

Contents

Acknowledgements vii

Manifesto for occupation
Hanneke van Bruggen, Nick Pollard, Sarah Kantartzis ix

Foreword by Sridhar Venkatapuram xiii

Foreword by Elizabeth Townsend xv

Prologue to Volume 1: Theoretical views and shifting perspectives xvii

About the authors xix

Introduction to Section 1 1

1. Social Inclusion
Hanneke van Bruggen, Nick Pollard, Sarah Kantartzis 3

2. Introducing occupation
Sarah Kantartzis, Hanneke van Bruggen, Nick Pollard 24

3. Occupation-based approaches for social inclusion
Nick Pollard, Sarah Kantartzis, Hanneke van Bruggen 36

Introduction to Section 2: Theoretical views 55

4. Getting back my ability
Tim Diggles 57

5. Emancipatory occupation:
Labour as the conceptual basis for occupation-based social practices
Aline Godoy, Luciana Cordeiro, Cassia Baldini Soares 61

6. Reflections on occupation transforming citizenship
Hetty Fransen-Jaïbi, Inés Viana-Moldes, Nick Pollard, Sarah Kantartzis . 75

7. Facilitating inclusion through occupation-based community development
Roshan Galvaan 91

8. Social transformation in theory and practice:
Resources for radicals in participatory art, occupational therapy and social movements
Gelya Frank 107

9. Advancing understandings of inclusion and participation through situated research
Robert B. Pereira and Gail E. Whiteford 129

Introduction to Section 3. Shifting perspectives..147

10. Opening Doors
Ellen Ferguson, Mary Jardine, Elizabeth Firth 149

11. Social enterprise and occupational therapy: New ways of working and modernisation of the profession in Scotland
Gillian Funai...156

12. The Taieri Blokes Shed: A place of productivity and belonging
James Sunderland, Linda Wilson, and the Membership of the Taieri Blokes Shed 167

13. Decolonising imposed occupation: A preventative strategy for foetal alcohol spectrum disorder
Lizahn Gracia Cloete, Maria Konstabel, and Eve Madeleine Duncan...181

14. Promoting positive collective occupations in African settings: Exploiting the latent potentials for social inclusion and well-being
Tongai Fibion Chichaya 201

15. Including people with vision impairments in museums
Beaux Guarini and Alison Wicks 217

Index 231

Acknowledgements

We would like to thank all the contributors and the people who have worked with them, and with us, to make 'And a seed was planted…' possible. Putting together such a diverse collection of material translated from so many languages and with authors in locations across the world is always challenging, and always worthwhile., Two of our contributors, Linda Wilson and Ellen Ferguson, did not live to see their work published, and we would like to dedicate this project to their memories. There are lots of ways in which we have had help and contributions from our colleagues, friends and families from coffee and a bit of space to work in, to advice, for which we are grateful. We would especially like to thank everyone for persevering with us to publication.

Nick: I would like to thank Linda, Molly, Joshua, Daisy and Olivia for their patience and toleration during this project, including some unusual 'holidays', to facilitate meetings. Thanks also to the Occupational Therapy, Vocational Rehabilitation and Dietetics team and students at Sheffield Hallam University (past and present) for their continued support and interest in this work.

Sarah: Thank you to Christos, Katerina and Harry for your patience and understanding, and to our grandchildren, Lucas and Francesca, that arrived during this project and who give so much love and never ending joy! Thank you also to colleagues at Queen Margaret University Edinburgh for your continual support.

Hanneke: Thank you Sarah and Nick for working together and taking the long road together with all the contributors to the end of this project. Thanks also to Hotze, who patiently listened to me and continued to support me. Thanks to my daughters, Mieke, Floortje and Sanne, who still tolerate that their mother is sometimes "absent" because she "has to" work.

Manifesto for occupation

Hanneke van Bruggen, Nick Pollard, Sarah Kantartzis

Health through occupation

Occupational therapy is about enabling people to do activities that are necessary and important to them and through these to participate in the society of which they are part. 'Occupation' means anything a person *does*. The significance of doing is often overlooked because it is so fundamental to human existence. All our human stories are accounts of things we have done, to become who we are, and the expression of our belonging in a world with others. Through our doing we have constructed, and continue to reconstruct what we do, where, when, how, why and with whom. Occupation, or simply 'doing', is something common to all people everywhere, at all stages of life. It is important not only for what each of us can do in our lifetimes, but also for the kind of world we are building for the future.

There is a fundamental relationship between health and occupation. Through our occupations we are able to orchestrate our lives in ways that enable us not only to survive, but also to develop our potential and express our skills, while creating and maintaining our connections with others. Through our occupation we can develop and maintain our families, neighbourhoods and communities as sources of belonging, opportunities and common action. Occupation therefore is not only important to each individual, but also, through our collective occupation we develop the kind of lives that we live together. Occupation is an essential factor in life quality, and in the experience of being human.

However, occupation does not always lead to such positive and health supporting outcomes, and there are many challenges to meaningful and purposeful occupation for some people. These include disability; illness, trauma and disease; differences in access to food, water, shelter, transport, utilities; relative poverty; differences in social status and citizenship rights; differences in legal status; the economic and social consequences of war and other forms of conflict, climate and climate change; pollution; the planning and development of built structures; the effects of social change arising from shifts in population such as ageing, migration or resulting from disease such as HIV/AIDS; the consequences of disaster; personal tragedy; poor government; economic restructuring. The list is not comprehensive, and the factors can be combined in multiple forms with localised and specific effects.

Our concern is that the link between occupation and health has been consistently overlooked. In occupational therapy there has been an ongoing focus on the impact of illness, disease and trauma on the individual. There has been less attention paid to the social determinants of health and to the impact of social exclusion. Health promoting occupation is a key element in public health and in preventing ill-health. Overlooking this has restricted working with the potential of occupation to express and support human flourishing and develop healthy communities.

We argue that the expression of human health is more than an index of outcomes or therapeutic interventions. We support a view of health as not a stable and normative concept but as unbounded and potentially ever extending, incorporating notions of people's flourishing, the ongoing satisfaction of needs and the development of their potentials as fully included members of the society in which they live. We are calling for a discussion about the value and importance of occupation, not just for occupational therapists alone, but for everyone in health and social care and human sciences. We are calling for a rethink of the way health outcomes relate to personal and collective experiences and human values which are based in the understanding of doing. We need to work with others in reclaiming the value of occupation for all and as an important part of public health.

We are also concerned that the idea of occupation is bigger than can be realised through the profession of occupational therapy. Access to health promoting occupations can be a goal for social changes. These occupations have the potential to be owned by everyone, as they are concerned with how we live together and can be based in shared experiences. However, the knowledge and experience that is common to all is not always valued simply because of its common ownership, so there is a role for some people to critically explore ways to make this value more evident. Again, this should engage both those who are occupational therapists and people who are willing to work with them. The future of evidence for the transformative power of occupation is through co-production, participant action, and the sharing of the discussions about it with others.

A call for change

In order to promote health through occupation we need to work to address the multiple factors that influence people's possibility to engage in health promoting occupation. We need to work together to move forward, to create opportunities for all, to achieve individual and societal flourishing. We need to work in partnership, across sectors, disciplines, political and social divides to create the conditions for change in our education, practice and research. To do this we must:

- Build and maintain active dialogues, and negotiate alliances and strategies with disadvantaged and excluded groups and individuals, disability groups and carers' organisations, practitioners and researchers.
- Effectively campaign for health promoting occupation including participation rights across all levels of disability and social barriers
- Develop different forms of action from protest to social enterprises which exemplify and are underpinned by health-promoting occupation
- Challenge the acceptance of social and the resulting health inequalities, through occupation-based practices and particularly those that incorporate sustainable and inclusive economic growth

Call for contributors

This call for change requires multiple partnerships with many and diverse actions. In considering our own potential contribution to this process we consider that it may be useful to develop a book that will provide both theoretical discussions but also discussion of practical and specific projects and actions. We intend that the book will set out examples of practice, narratives, research and theory which explore, explain and promote the connection between occupation-based practices, social inclusion and health. Our intention is to solicit contributions from a wide range of stakeholders, individuals and chapter-writing teams, including: lay persons, service users, administrators, students, professionals, building a 'tapestry' of experiences and ideas that is not only a textbook but a manual for practice, accessible to all. It will address:

- Understanding the importance of occupation in people's lives and its links with the social determinants of health, public health and prevention.
- Why occupation based practice and occupational therapists? Towards a wider awareness of occupation, and making sense of what occupational therapists might offer community groups.
- How occupation based practice fits in wider perspectives of social inclusion work
- Moving from occupational therapy practice based around individuals to occupation based practice with groups and communities
- The particular characteristics of occupation based practice, including:
- Identifying significant variations with occupational therapy practice in traditional settings, including professional boundaries, compartmentalization of responsibilities and being a community member;
- Recognising change – critical moments and turning points;
- Managing risks and dependency;
- Professionalism and power with vulnerable people as colleagues;
- Managing delegation and responsibility for sustainability;
- Common sense, tacit knowledge and articulating occupation;
- Project and change management, progress and timescales
- Strategies for identifying outcomes for funders, partners and managers;

Thank you

Foreword

The argument that the purpose of politics and the polity is to enable citizens to pursue flourishing lives is most often linked to Aristotle, the ancient Greek philosopher (330 BCE). Centuries of discussions and debates have taken place and still continue regarding various aspects of this argument such as what is a flourishing life, who is included as a citizen, what are the boundaries of politics, what are good processes for governing a polity, and so forth. There has also been much discussion about whether this argument can be reconciled with various religions, including Christianity, as well as the possibility of such an argument in other societal political traditions. For example, tall pillars erected during the reign of the first Buddhist emperor Ashoka (220 BCE) identify various entitlements of citizens and instructions for living a good life.

While it may not be apparent to people outside, academic political philosophy in the Anglo-American world has been thriving over the past few decades because various philosophers have revived the direct conversation with Aristotle and Ashoka by putting forward what they argue to be theories of a good and just society for the modern world. In some cases, individuals have put forward a theory of a just world, or global justice. The person often credited with instigating this activity is John Rawls (1921-2002). In 1971, in his book, *A Theory of Justice*, he laid out critiques of various secular approaches to a good society and then put forward a careful argument for the purpose of some basic social institutions, what citizens are entitled to, how they should engage with each other in mutual cooperation, and so forth.

One of the curious and frustrating things about Rawls's stupendous effort is that he did not give sufficient consideration to health. The state of one's physical and mental functioning directly affects what one can be and do on any given day as well as what plans one can make and the life one can pursue. So how can something so important not be included in the consideration of what public institutions are meant to do, and how fellow members of society should treat each other? One plausible explanation is that Rawls, like many other individuals, particularly in the United States, believed that health is a 'natural good.' Health is seen as something that luck /nature gives to some people or takes away. Health is also something that individuals control through their personal behaviours. And, society addresses poor health through provision of sufficient income to individuals that will allow the purchase of adequate 'healthcare' to return them back to normal functioning. And, without going into much detail, Rawls thought that people who are born severely impaired or who will never return to 'normal' should be dealt with by charitable institutions – not our justice promoting institutions. Given his quite monumental project to articulate a theory of a just and well-ordered society, he was focused on the 'typical' or 'ideal' individual that is able bodied and interested in pursuing a flourishing life. Similarly, he wanted to focus on one society before thinking about a world with many societies, some of which may not even share some of the basic tenets of his just society.

Rawls's theory has received enormous scrutiny resulting in both criticism and praise. Nevertheless, across the discipline and world over, he is credited with bringing back our philosophical attention to the idea of social and global justice, or the question of a good society. Other philosophers have responded to Rawls, and all theories previous to his, by offering their own alternatives. They all start from the point that all human beings are morally equal and value freedom. And from here, different theories focus on what individuals are entitled to from their social environments including public institutions as well as how people should treat each other. Now, while this has been going on in academic literature, it is not hard to see that the same questions are in play in 'real world' politics across the world. Who is included in a society? What are they entitled to? Which institutions are required and which are not? What makes a good institution? How should citizens treat each other?

It is against this background that it is profoundly exciting to see Occupational Science seeking to identify its moral or ethical mission. One could situate Occupational Science as part of health institutions that constitute basic social institutions. That is, Occupational Science is part of a basic social institution whose primary purpose is social justice, or enabling individuals to pursue flourishing lives. Or, more courageously, Occupational Science could aim to stand on its own and assert that it seeks to enable flourishing lives everywhere—within and outside health institutions. Nevertheless, in either case, linking a science to a moral mission requires rigorous and careful reasoning that cuts across the sciences and humanities. And importantly, it requires a clear engagement with a conception or theory of social justice, or a good society. The present volume reflects the kind of deep empirical engagement and mutual reflection between Occupational Science and social justice philosophy we need right now.

I personally feel enormous pride and delight that Occupational Science academics and practitioners have found something helpful in my argument for health justice, and the capabilities approach more generally. While I invite and look forward to further engagement, I also want to encourage a much wider engagement with all the other philosophical approaches to social and global justice. The idea that there is a group of people who believe in and aim to help individuals, particularly those that are marginalized in a society, to be and do things in their lives that they value, should be more widely known and appreciated. Philosophers will benefit from knowing that it is not just a theoretical argument, but embodied in the work of Occupational Science practitioners. And Occupational Science will likely benefit from seeing all the variety of conceptions of justice and how philosophers reason and justify arguments for equity. The present volume represents the start of such an engagement, and I hope, will initiate a new phase in both Occupational Science and in our broader reasoning about social and global justice.

Sridhar Venkatapuram
London

Foreword

What an accomplishment! With *And a Seed was Planted* the European editors and a global array of authors have created a unique book about transforming societies day by day. Here is a book full of ideas and examples for globally minded persons who are committed to engagement 'with' versus doing 'to' others in promoting health, well-being, and justice around the world.

And a Seed was Planted offers a collection of very interesting approaches to complex, global issues based on citizen participation, not relying on top down governmental action. The projects are socially minded with awareness that policies, economics, rituals, and other social structures are at the root of social exclusion, inequity, poverty, and other conditions that persists to this day across parts of Europe, Asia, Africa, South, and North America. It's interesting to consider that some readers may find the approaches described here as ordinary because they are based on engaging people in day-to-day occupations like gardening and employment. Yet these are radical approaches because they challenge the status quo for marginalized or vulnerable groups, like the persons with visual impairments or refugees, whose participation in daily life is restricted beyond their individual conditions. Transformation is of concern here particularly in times and places where disabled people and others face restricted participation, including their lack of voice and choice in health and social services.

This book should attract any practitioner who engages participants in projects with aims for transforming societies anywhere in the world. Hopefully occupational therapists will be especially pleased to see projects that, to me, illustrate the untapped potential of this profession to create an occupationally just world. In seeing occupational therapy's potential with the examples and projects in this book, readers may imagine new ways to link day-by-day life with health, well-being, and daily life.

As an occupational therapist with 50 years experience, I celebrate the book's reclamation of engagement in occupation – action beyond talking – and the commitment to practices that illustrate funding and approaches outside as well as inside medical systems. Despite global job pressures, from salaries and job descriptions to standardized protocols and evidence-based practice based on individualistic, biomedical priorities, the authors present an array of ways in which occupational therapists can break away. Community occupational therapy, government policy-based occupational therapy, justice-oriented occupational therapy, occupational therapy leadership, and related ideas are all championed and legitimized through the authors' stories.

Why am I so enthusiastic? Clearly I love the ideas and practice examples in *And a Seed was Planted*. I also love the accessibility of these in seven clearly organized sections. Section 1 nicely introduces Social Inclusion, Occupation, and Occupation-Based Social Inclusion, plus a story by an artist with a difficult life. The book is more than a collection of practice stories with Section II illuminating *Theoretical Views* related to projects, and Section III on projects that profile *Shifting Perspectives*. Section IV (*Learning Inclusion*) and Section V (*Projects*) together include 12 chapters of wonderful examples of occupation-based social inclusion practices. Beyond the neatness of the book's structure, I also love *Occupation-Based Social Inclusion* because the projects illustrate the intent of the 1948 Declaration of Human Rights (United Nations) with its naming of education, housing, employment, and other everyday sites for doing human rights and justice. Amartya Sen (2009) might see the projects described here as real life ways to reduce what he called 'inclusionary incoherence', referring to gaps between ideas like justice, and everyday realities.

Finally, congratulations are due to the team that made *Occupation-Based Social Inclusion* possible. After what must have been many hours of collaboration, translation, and editing, the editors and authors can be proud of their invaluable gift to the English-reading world. With their efforts, English-readers are privileged to learn about innovative approaches to occupation-based social inclusion around the world.

Elizabeth Townsend, PhD, OTRegPEI, FCAOT
Professor Emerita, Dalhousie University
Liz.Townsend@Dal.ca
Adjunct Professor, University of Prince Edward Island
etownsend@upei.ca

Prologue to Volume 1
Theoretical views and shifting perspectives

Occupational therapy originated in social reform, but early in its history became allied with medicine, a biomedical perspective and a focus on individual health. Over the last two decades the profession has recognised the value of the work of its pioneers and argued for principles such as occupational justice and the right to health-promoting occupations, social inclusion, and for forms of involvement based in the community which centre around people doings things together for social change. In *'And a seed was planted...' Occupation based approaches for social inclusion* the Editors have set out to show how these ideas are being put into practice internationally.

This is the first volume of this three-volume set. It opens with three chapters in which the Editors offer an introduction to the main concepts discussed throughout the set – social inclusion, occupation including the links between occupation and health, and approaches to occupation-based social inclusion.

The following chapters are organised in two sections, Theoretical Views and Shifting Perspectives. With contributions from Africa, Australasia, Europe, South America and the United States of America, authors draw on ideas such as critical theories and citizenship which until recently have been unfamiliar territory for occupational therapists. Further chapters explore perspectives of practice from the global South, the viewpoints of service users, and shifting institutional and community practices.

About the authors

Dr Tongai F. Chichaya lectures in Occupational Therapy, at Bournemouth University, England

Lizahn Gracia Cloete BSc(OT),MSc(OT),PhD(OT) is with the Division of Occupational Therapy, Faculty of Medicine and Health Sciences, Stellenbosch University, South Africa

Luciana Cordeiro, PhD is Associate Professor, Faculty of Medicine, Federal University of Pelotas, Brazil

T. Diggles is retired but still making art using photography, words, and drawings. He is Chair of Stoke-on-Trent based arts organisation The Cultural Sisters Core Group, and a member of the Photographers' Collective North Staffordshire, England

Eve Madeleine Duncan, BAHon(psych), MscOT, Dphil (psych), is with the Division of Occupational Therapy, Faculty of Health Sciences, University of Cape Town, South Africa

Miss Ellen Ferguson service user. Unfortunately Ellen has passed away since contributing to this book

Elizabeth Firth is an occupational therapist technical instructor in mental health

Hetty Fransen-Jaïbi is with the Division of Occupational Therapy, École Supérieure des Sciences et Techniques de la Santé de Tunis, University of Tunis, Tunisia

Gelia Frank is a Professor and cultural anthropologist on the faculty of the Departments of Occupational Science & Occupational Therapy and Anthropology at the University of Southern California

Gillian J. Funai, Bsc (Hons) Occupational Therapy is a Highly Specialist Occupational Therapist with NHS Tayside, Scotland

Roshan Galvaan, Professor, Division of Occupational Therapy, Department of Health and Rehabilitation Sciences, University of Cape Town, South Africa

Beaux Guerini is a PhD candidate at the Faculty of Arts and Design, University of Canberra, Australia

Mary Jardine is an occupational therapist

Sarah Kantartzis is a Senior Lecturer in the Division of Occupational Therapy and Arts Therapies, Queen Margaret University, Edinburgh, Scotland

Taieri Blokes' Shed was established in 2008 as a place for retired men in Dunedin, in Aotearoa/New Zealand to have a social outlet and engage in projects which provide value and enhancement to the local community. The blokes' shed has over 50 members, and was one of the first in the South Island.

Robert B. Pereira is Care Coordinator, Hospital Admission Risk Program, Barwon Health, Geelong, Victoria, Australia, and Adjunct Associate Professor, Discipline of Occupational Therapy, School of Public Health and Nutrition, Faculty of Health, University of Canberra, Bruce, Australian Capital Territory, Australia

Nick Pollard is a Senior Lecturer in Occupational Therapy at Sheffield Hallam University.

Cassia Baldini Soares, RN, MPH, PhD is Associate Professor, Department of Collective Health Nursing, School of Nursing, University of São Paulo, Brazil

James Christin Sunderland MOccTher, PGDipp OccTherPrac, BA, NZROT is with The School of Occupational Therapy, Otago Polytechnic, Dunedin, New Zealand

Hanneke E. van Bruggen, Hon. Dscie, Bsc OT, FWFOT, is Director of Facilitation and Participation of Disadvantaged Groups (FAPADAG), The Netherlands, Senior Lecturer, Ivane Javakhishvili Tbilisi State University (TSU), Georgia, Adjunct Professor, Dalhousie University, Canada, and Honorary Research Fellow in the school of Health Sciences in the University of Kwazulu-Natal, South Africa

Aline Godoy Vieira, PhD is a Collective Health researcher., School of Nursing, University of São Paulo, Brazil

Inés Viana-Moldes is with the Department of Health Sciences, Campus de Oza, Coruña, Spain

Gail E. Whiteford is Principal, Whiteford Consulting, Port Macquarie, New South Wales, Australia,and Adjunct Professor, Discipline of Occupational Therapy, School of Public Health and Nutrition, Faculty of Health, University of Canberra, Bruce, Australian Capital Territory, Australia

Linda H Wilson, PhD, MSc, DHA, NZROT, NZCAET, was a senior academic in the Department of Occupational Therapy, Otago Polytechnic, Dunedin, Aotearoa/ New Zealand. The first occupational therapist from her country to be awarded a Fulbright scholarship, she was instrumental in the development of the profession. She passed away in 2017.

Dr Alison Wicks is Adjunct Associate Professor at the University of Canberra, Australian Capital Territory, Australia

Section 1
Introduction

In 2014, the editors of this book wrote a manifesto for occupation (see page ix) with a call for change to promote health through occupation, to challenge the acceptance of social and the resulting health inequalities through occupation-based practice, and to develop different forms of action from protest to social enterprises which exemplify and are underpinned by health-promoting occupation. Now, even more than before, we see the need to work in partnership, across sectors, disciplines, political and social divides to create the conditions for change in our education, practice and research.

What the writers in this volume (and scholars in general) mean by inclusion and exclusion and the specific groups and social problems they refer to varies by context. The context-dependency of social inclusion is more than a question of labelling. 'Many synonyms – solidarity, cohesion, social capital, integration – are in use in different settings. But it is also the case that the conception of belonging, membership, and citizenship that undergirds such terms draws upon history and culture of particular places' (Silver, 2015, p.3).

In the first chapter of this introductory section we will briefly look at the concept, the history, the context and the contemporary relevance of social inclusion. The second chapter will then offer an introduction to the concept of occupation and the links between health and occupation. In the third and final chapter of this section, approaches towards social inclusion in general and related to occupations will then be described and illustrated with examples of the chapters which have been contributed by authors from throughout the world.

Reference

Silver, H. (2015) *The Contents of Social Inclusion.* DESA Working Pager no. 114. New York: United Nations

Chapter 1
Social Inclusion

Hanneke van Bruggen, Nick Pollard, Sarah Kantartzis

Inclusion

Inclusion brings diversity and creates problems of definition and complexity. This arises from the confluence of cultural and socioeconomic differences, differences in access to resources, geographical and infrastructure differences, different political systems and even time zones. The concept lacks universality in the way it has been defined and employed and it lacks a coherent theoretical core (Buckmaster & Thomas, 2009). Social inclusion is often used interchangeably with the terms social cohesion, social integration, and social participation, (although these can be quite different things) positioning social exclusion as the opposite. The latter is a contested term that refers to a wide range of phenomena and processes related to poverty and deprivation, but it is also used in relation to marginalised people and places. The discussion hereafter is largely based on literature from the northern hemisphere where the concept of social inclusion/exclusion originated. It is restricted primarily to the English language. We are aware that there is considerable literature in other languages that we have not taken into account.

History

Acts and practices of including or excluding others as aspects of systems of stratification may be as old as much of humanity itself. Certainly, most societies display some degree of taboos and customs concerning forms of both social rejection and social acceptance (Radcliffe-Brown, 1952).

A very early form of social exclusion is evident in the role of ostracism (a method of temporary banishment by popular vote without trial or special accusation practiced in Athens, Greece, during the 5th century BC (Merriam Webster Dictionary, 2016), when the provision of an official mechanism to institutionalise ostracism was enacted. The law of ostracism was instituted as a means to protect the young democratic institutions from the revival of tyranny (Allman, 2013).

Whilst the Ancient Greeks are universally renowned for asserting citizenship rights and the dignity of the individual, these were only extended to Greek males - women and non-Greeks were considered inferior. Furthermore in ancient Greek society the pursuit of physical and intellectual fitness was essential; there was little room for people with any form of flaw or imperfection. However, both the Greeks and Romans developed 'scientifically' based treatments for people with acquired impairments. Aristotle, for example, attempted to study deafness and Hippocrites tried to cure epilepsy (Barnes, 1997).

Forms of social exclusion have often concerned differences. Sometimes these have been in terms of perceived disability or because of the fear of the spread of disease, as might be evident with the historical treatment of people with conditions such as leprosy, who were frequently housed in colonies outside cities or on islands. However, it was recognised that they had to be cared for as a Christian duty, and such care was regarded as a path to holiness (Porter, 1997).

With regard to the confinement of people with mental health problems in the 19th century, an interweaving range of social and economic factors may be seen as contributing to these exclusionary processes. Porter (1990) argued that their incarceration was not due to a fear of social contamination but because it became possible to run a madhouse as a profitable business. He disputed Foucault's (1972) claim of an age of confinement starting in the 18th century, but suggested that the development of large institutions in the 19th century were largely due to state bureaucracies acting *despite* the protests of some doctors. People of all classes were confined in the charitable and state institutions developed in the 19th century. Previously madhouses were subsidised mostly by people with sufficient means to afford to pay a madhouse keeper to maintain a family member who was an embarrassment, while pauper lunatics might be subjected to the more precarious regimes of neighbours or workhouse masters (Walton, 1981). Porter (1997; 1990) and Jay (2003) reported the public social concerns that led to the reformation of madhouse keeping, the development of moral treatments and the regulation of asylums. Many people continued to feel that the best place for people with mental health issues was with the family.

If religious duty was in part responsible for the establishment of hospitals, leper colonies and early psychiatric care, religion has also been used as a marker of difference, emphasised in order to promote the interests of one group over another. In Spain, for example, the gradual reconquest of the Iberian Peninsula from the Muslims who had invaded in the early 8th century, began primarily as a territorial conflict. In fact, Christians and Muslims fought both with and for each other, and both they and the Jewish community lived in a degree of mutual tolerance but with separate customs and types of participation in the economy and religious observances (Kamen, 1997). Earlier, in Northern Africa, where Jews and Muslims had established a mutual tolerance, Christianity began to spread through a series of schismatic movements, which at the same time aimed to preach to and convert parts of the local population. This process of conversion was aimed at dividing those who might more easily be converted from other sections of the population. Jews were seen as more amenable to proselytising, on the basis that Jesus was the messiah foretold in the scriptures (Oliver, 1999).

However, by the 11th century the Catholic reconquista had acquired the characteristics of a holy war (Runciman, 1965), and by the 13th century Christian monks and town councils were beginning to treat the people who had converted to Christianity with suspicion. Kamen (1997) suggests that much of this persecution seems to have arisen through the popular resentment of Jewish financial success, particularly in urban areas where Jewish traders and financiers tended to live. In rural areas people seemed to be more accepting of religious difference. Demands for their expulsion seem to have had religious motives following accusations that recent converts continued with their former religious rites. Increasingly the toleration of Jews, Muslims and of the converted New Christians began to break down, so that by the reign of Ferdinand and Isabella (1479-1516), under whom the reconquest of Spain was completed, the process of inquisition, or investigation into religious sincerity or heresy, began.

The reconquista was coterminous with a series of crusades, which originated largely in Germany and France, but involved some popular mass movements from all over Europe. Jewish merchants were often a source of loans to knights and princes in the medieval conflicts which took place throughout the continent. Borrowers realised that persecution was more cost effective than repayment of their debts, and this was combined with the characteristics of religious fervour. As crusades moved through eastern Europe on their way to Palestine, Jewish communities were often plundered and massacred to meet the costs of a marching army. None of the crusading movements maintained their religious character for very long, and many of the mostly Norman nobility involved saw them opportunistically as providing lands and wealth that might be unobtainable through inheritance at home. Crusading armies were composed of many different nationalities and often fraught with internal rivalries over status and command. By the time they had arrived in the East discipline and order had often broken down. The victims of their lust for wealth were as likely to be local orthodox Christians as local Muslims. The conflict was not continuous, however the Europeans failure to adapt to local lifestyles and their consequent susceptibility to diseases meant a constant demand for migrants, with the result that colonies struggled to survive and failed to integrate.

The long term consequences of these invasions, their brutalities and their inward looking colonisation can still be felt in the Islamophobia of the present; they contrast with the assimilation of culture which had occurred through the Muslim invasion of Spain, and the influence which occurred through the Islamic scholarship made available to Europeans in the reconquest period. However, in Spain the subsequent Inquisition resulted in persecutions of converted Jews and Muslims, and included the burning of Arabic texts. Through the early 17th century many people were displaced, or migrated to North Africa. Moriscos (people who were formerly Muslim) were often sold into slavery (Kamen, 1997).

Cultural difference has also long been an element in social exclusion and not infrequently linked to religious differences. An example which was particularly important in the pattern of British colonisations is that of the plantation of Ireland which began in the 16th and 17th centuries. The defeat of rebel catholic Irish earls in the late 1500s and their flight from Ireland in the early 1600s made their lands available to colonisation in the form of plantations which were rented to English, Scottish and other largely Protestant groups of settlers. Large numbers moved to Ireland, establishing a pattern whereby native Irish people were thrown off the land, as the settlers returned a higher profit for their landlords (Lydon, 1998). Comparisons might be drawn between these activities and the pattern of colonisation in the early days of European influence in America, where the plantation model was also adopted by English companies hoping to make profits by encouraging people to settle in new territories. Philbrick (2006) details how the Native Americans at first aided the new colonists, showing them how to adapt to their new environment with advice on agricultural techniques and food sourcing that enabled them to survive their first winter. However, this co-operation and tolerance soon deteriorated, and the first generation born in America came into conflict with Native Americans as they sought to expand their land ownership. This quickly hardened into a racial conflict, in which Native Americans were targeted with attempts to eradicate them through disease, the wholesale massacre of communities, and the export of prisoners for slavery. Native American communities eventually recognised that their only chance of survival was to drive the English back to the sea, but exploiting differences between the various groups enabled the settlers to defeat them.

The fragility of mutual tolerance between very different groups is also evident here. Although the Native American communities engaged in a somewhat ritualistic conflict from time to time, the emphasis of their society appears to have been mainly concerned with coexisting with their environment. However, they lived in a number of communities with different languages, sometimes quite different cultures and in many accounts of colonisation these differences have made people amenable to exploitation and division which eventually become a focus for practices of exclusion, and situations in which they were drawn into more serious conflict with each other. In addition, cultural differences make it possible for one group to regard the other as somehow less than human. In the case of Native Americans it was their responses to provocations, in particular some of their practices with regard to the torture of prisoners (Philbrick, 2006) – that in some groups was a ritualistic endurance of pain expected of a warrior (Debo, 1995) – which enabled the settlers to justify how they could be enslaved, or treated as vermin.

Although slavery as a practice was very widespread and the slave trade had already been long established in Africa before the colonial era, it was due to a disregard of humanity which came with European colonisation for profit that made it conceivable to operate slave systems in the Americas on a vast scale. The consequences have reverberated around the world in terms of a continuing inequality, and from which civil rights and black consciousness have themselves been a key part of the philosophical basis for liberation movements for other groups, such as people with disabilities. Ultimately in modern times cultural differences have been exploited to the extent that people have been processed industrially through death camps, even though populations have lived in proximity for hundreds of years; or in other regimes subjected to generations of humiliation through systems of segregation such as South African apartheid and the institutionalised racism practised in Guatemala in the last century (Hale, 2006).

In some instances there have been successful attempts to resist the dangers of colonial invasion. One of these might be Japan, whose governments kept foreigners at a distance through the operation of restrictions on contact and trade. This was initially due to the fear of Chinese influence, but it applied to other contacts with British, Portuguese, Russian, French and Dutch traders and naval expeditions, until eventually in the 19th century it became evident that it was impractical to continue because of Japan's defence needs (Cullen, 2003). The foreign threat was potentially of destabilisation, and Japanese society valued its status quo, even if there were internal disputes and problems. Aoyama (2012) describes how the perceived threat of Russian expansion into disputed areas in the North of the Japanese archipelago altered a policy of colonisation and exploitation towards the aboriginal Ainu people living there into one of forced and systematised assimilation and the denial of their culture.

All of these examples of social exclusion have a long historical taper into the present. The reduction of the native Irish population in the 16th and 17th century continued in successive centuries with many people migrating in search of seasonal agricultural work and industrial work in Britain, or emigrating to America where they made up some of the communities of urban poor (Riis [1890] 1997). In Britain, many such migrants were criminalised for the petty offences they often committed for survival who were transported as prisoners to Australia during the 18th and 19th centuries (Linebaugh, 1991; Hughes 1987), and later as economic migrants. Whereas the rest of Britain had achieved its industrial revolution sometime in the 19th century, Ireland continued to struggle economically well into the 20th century. In the north, policy in Ulster failed to address the needs of large, mostly catholic, sections of the community. This exacerbated the traditions of sectarianism, which dated from the colonisations of the 17th century by Scots and English settlers. Eventually the scale of migration was such that the economy of Ireland was partly sustained by its diaspora sending its wealth back to the 'old country' (Wright, 1992).

The tension between England and its Northern Irish province has in the past drawn comparisons with apartheid in South Africa and French colonialism in Algeria (Wright, 1992). Although he was writing before the conclusion of the peace settlement in Ulster, Wright explored the historical perspective of a range of colonial conflicts and warned that the problems of achieving reconciliations were complex and multilevel, requiring a political will to recognise the extent of the issues as well as community actions.

The legacy of the Algerian civil war and French colonisation in North Africa led to considerable numbers of migrants living in some of the larger cities in France. This gave a colonial context to the discussion of the concept and terminology of social exclusion/inclusion which figured prominently in French policy discourse in the mid-1970s (Bigea, 2016). This was an interesting development as in 1974 France had suspended non-European immigration, with the consequence that the Algerian and other North African people working in France settled in what became known as *les banlieues* - cheap social housing situated in city suburbs. Previously many of these workers had only lived temporarily in France, but the legislative changes meant that they might not be able to return to their jobs if they went home for a short period, instead they brought their families to live with them.

Beaman (2015) contends that French republican ideology does not recognise difference but assumes that everyone in the Republic is French. In its intention this confers equality on everyone who is French irrespective of their ethnic or cultural origin, but policy does not match the experience of cultural and ethnic difference. Parts of France have a very diverse population. Being French involves many characteristics, and Beaman (2015) found that people made a distinction between the apparent legal inclusion and the cultural experience of exclusion. Bigea (2016) argues that the inherent failure which arises from this policy to recognise the experience of difference has led to both the rise of extremism and disaffection in the Muslim communities and the strengthening of the far right wing Front National.

While the concept of social inclusion was later adopted by the European Union in the late 1980s as a key concept in social policy and had, in many instances, replaced the concept of poverty; for immigrant groups it came to mean an approach which was largely about integration, where the responsibility for the process was transferred to migrant populations. People coming into just over half the European Union countries found that they had to learn the language and pass tests on citizenship, or pass informal interviews (Goodman, 2010), perhaps a practical process but one which also involves the redefinition of one's identity and the socialisation and remodelling of one's otherness into assimilable form. How this affects individuals depends very much on their circumstances. The absence of border controls facilitates movement and perhaps allows people to construct themselves as broadly European, or in combinations of regions, nationalities and localities to which they feel they may belong irrespective of their actual origins. Yet many people still find they are different, at the bottom of a ladder which has already been pulled up (De Roo et al, 2016), and in which they have to pass the tests in order to integrate into a society which sets the agenda. This is a complex issue. Byrne (2016) points out that for some migrants to the UK testing may be intended to demonstrate a policy of tighter controls and a narrower perspective of culture, but is experienced positively by migrants as part of the passage to becoming a citizen.

As this book was under preparation a further development unfolded in the story of migration in Europe, with the 'refugee crisis' of 2015 and onwards, and while such population shifts are not unusual in history as we have seen, the long term contemporary implications are still to unfold.

Les exclus

The concept of social exclusion, as it appeared in France and Europe in general, was tied to the effect of the failure of integrative institutions. The concept has its roots in the functionalist social theory of Emile Durkheim (O'Brien & Penna, 2008). Writing at the turn of the 20th century Durkheim was concerned with how social order and stability could be maintained in a society where social dislocations accompanied the transitions from an agrarian to industrial society. His policy recommendation was the creation of 'corporative organisations' or community betterment groups, whose purpose would be adjusting people's social identities to conform with changes in the economy. That raises the question of how can we include people and groups into structured systems that have systematically excluded them in the first place. In a Durkheimian sense, this implies assimilation to the dominant culture.

The publication of *Les exclus* by René Lenoir in 1974 was a milestone in the emergence of social exclusion as a concept. His main concern was his estimate that one in ten inhabitants of France were being left aside by the country's economic and social development. As we have already explored, the republican ideology of France with regard to the inclusion of its citizens may have been monolithic. In July 1998 a law was approved in France to prevent and combat social exclusion through guaranteed universal access to fundamental rights. This law mandated coordinated interventions in at least ten spheres: employment, training, social enterprise, minimum substance income, housing, health, education, social services, culture and citizenship (for example, helping the homeless to vote) (Loi 98-657, du juillet 1998).

In the French republican tradition, a great deal of weight is placed on citizenship and on the importance of social solidarity. In this tradition, social exclusion is conceived not simply as an economic or political phenomenon, but as a deficiency of solidarity, a break in the social fabric (Silver, 1994). The concept of citizenship and social integration which underlies the notion of social exclusion in this French tradition is difficult to grasp for people working within a liberal individualist tradition, which permeates Anglo-Saxon thinking. It sees citizenship as a social contract based on the possession of equal rights by all individuals, and views social integration in terms of freely-chosen relationships between individuals, rather than a relationship between the individual and society (Silver, 1994). But this sharp conceptual divide has not prevented the wider adoption of the term and a broad approach to tackling it in the policy and rhetoric of the European Union. The main architect for its spread was Jacques Delors, President of the European Commission in the 1980s, who sought to promote a social dimension to European integration. In 1997 the European Social Protocol, which guaranteed the fundamental social rights of workers, was incorporated into the Amsterdam Treaty in which the Union committed itself to establish a common area of freedom, security and justice. The European Social Inclusion Strategy was part of the 2000 Lisbon Strategy which aimed to make a decisive impact on the eradication of poverty by 2010 (Buckmaster & Thomas, 2009). Due to the economic downturn, social inclusion in Europe has shifted from a broad matter of social and economic functioning to a narrower concern with employment and the sustainability of benefit systems (Daly & Silver, 2008).

The concept of social inclusion gained widespread applicability after the World Summit for Social Development (1995) as a result of which, increasing attention has been paid to the possible relevance of the concept to social policy analysis in developing countries (Kabeer, 2000), and it was widely adopted by development agencies and in development studies as another way of understanding and reducing poverty. Given its roots in northern policy discourse, there is a danger that this conceptualisation of social inclusion will promote a tendency to assess southern realities in terms of the extent to which they converge or diverge from some 'standard' northern model (Kabeer, 2000). The relevance to less economically developed countries continues to be questioned to the extent that most definitions take for granted strong governance, a welfare state and a largely established formal economy. Yepez (1994) questioned the value of speaking about social exclusion in countries where people have never been integrated through a welfare state system. At the same time there is the danger that exclusion may be used as a screen to hide extreme poverty and as a blaming label to make the poor responsible for their condition (Mathieson, 2008).

Understandings of inclusion and how they are enacted may not always be positive. Assimilation often means acculturation or the end of group practices, solidarity and beliefs. Languages become extinct and tribes can no longer maintain their social and cultural practices. Inclusion sounds good but without questioning the determining conditions and interests there can sometimes be a pressure for minorities to conform inappropriately to the majority's needs.

Social exclusion is frequently defined in relation to social inclusion. This signifies the importance of being "included" as part of society (European Foundation, 1995, p.4). This view is also implied in the DFID/World Bank (2005) definition of social inclusion. This dualistic or binary logic has been criticised by several authors on various grounds (O'Reilly, 2005; Hanney, 2002; Jackson, 1999). O'Reilly (2005, p.84), for example, argues:

> 'The language of inclusion and exclusion implies a binary logic, that one is either included or excluded... (however) people are included or excluded in relation to some variable. The question of inclusion, therefore, is best conceptualised as a sort of sliding scale rather than as a binary function, so that inclusion and exclusion are the extreme poles of a continuum of relations of inclusion/ exclusion.'

The concept of social inclusion is often meant to include only the excluded. This requires that the excluded have first to be identified. This leads to the question as to how much inclusion for the excluded is needed (before a certain result/state/desired place is obtained), and where the actual tolerance limits for inclusion are placed. Who is to be the beneficiary of less exclusion/more inclusion, and what are the mechanisms for this to be enacted? (Oyen, 1997). All these questions and many more need to be answered before we can start using the concepts of social exclusion and social inclusion as valuable tools in occupation-based practice.

Context of social inclusion

The place where one lives contributes to social inclusion, identity and access. Places of residence vary in resources, facilities and social composition. Border controls, immigration and naturalisation laws are just some of the spatial exclusionary mechanism with social, economic, political and cultural effects. Social inclusion and exclusion are context dependent concepts in at least three senses.

Firstly, the paradigm of an inclusive society varies by political philosophy (Silver, 1994). Political liberals envisage social inclusion as a consequence of state-guaranteed freedoms to exchange property, ideas and make cross-cutting networks. Republican political ideas in the French tradition stress the social bond, the solidarity of equality to achieve the collective good. Social Democrats emphasise the social rights of citizens to a decent minimum standard of living in return for active contributions to society (Silver, 2015). A more inclusive interpretation of social inclusion is identified through social justice ideology. Here acts of community engagement and participation are foregrounded (Gidley et al, 2010). Religious paradigms generally are built on a community of believers who submit to one or more divinities and their rules. Social inclusion is conceived in many different ways depending on the ideology through which the concept is addressed (Silver, 2015).

Secondly, the different histories, cultures, institutions and social structures in different places make some dimensions of social inclusion - economic, social or political - more important than others. For example, in some European countries class conflicts tend to be emphasised, while in India the exclusion of lower castes is an issue, and in the histories of United States and South Africa racial cleavages are more present. Formal citizenship excludes non-citizens from most rights and obligations of the nation. National conceptions of social inclusion are often embedded in the law and other institutions that regulate entry, such as schools, official languages, recognised religions and so on. National contexts shape the policy approaches to social inclusion in economic, social and political life (Silver, 2015).

Thirdly, the neighbourhood, where someone lives, shapes access to resources and opportunities, ultimately affecting one's health, education and economic outcomes (Silver, 2015; Marmot, 2013). Growing up in a poor neighbourhood can have an impact on verbal and cognitive development, well-being, employment and income and it increases exposure to crime and violence (WHO, 2008). As a consequence there can be strong social and economic pressures within communities for people to move in search of better opportunities, and for other people to be displaced as they are unable to maintain their social position. Differences between neighbouring communities can intensify over a complex range of factors linked to opportunities and access to resources; investment is withdrawn from those communities with less to offer the economy. Much of today's global political disruption can be linked to the demographic, spatial, economic, and knowledge transitions that are transforming societies (World Bank, 2013). Complex demographic transitions have significant social impacts. Globally, the youth cohort is the largest in history, living mostly in developing and conflicted countries. This phenomenon requires action to include young people in services, markets and social and cultural spaces. Additionally, migration is likely to become a more dramatic demographic process than fertility or mortality. Urbanisation was one of the biggest transitions of the previous century, and it will continue to unfold in the present one. Cities are increasingly polarised between people who have access to basic services and people who do not.

The context-specific and complex nature of social inclusion/exclusion also results in different countries being at different stages in overcoming social exclusion. While inclusion is usually a desirable object the application depends on the context.

Social in/exclusion and health

The Social Exclusion Knowledge Network of the Commission on Social Determinants of Health (WHO, 2008) defines social exclusion as consisting of dynamic, multidimensional processes driven by unequal power relationships interacting across four main dimensions – economic, political, social and cultural – and at different levels including individual, household, group, community, country and global.

It results in a continuum of inclusion/exclusion characterised by unequal access to resources, capabilities and rights, which leads to health inequities. In this definition, 'resources' refers to the 'means' that can be used to meet human needs and 'capabilities' to the relative power people have to use the resources available to them. This definition of social exclusion focuses on multifactorial relational processes driving differential exclusion. Poverty, exclusion and stigmatisation are a reality for millions of people, resulting in illness and poor well-being. People at risk of social exclusion from society are more likely to die prematurely due to unhealthy occupations and lifestyles as well as poor living and working conditions (WHO, 2008), and these do not simply affect the person in the present, but over their full lifetime and impact upon the lives of subsequent generations. There is a broad consensus that health in general, and health inequalities in particular are strongly related with socio-economic determinants and that the degree of marginalisation influences the well-being of individuals and groups (Marmot, 2013; WHO, 2008). Mortality rates tend to be lowest in countries that have smaller income differences and thus have lower levels of relative deprivation/ poverty. The existence of wide- and widening- socioeconomic differences in health shows how extraordinarily sensitive health remains to socioeconomic circumstances (Wilkinson & Pickett, 2010). In a Neoliberal focus, unemployment, inequality, and poverty have become increasingly blamed on individuals rather than on structural constraints (Passas, 2000). Neoliberalism and its repercussions have led to many changes at the state-level, the international-level, and the individual-level. Such changes include the dismantling of the welfare state, the growing reality of global inequality, and the individualisation of all actions.

Ensuring healthy lives and promoting wellbeing for all at all ages is impossible without also a consideration of mental health. Inequality within and among countries cannot be fully addressed unless we recognise that nearly a quarter of the world population - the number who experience a mental illness each year - experience systematic discrimination in most areas of life (Thornicroft & Patel, 2014). The fundamental point is that mental health is an integral part of health (WHO, 2016a). Mental and substance use disorders are the leading cause of disability worldwide; about 23% of all years lost because of disability are caused by mental and substance use disorders (WHO, 2016b).

One of the approaches to secure population health improvement is promoting social inclusion policies and strategies (Marmot, 2013; UN DESA, 2009; WHO, 2008).

Social inclusion and disability

Social inclusion is recognised as a general principle (article 3), a general obligation (article 4) and a right (articles 29 and 30) in the United Nations Convention on the Rights of Persons with Disabilities (CRPD) (United Nations, 2006). The convention embraces the diversity of human experience and advocates for the full inclusion and participation of people with disabilities in society. It is also an explicit goal for community-based rehabilitation (CBR) services in many countries (WHO, 2010). The World Health CBR guidelines have a strong focus on empowerment through facilitation of the inclusion and participation of disabled people, their family members, and communities in all development and decision-making processes. However, the European Disability Forum's (EDF, 2014) alternative report highlights that the overall purpose of the UN CRPD - to promote, protect and ensure the full and equal enjoyment of all human rights and fundamental freedoms by all persons with disabilities - has not been realised today in the European Union. Freedom of movement, as one of the key principles and rights of all EU citizens, is not being met for persons with disabilities or their families in the EU. Persons with disabilities are still discriminated against in many areas of life and since the financial and economic crisis, are experiencing increased poverty and social exclusion. Also, a UN report (2016) highlights Government failure to uphold disabled people's rights in Great Britain, in particularly tightening of criteria to access social care and the closure of the Independent Living Fund, disproportionately affected persons with disabilities and hindered various aspects of their right to live independently and be included in the community.

The Sustainable Development Goals (SDGs), adopted by the General Assembly at the United Nations Headquarters on 25 September 2015, contain seven explicit references to persons with disabilities, including in relation to health, education, employment, accessible cities and transport and disaggregation of data (UN, 2015b). For many of the SDG targets there is need for urgent action for inclusion of persons with disabilities (poverty, social protection, health coverage, violence against women, sexual and reproductive health, access to water and sanitation, resilience to disasters, birth registration). In the first year of the implementation of the 2030 Agenda it seems that the global political and economic environment for its implementation has become even worse (Reflection group on the agenda 2030, 2016).

Whether these reforms result in better lives for people with disabilities is still yet to be seen. The assumption that the path to social inclusion is unidirectional, involving people with disabilities making a journey to mainstream contexts without any expectation that non-disabled people need to make the return journey, should be challenged. Community participation for people with disabilities almost invariably implies assimilation into mainstream culture. Rather, it should involve mainstream culture seeing itself through other's eyes (Milner & Kelly, 2009).

Social inclusion is at risk of being an ideology and may lead to ineffective strategies; it is still mainly defined as the acceptance and achievement of the dominant societal values and lifestyle, which may lead to moralistic judgements (Cobigo et al, 2012). Persons with disabilities can experience mainstream social values as oppressive (Milner & Kelly, 2009; Schneider & Bramley, 2008). Certain patterns of social inclusion may undermine minorities' ways of living and suppress cultural diversity or can lead to an unwanted imposition of uniformity (UNRISD, 2015). This is not only applicable for persons with disabilities, but for all kinds of minority groups, such as First Nations, or LGBTQ people.

Five key attributes of social inclusion emerged in a participatory action research study by Milner & Kelly (2009) with 28 young adults with disabilities as important qualitative antecedents to a sense of participatory membership and belonging: self-determination, social identity, reciprocity and valued contribution, participatory expectations and psychological safety.

Broadening our understanding of inclusion in ways that accommodate qualitative indicators has benefits for all partners. When people without disabilities experience being 'out of place' or are confronted by disability art or moments of collective agency of persons with disabilities, they are permitted glimpses of the 'alternative imaginings' of community, permitting those on the 'inside' of society a chance to listen to and learn from communities on the 'outside' in a collective endeavour to construct inclusive ways of being together (Milner & Kelly, 2009).

From a position of recognition we now move to constructing inclusive ways of being together through participating in occupations and local communities. A good example of being together was Latin America's first Paralympics in 2016, which will be remembered as the peoples' games where the people of Rio turned out in their droves to support athletes of all countries. More countries than ever before won at least one Paralympic medal, and for the first time ever an Independent Paralympic Athletes team took part featuring two refugee athletes.

Social inclusion in what?

Because the concept is based on an assumed mainstream society, to which the excluded are held to aspire, the criteria for integration and membership are the acceptance of the dominant values and way of life. Partly as a result of this, the question, inclusion into what? (that is, inclusion into what sort of society?) tends to be neglected. Rather than challenging the status quo and raising questions as to how society/community might be made more inclusive the concept can, in a weakened form, serve to normalise and unquestioningly strengthen existing arrangements.

Our concern should not only be with the groups or conditions that are excluded, but also with the socio-economic rules and political powers that create excluded groups and conditions, and the social groups who benefit by this.

There is no agreement in the literature about how and where social inclusion can be enacted or applied, and it seems to be dialectic to include more people into social systems stratified by exclusion even while trying to transform these systems. It remains at best a wrestling match between 'the imperatives of revolution and the pragmatics of reform' (Labonte, 2004, p.121).

However, there is in general more or less consensus of what is required to address exclusionary processes:

* Create the conditions necessary for entire populations to not only meet but go beyond basic needs through access to education, health care, labour markets and community resources
* Enable participatory and cohesive social systems, opportunities for social participation
* Value diversity, freedom from discrimination
* Guarantee peace and human rights
* Sustain environmental systems (UN 2015a; Labonte et al, 2011; SEKN, 2008)

In general participation in social activities is seen as social inclusion. Sen (2001, p.74) writes,

> 'Inclusion is characterized by a society's widely shared social experience and active participation, by a broad equality of opportunities and life chances for individuals and by the achievement of a basic level of well-being for all citizens.'

This shared vision about what it means to be included in society is crucial, as it underlines support for inclusionary measures.

Social inclusion and participation

The idea of participation is central to many attempts to define social inclusion. However, a number of authors have gone further than this and argued that participation, rather than inclusion, should be the main focus of efforts to address social exclusion. Such authors suggest that it is the more active logic of participation, rather than the relatively passive logic of inclusion, that is most likely to address the problem of exclusion.

This has probably been described most directly by Heinz Steinert (2003), who argues that the concept of inclusion implies the necessity to conform with dominant social norms and demands. In contrast, he argues, an approach based around participation assumes the need, necessity and democratic right to participate to a degree and in ways that are constantly negotiated and contested. Steinert's definition of social exclusion therefore focuses directly on participation:

> 'Social exclusion can be understood as the continuous and gradual exclusion from full participation in the social, including material and symbolic, resources produced, supplied and exploited in a society for making a living, organising a life and taking part in the development of a (hopefully better) future' (Steinert & Pilgram, 2003, p.5).

He identifies political, economic, social and cultural exclusion as arising, respectively, from deficiencies in citizenship, lack of resources, isolation and deficits in education. Participation can be thought of as active citizenship.

Participation is, like social inclusion, a rich concept that means different things to different people in different settings. Arnstein (1971, p.3), through 'The Ladder of Citizen Participation', noted that there are citizen participation variants ranging from nonparticipation, tokenism to total citizen control. Depriving people of resources is tantamount to incapacitating them when it comes to participation. In some cases, participation has been viewed as an attempt to deprive the marginalised members of society of equal access to resources and job opportunities (UNHRC, 2014).

> 'At the core of most definitions of social inclusion lies the concept of full participation in all aspects of life, while exclusion refers to the conditions (barriers and processes) that impede inclusion. Participation is most significant as it denotes an active involvement in the process, not merely having access to society's activities, but engaging in them, and building and maintaining a social network. Participation also creates a sense of responsibility towards others, a community or an institution, and influences decisions or enables individuals to have access to the decision-making processes' (United Nations Department of Social and Economic Affairs (UN DESA), 2009, p.12).

Social inclusion as a process and in the context of development

The 1995 World Summit for Social Development (WSSD) in Copenhagen affirmed that social integration was one of the key goals of social development and that the aim of social integration was to create a 'society for all' (UN DESA, 1995). The Summit recognised that the extent of social integration was an important determinant of, and was significantly affected by, poverty and unemployment. There was wide consensus that global threats require a multidimensional response, including efforts to address the social side of the macro-economic equation, particularly in light of the widening gap between the rich and poor, and the deteriorating conditions in which many people struggle to survive. Social integration is used in the World Summit on the basis of the promotion and protection of all human rights, as well as on non-discrimination, tolerance, respect for diversity, equality of opportunity, solidarity, security and participation of all people, including disadvantaged and vulnerable groups and persons.

'Social inclusion is understood as a process by which efforts are made to ensure equal opportunities for all, regardless of their background, so that they can achieve full potential in life. It is a multi-dimensional process aimed at creating conditions which enable full and active participation of every member of the society in all aspects of life, including civic, social, cultural, economic, and potential activities, as well as participation in decision making processes' (UN DESA, 2009, p.3).

Recent political developments, such as austerity measures cutting benefits, diminishing health and education services, and making jobs more temporary as well as the immigration crises, stress the contemporary relevance of social inclusion and have drawn public attention to the corrosive effects of deep inequalities in both the global North and the global South (UNRISD, 2014). Social inclusion is a significant factor in development and requires policies that recognise the importance of societal levels of analysis, not simply economic or individual indicators.

The global sustainable development goals (UN, 2015a) as well as the WHO global strategy on people-centred integrated health services (WHO, 2015) focus on inclusion, community engagement, empowerment, in/equalities and in/accessibility. Local participation in community development has become a central theme in the international movement for inclusionary development. Yet underneath this public embrace lies notable uncertainty about what exactly local participatory development means, what it can achieve, and how well service providers know how to support it. Participatory programmes are expected to enhance civic capacity, empower marginalised communities, increase government accountability, improve service delivery, reduce poverty, and more. However, participation is often costly for the poor, both in terms of the political risk it entails and the time and resources they are asked to invest in development programmes from which they may not benefit.

The world is undergoing important social transformations driven by the impact of globalisation, global environmental change and economic and financial crises, resulting in growing inequalities, extreme poverty, exclusion, migration, violence and the denial of basic human rights. These transformations demonstrate the urge for innovative solutions conducive in all sectors to universal values of peace, human dignity, gender equality, health equity, distribution of power and non-violence and non-discrimination (UNESCO, 2015; UN, 2015a)

Approaches to social inclusion

Strategies to address social inclusion require attention to three cross-cutting processes: recognition of diversity, redistribution of resources and justice, and representation of political voice (UN DESA, 1995). Recognition can be understood in two ways: inter-subjectively and institutionally. In relation to inter-subjectivity, Honneth (2001) and Taylor (1994) state that misrecognition and denied recognition are forms of oppression and lead to a negative self-image. Groups which experience repeated stigmatisation internalise negative self-images. Honneth distinguishes three fundamental recognition relations. Firstly, love relationships: these are typically bonded to the institution of families and enable us to gain a basic confidence; secondly legal relationships that enable us to understand ourselves as autonomous individuals and thereby make possible self-respect; and thirdly, relations of solidarity, relationships in which individuals express appreciation for each other's practices and lifestyles. Such relationships are necessary for self-esteem.

Nancy Fraser (2000) argues that being misrecognised is being denied the status of full partner in social interaction, as a consequence of institutionalised patterns of cultural value. Misrecognition arises when institutions structure interaction according to cultural norms that impede parity of participation. For example, women cannot participate in the labour market and politics on equal terms as men, because of care responsibilities which are the result of the internalised norm that care activities are considered female activities. Nonrecognition or misrecognition can inflict harm and can be a form of oppression (Fraser, 2000).

These two approaches to recognition can be distinguished as 'inter-subjective' recognition (Honneth, 2001, Taylor et al, 1994) and 'institutional' recognition (Fraser, 2000). Both are fundamental to social inclusion. Inter-subjective recognition issues are not only important to the achievement of institutional recognition, they are also important to the achievement of redistribution. Issues related to recognition are integral to working towards social inclusion.

Legal and symbolic recognition of minority rights and cultural practices is central to questions of identity and diversity. It does not, however, always lead to a reduction in inequalities in access to services or in well-being (Hopenhayn, 2008). Promoting equality of rights and opportunities for disadvantaged groups requires redistribution of resources as well as legal recognition of difference (Fraser, 1995).

Representation and participation in decision making is a human right and of value in itself. It is also a means of ensuring redistribution of public resources to disadvantaged groups. Participatory processes focus on both formal political representation as well as broader consultative processes as well as full participation in occupations.

Social inclusion could be considered as a means to understanding and responding to disadvantage (Perkins, 2010). This disadvantage can take many forms, including marginalisation, discrimination, segregation and abandonment (Daly & Silver, 2008). However, how this disadvantage is addressed in occupation-based practice is of ongoing debate and will be partly demonstrated in the chapters hereafter. Social inclusion promises to be a new, 'multidimensional' approach to the problems of poverty, disadvantage, and social polarisation, an approach that takes the economic, health and social into account, and focuses on processes as well as outcomes.

Social inclusion enables human freedom and involves having opportunities for personal development, wellbeing and a minimally decent life (Sen, 1992). Exclusion constrains the development of basic functionings and the complex capabilities required for full participation in community life (Sen, 2000). However, a capabilities approach may be criticised for focusing too much on individual agency rather than the broader structure it takes place within (Lister, 2004). Baser and Morgan (2008) define a capability as the collective skill or aptitude of system or community to carry out a particular function or process either inside or outside the system. Capabilities enable a group or community to do things and to sustain itself. Baser and Morgan (2008) have grouped these collective skills into five core capabilities that contribute to the overall capacity and sustainable and inclusive development of a system or community. Empowerment is critical to capacity development and is a key element of the core capability to commit and engage. The other core capabilities are to: generate development results; relate; adapt and self-renew; and balance diversity and achieve coherence. All five capabilities are necessary to ensure the optimum capacity (including inclusive issues) of a community.

Labonte (2009) argues that 'forcing' the inclusion of groups into the society that has historically and politically excluded them, without critically examining structures and hierarchies, may perpetuate oppressive hierarchies and health inequities. Labonte points out that uncritical application of social inclusion discourse can divert attention away from hierarchies of exclusion and those who benefit from them. Social inclusion is focused on transformational social change and creating a just and equal society. A combined focus on social inclusion and exclusion is required to create the social conditions for equal citizenship and to address the structural inequalities sustaining exclusion (Labonte, 2009).

Social inclusion is multi-dimensional, and should be approached from various angles. The following five dimensions of inclusion may be considered as incremental steps to social inclusion:

1. *Visibility*: to be noticed; to be recognised
2. *Consideration*: one's concerns and needs are taken into account by policy makers
3. *Access* to social interactions; people must be able to engage in society's activities and social networks in their daily life, including economic, social, cultural, religious, and political activities
4. *Rights*: rights to act and claim (including right to be different, 'identity'), right to access quality and accessible social services (housing, education, transport, healthcare, etc.), right to work, right to participate in the cultural life
5. *Resources* to fully participate in society: social and financial resources are key; other important aspects also need to be taken into account in the possibility to fully participate, such as time, energy, spatial distance, power ... (UN DESA, 2009)

Achieving 'inclusion' is rarely a simple process of increasing incomes or enhancing access to economic opportunity or services; nor can it be addressed only through specific interventions in a single sector (health, education). It requires more complex change in social structures, institutions, relations and norms (institutions); and attention to intersecting forms of disadvantage across economic, social, political and environmental spheres (intersections) (UNRISD, 2015). It is concluded that health inequalities cannot be tackled by the health system alone but only together with inter-sectoral cooperation and multidisciplinary approaches.

Finally, social inclusion is intuitively understood to be a worthy objective; however, the call for social inclusion is paradoxical in that it both expresses a genuine desire to tackle the consequences of social inequality and yet at the same time could become co-opted as a modern form of moral and social strategy which reproduces and legitimises the prevailing socio-economic order. On the one hand it offers the promise of emancipation through the resolution of social exclusion and yet it simultaneously becomes another way in which the disadvantaged are subject to social, moral and economic regulation. To ensure that social inclusion does not become a buzzword, vigilance is needed to the context in which inclusion policies are implemented, and the possible consequences of their adoption as a moral imperative. Uncritical use of social inclusion can blind us to the use, abuse and distribution of power.

The above described cross cutting processes and the chapters hereafter reflect the multi-dimensional aspirations and discussions around social inclusion.

References

Allmann, D. (2013) The Sociology of social inclusion. *Sage Open*, 3, 1-16

Arnstein, Sherry. R. (1971) A ladder of citizen participation. *Journal of the Royal Town Planning Institute*, 35, 4, 216-22

Aoyama, M. (2012) Indigenous Ainu occupational identities and the natural environment in Hokkaido. in N. Pollard and D. Sakellariou (Eds.) *Politics Of Occupation-Centred Practice*. Oxford: Wiley-Blackwell (pp. 106-127)

Barnes, C. (1997) A legacy of oppression: A history of disability in western culture. in Barton, L and Oliver, M (Eds.) *Disability Studies: Past Present and Future*. Leeds: The Disability Press (pp. 3– 24)

Baser, H., Morgan, P. (2008) *Capacity, change and performance study report*. ECDPM Discussion Paper 59B. European Centre for Development Policy Management, Maastricht, the Netherlands

Beaman, J. (2015) Boundaries of Frenchness: Cultural citizenship and France's middle-class North African second-generation. *Identities* 22, 1, 36-52

Bigea, G. (2016) France: The French Republican model of integration. A potential driver for extremism. *Conflict Studies Quarterly*, 16, 17-45 [Accessed 25 November 2016 at http://www.csq.ro/wp-content/uploads/CSQ-_16.pdf]

Buckmaster, L. and Thomas, M. (2009) Social Inclusion And Social Citizenship – Towards A Truly Inclusive Society. Research paper No. 08 2009–10 Australian Government. [Accessed 25 November 2016 at http://www.aph.gov.au/About_Parliament/Parliamentary_Departments/Parliamentary_Library/pubs/rp/rp0910/10rp08]

Byrne, B. (2016) Testing times: The place of the citizenship test in the UK immigration regime and new citizens' responses to it. *Sociology*, [Accessed 30 November 2016 at http://soc.sagepub.com/content/early/2016/02/02/0038038515622908.full.pdf+htmlDOI: 0038038515622908]

Cobigo, V., Ouellette-Kuntz, H., Lysaght, R. and Martin, L. (2012) Shifting our conceptualization of social inclusion, *Stigma Research and Action*, 2, 2, 75–84

Cullen, L.M. (2003) *A history of Japan, 1582-1941: Internal and external worlds*. Cambridge: Cambridge University Press

Daly, M. and Silver, H. (2008) Social exclusion and social capital: A comparison and critique, *Theory and Society*, 37, 6, 537–566

Debo, A. (1995). *A history of the Indians of the United States*. London: Pimlico

De Roo, P., Braeye, S. and De Moor, A. (2016) Counterbalancing the integration policy for migrants through social work. *International Social Work*, 59, 2, 210-223

DFID/World Bank (2005) Summary Report. Citizens with(out) Rights: Nepal gender and social exclusion assessment. Kathmandu: DFID/World Bank.

European Disability Forum, EDF. (2014) *Alternative report on the implementation of the UN convention on the rights of persons with disabilities*, Brussels [Accessed 2 December 2016 at http://www.icps.org.uk/images/pdf/2015%2003%2004%20EDF%20Alternative%20 report%20final%20ACCESSIBLE.pdf]

European Foundation for the Improvement of Living and Working Conditions, (1995) Public Welfare Services and Social Exclusion: The development of consumer oriented initiatives in the European Union. Dublin: European Foundation

Foucault, M. (1972) *Histoire de la folie a l'age classique*. Paris: Editions Gallimard

Fraser, N. (1995) From redistribution to recognition? Dilemmas of justice in a 'post-socialist' age', *New Left Review*, 1/212

Fraser, N. (2000) Rethinking recognition, *New Left Review*, 3, May-June, 107–20

Gidley, J.M., Hampson, G.P., Wheeler, L. and Bereded-Samuel, E. (2010) Social inclusion: Context, theory and practice, *The Australian Journal of University-Community Engagement*, 5, 1, 6-36

Goodman, S.W. (2010) *Naturalisation policies in Europe: Exploring patterns of inclusion and exclusion, EUDO-Citizenship Comparative Report*. Florence: European University Institute. [Accessed 2 December 2016 at http://eudo-citizenship.eu/docs/7-Naturalisation%20Policies%20in%20 Europe.pdf]

Hale, C.R. (2006) *Mas que un Indio (More than an Indian): Racial ambivalence and neoliberal multiculturalism in Guatemala*. Santa Fe: School of American Research

Hanney, L. (2002) Review of social inclusion: Possibilities and tension (edited by Peter Askonas and Angus Stewart). *Contemporary Sociology*, 31, 3, 265-67

Honneth, A. (2001) Recognition or redistribution? Changing perspectives on the moral order of society', *Theory, Culture and Society*, 18, 43–55

Hopenhayn, M. (2008) Recognition and distribution: Equity and justice policies for disadvantaged groups in Latin America. in A.A. Dani and A. de Haan (Eds.) *Inclusive States, Social policy and social inequalities*. The World Bank [Accessed 1 December 2016 at https://elibrary. worldbank.org/doi/abs/10.1596/978-0-8213-6999-9]

Hughes, R. (1987) *The fatal shore*. London: Collins Harvill

Jackson, C. (1999) Social exclusion and gender: Does one size fit all? *The European Journal of Development Research*, 11, 1, 125-146

Jay, M. (2003) *The Air-Loom Gang: The strange and true story of James Tilly Matthews and his visionary madness*. London: Bantam Press

Kabeer, N. (2000) Social exclusion, poverty and discrimination: Towards an analytical framework, *IDS bulletin*, 31, 4, 83-97

Kamen, H. (1997) *The Spanish Inquisition: An historical revision*. London: Weidenfeld and Nicholson

Labonte, R. (2004) Social inclusion/exclusion: Dancing the dialect, *Health Promotion International*, 19, 1, 115-121

Labonte, R. (2009) Social inclusion/exclusion and health: dancing the dialectic. in: D. Raphael (Ed.) *Social Determinants of Health: Canadian Perspectives*. 2nd edition. Toronto: Canadian Scholars' Press (p. 269-279)

Labonte, R., Hadi, A. and Kauffmann, X E. (2011) *Indicators of Social Exclusion and Inclusion: A critical and comparative analysis of the literature*, Exchange working paper series, Globalization and Health Equity Research Unit, Institute of Population Health, University of Ottawa

Lenoir, R. (1974) *Les exclus: un français sur dix.* Paris: Editions du Seuil

Linebaugh, P. (1991) The London Hanged: Crime and civil society in the eighteenth century. London, NewYork: Verso

Lister, R. (2004) A politics of recognition and respect: Involving people with experience of poverty in decision-making that affects their lives. in J. Andersen and B. Siim (Eds.) *The Politics of Inclusion And Empowerment.* New York, NY: Palgrave

Loi 98-657 (1998) La Loi relative a lutte contre exclusions, No 98-657, Loi du 29 juillet 1998: Journal Officiel du 31 juillet 1998 [Accessed 2 July 2016 at https://www.legifrance.gouv.fr/affichTexte.do?cidTexte=JORFTEXT000000206894&categorieLien=id]

Lydon, J. (1998) *The Making of Ireland.* London: Routledge

Marmot, M. (2013) *Health Inequalities in the EU* [Accessed 1 December 2016 at http://ec.europa.eu/health/social_determinants/docs/healthinequalitiesineu_2013_en.pdf]

Mathieson, J., Popay, J., Enoch, E., Escorel, S., Hernandez, M., Johnston, H. and Rispel, L. (2008) Social *Exclusion, Meaning, Measurement And Experience And Links To Health Inequalities, A Review Of Literature.* Lancaster University, UK

Milner, P. and Kelly, B. (2009) Community participation and inclusion: People with disabilities defining their place, *Disability and Society*, 24, 1, 47-62

O'Brien, M. and Penna, S. (2008) Social exclusion in Europe: Some conceptual issues. *International Journal of Social Welfare,* 17, 84–92

Oliver, R. (1999) *The African Experience.* London: Phoenix

Oyen, E. (1997) The contradictory concepts of social exclusion and social inclusion. in, C. Gore and J. B. Figueiredo (Eds.) *Social Exclusion and Antipoverty Policy.* Geneva: International Institute of Labour Studies

O'Reilly, D. (2005) Social inclusion: A philosophical anthropology, *Politics,* 25, 2, 80-88

Passas, N. (2000) Global anomie, dysnomie and economic crime: Hidden consequences of neoliberalism and globalization in Russia and around the world. *Social Justice* 27, 2, 16-44

Philbrick, N. (2006) *Mayflower.* New York: Viking

Porter, R. (1990) *Mind Forg'd Manacles: A history of madness in England from the restoration to the regency.* Harmondsworth: Penguin

Porter, R. (1997) *The Greatest Benefit to Mankind: A medical history of humanity from antiquity to the present.* London: Harper Collins

Radcliffe-Brown, A.R. (1952) Structure and Function in Primitive Society. London: Cohen and West Ltd.

Reflection Group on the 2030 Agenda for Sustainable Development (2016) Spotlight on Sustainable Development, Report. [Accessed 20 November 2016 at www.reflectiongroup.org/sites/default/files/contentpix/spotlight/pdfs/Agenda2030_engl_160708_WEB.pdf]

Riis, J.A. ([1890] 1997) *How the Other Half Lives.* New York: Penguin

Runciman, S (1965) *A History of The Crusades.* Harmondsworth: Peregrine

Schneider, J. and Bramley, C J. (2008) Towards social inclusion in mental health? *Advances in psychiatric treatment,* 14, 131-138

SEKN (Social exclusion knowledge network) of the WHO, (2008) *Understanding and Tackling Social Exclusion,* final report, [Accessed 2 December 2016 at www.who.int/social_determinants/knowledge_networks/final_reports/sekn_final%20report_042008.pdf]

Sen, A. K. (1992) *Inequality Re-examined,* Oxford: Clarendon Press

Sen, A.K. (2000) *Social Exclusion: Concept, application, and scrutiny.* Asian Development Bank,

Office of Environment and Social Development [Accessed 2 December 2016 www.adb.org/sites/default/files/publication/29778/social-exclusion.pdf]

Sen, A. K. (2001) *Development for Freedom,* Oxford: Oxford University Press

Silver, H. (1994) Social exclusion and social solidarity: Three paradigms. *International Labour Review,* 133, 5-6, 537

Silver, H. (2015) *The Contexts Of Social Inclusion, DESA working paper nr.44,* [Accessed 2 December 2016 at http://www.un.org/esa/desa/papers/2015/wp144_2015.pdf]

Steinert, H. and Pilgram, A. (2003) *Welfare Policy from Below: Struggles against social exclusion in Europe,* Aldershot: Ashgate

Taylor, C., Appiah, K., Habermas, J., Rockefeller, S., Walzer, M. and Wolf, S. (1994) *Multiculturalism: Examining the politics of recognition,* Princeton University Press, Princeton

Thornicroft, G. and Patel, V. (2014) Including mental health among the new sustainable development goals, *BMJ,* 349, g5189

UN, (2015a) *Transforming Our World: The 2030 Agenda for sustainable development* [Accessed 2 December 2016 https://sustainabledevelopment.un.org/content/documents/21252030%20Agenda%20for%20Sustainable%20Development%20web.pdf]

UN Committee on the rights of persons with disabilities, (2016) Inquiry concerning the United Kingdom of Great Britain and Northern Ireland carried out by the Committee under article 6 of the Optional Protocol to the Convention [Accessed 2 December 2016 at http://www.disabilityrightsuk.org/news/2016/november/un-report-highlight-govt-failure-uphold-disabled-peoples-rights]

UN Department of Social and Economic Affairs (UN DESA) (2009) Creating an Inclusive Society: Practical strategies to promote social integration [Accessed 2 December 2016 http://www.un.org/esa/socdev/egms/docs/2009/Ghana/inclusive-society.pdf]

UN Educational, Scientific and Cultural Organisation, (2015) Rethinking Education? Towards a global common good [Accessed 2 December 2016 http://www.unesco.org/new/fileadmin/MULTIMEDIA/FIELD/Cairo/images/RethinkingEducation.pdf]

UN General Assembly, (2015b) Resolution adopted by the General Assembly on 25 September 2015 [Accessed 2 December 2016 www.un.org/ga/search/view_doc.asp?symbol=A/RES/70/1&Lang=E]

UN Human Rights Council (HRC) (2014) Factors that impede equal political participation and steps to overcome those challenges [Accessed 2 December 2016 at www.ohchr.org/EN/HRBodies/HRC/RegularSessions/.../A_HRC_27_29_ENG.doc]

UN Research Institute for Social Development (UNRISD), (2014) *Social Inclusion and the Post-2015 Sustainable Development Agenda* [Accessed 2 December 2016 at http://www.unrisd.org/unitar-social-inclusion]

UN Research Institute for Soocial Development (RISD), (2015) Dugarova E, *Social Inclusion, Poverty Eradication and the 2030 Agenda for Sustainable Development* [Accessed 2 December 2016 http://www.unrisd.org/80256B3C005BCCF9/(httpAuxPages)/0E9547327B7941D6C1257EDF003E74EB/$file/Dugarova.pdf]

Walton, J. (1981) The treatment of pauper lunatics in Victorian England: The case of the Lancaster asylum 1816-1870. in A. Scull (Ed.) *Madhouses, Mad-Doctors And Madmen: The social history of psychiatry in the Victorian era.* Philadelphia: University of Pennsylvania Press. (pp 166-199)

WHO, (2008) *Closing the Gap in a Generation* [Accessed 2 December 2016 at http://www.who.int/social_determinants/final_report/csdh_finalreport_2008.pdf]

WHO, (2010) *CBR guidelines* [Accessed 2 December 2016 at http://www.who.int/disabilities/

cbr/guidelines/en/]

WHO, (2015) *WHO Global Strategy On People-Centred And Integrated Health Services*, Geneva, Switzerland: WHO

WHO, (2016a) *Mental Health: Strengthening our response* [Accessed 2 December 2016 at http://www.who.int/mediacentre/factsheets/fs220/en/]

WHO, (2016b) *Fact File, 10 Facts on mental health* [Accessed 2 December 2016 at http://www.who.int/features/factfiles/mental_health/mental_health_facts/en/index3.html]

Wilkinson, R. and Pickett, K. (2011) *The Spirit Level. Why equality is better for everyone.* London: Penguin

World Bank (2013) The World Bank Annual Report 2013 [Accessed 2 July 2019 at https://openknowledge.worldbank.org/handle/10986/16091]

World Summit for Social Development, (WSSD)(1995) [Accessed 2 December 2016 at http://www.un.org/esa/socdev/wssd/text-version/]

Yepez, I. (1994) Review of the French and Belgian literature on social exclusion: A Latin American perspective. *Discussion Paper Series No.71.* Geneva, IILS

Chapter 2
Introducing occupation

Sarah Kantartzis, Hanneke van Bruggen, Nick Pollard

This chapter aims to introduce the concept of occupation as we (the editors) understand it, based on the literature, primarily from within the disciplines of occupational science and occupational therapy, but also, as part of the ongoing history of human beings incorporated in the underpinning theories of many disciplines. The second part of this chapter will consider more specifically links between occupation and health, before the final chapter in this introductory section will draw together the concepts of occupation, social inclusion and health as mutually influential aspects of our daily lives, and as explored in the chapters that follow.

The perspective on social inclusion taken in this book is an occupational perspective. This is not the narrow understanding of occupation used in discussions of people's employment, but is an understanding which encompasses the complex and dynamic doing of everyday life by us all, everywhere. Throughout history people have survived and developed their homes, communities and societies through their daily activities both individually and as groups (Diamond, 1999; Wilcock & Hocking, 2015). Through these ongoing iterative processes our present doing shapes what we are and will be able, permitted, need and want to do and how we perceive and experience that doing, give value to it, and develop our selves through it.

We therefore understand that occupation, this multidimensional doing of people through time and space, is core to the processes of social inclusion, especially given that some societies are experiencing super-diversity (Vertovec, 2007) due to the influences of migration and post colonial transition. Our occupation is not only fundamental to our own development but also shapes, blocks, permits, recognises and rewards, devalues and destroys others' potential and possibility for doing, both through our day to day occupational interactions at a micro and meso level, but also through the macro, structural conditions we construct and maintain (Berger & Luckmann, 1966). To illustrate and understand further the processes by which social inclusion may be facilitated through occupation is a primary objective of this publication. We aim to shine a spotlight on the often taken for granted, unspoken, occupation of our everyday lives, and to explore its power for individual, collective and societal transformation.

The chapters in the book reflect the extent and depth of many of the current discussions around the nature and purpose of occupation in the occupational science literature and occupational therapy practice. However, and as we stated in our manifesto which served as the call for this book, we do not believe that occupation is the 'property' of any one academic discipline or profession. While occupational science and occupational therapy may have particular knowledge and skills in relation to occupation, we wish to illuminate occupation as a central element of inclusive processes, and the possibilities of occupation for all interested and engaged with these processes. Therefore, within this chapter we will present some further discussion of occupation itself, to situate some of the multiple perspectives of occupation in relation to health and inclusion presented in the following chapters.

Introducing occupation

Given the multiple languages underpinning the writings in this book, although all texts are ultimately presented in English, a useful starting point for this discussion is that occupation is not a universal concept linguistically. Occupational therapy was founded in the United States of America and the concept of occupation, as understood by this profession, has been exported around the world. However, the translation and conceptualisation of occupation in languages other than English is almost universally problematic, particularly in those languages which do not share Latin roots.

In part, this is due to the complexity of the term. The Mirriam-Webster dictionary (2016) suggests that occupation may be used in three main ways. The first is when used in relation to 'an activity in which one engages' or the 'principal business of one's life'. It is also used in relation to holding or filling a particular function or filling time and/or a physical place (e.g. she occupied the entire bench). The third use relates to the seizure of a place or area (e.g. the army occupied the entire city). These definitions refer to the use of the word as a noun; however, occupation can also be used as an adjective (occupational) and an adverb (occupationally). This rich and complex conceptual and grammatically structure of the term was important for the founders of occupational therapy as choosing it to name the new profession signified their understanding that what we do (our occupation) is complex and can promote our health. They primarily used it to signify 'engagement' in an occupation, while the idea of occupying time and place in purposeful ways was also of key importance (Dunton, 1919). This use was similar to the use of the term in the wider literature (and probably the daily conversations of the time) by 19th century English authors such as Charles Dickens and Jane Austen. Both used the term to refer to any form of task or activity, signifying the importance of how people use their time beyond paid employment, while also suggesting that occupations vary with gender and social stratification, and that some may be more useful than others, or at least are perceived as such.

As occupational therapy expanded around the world, with a good deal of the early professional literature written in English, the need to develop translations of the term occupation into other languages became evident. A number of National professional associations translate occupation as *ergo*. However, ergo (originating in Ancient Greek rather than Latin) carries different meanings. For example, in Modern Greek ergo (pl. = erga) is defined as: any activity with some aim (e.g. an ambitious ergo/work, we want erga/works); important activities (e.g. one's life ergo/work); construction activities (e.g. there are erga/works on the national road); and an artistic creation (e.g. a work of art, a theatre work) (www.the freedictionary.com). As can be seen, it does not imply a purpose of fulfilment for the individual person (engagement), or an occupation of time and place. Also, grammatically ergo cannot be used to construct terms such as *occupational behaviour* as in English.

That occupation as an English term with its multiple grammatical forms is not directly translatable into other languages is an indication of the complex and diverse contexts within which languages develop. It indicates the contextual differences in appreciation of what is the nature of everyday activity and what is important to do and achieve through our everyday occupation (Zango Martin et al, 2015; Kantartzis & Molineux, 2011). Some of these cultural differences in understandings of everyday activity are evident in the chapters that follow, while the restrictions of attempting to present in English concepts developed in other cultures and expressed in those languages are important considerations for the reader.

While there are diverse representations of occupation, core to contemporary understandings is that occupation is powerful and shapes people's lives. Traditionally, occupational therapy in the Western world has focused on the relationship between occupation and the individual, reflecting Western individualism and the bio-medical model of health. In other parts of the world, for example in South America, understandings of occupation have been also, and sometimes primarily, focused on social occupation, the occupation of groups and communities (Guajardo & Mondaca, 2016; dos Santos & Gallasi, 2014). Increasingly, throughout the world, occupation is seen to be important at all levels from micro to macro, and these views will be introduced here, reflecting also the complex multidimensional understandings of social inclusion.

Regarding the relationship of occupation and the individual, within the occupational science literature occupation is understood to be a complex process of 'doing, being, becoming and belonging' (Wilcock, 2006, p.xi) for the individual, reflecting wider understandings of well-being, particularly of eudemonic wellbeing and contemporary understandings of flourishing (Robinson et al, 2012; Ryff & Singer, 2008).

The importance of what an individual does, including both the moment to moment experience and the outcomes of that doing, have been recognised throughout history. This relates to both engagement in specific occupations as well as the overall construction of a life worth living over time. Regarding engagement in specific occupations, Ancient Greek practices to promote health included engagement in athletics and theatre, while in the East Tai Chi and other martial arts reflect these concerns. The history of religious belief as well as of traditional rituals (Turner & Bruner, 1986) recognise the experiential importance of such practices. Occupational therapy was founded primarily on the understanding of the healing potential for the individual of their engagement in specific occupations. It is commonly understood that certain named occupations, for example, those which are arts-based, sports, cooking, singing and dancing, offer particular, positive and affirming experiences for the participant(s) which are not only related to the result or outcome, but also during the process of engaging in them. In this book Diggles' narrative of engaging in photography-based art projects, demonstrates this subjective experience (chapter 4), as does the engagement in constructive work by the members of the Taieri Blokes Shed (see Sunderland et al, chapter 12).

However, occupation is not only about the experience of engagement in a named activity, bounded in time and place, but is part of an ongoing process of living a life. This process is part of each person's story of who they are, where they come from and what they might be. Ideas about the kind of life that one is able to (and should) live have been an important part of philosophical discussions for thousands of years. Eudomonic theories of well-being originate in Aristotle's work 'Nichomacean Ethics' that discussed the nature of a life well lived. Here, Aristotle states that the 'ergo' (work) of man (sic) is actualisation, achieved through a combination of practical wisdom and moral virtue. A similar understanding of the importance of the nature of the whole of ongoing day to day living in enabling the construction of a healthy life is evident in the Moral Treatment movement in 18th and 19th Century Western Europe and United States, which promoted the active engagement of the person with mental illness in a well regulated round of daily activities. The Moral Treatment movement, as also the Arts and Crafts movement, both of which formed part of the philosophical and theoretical underpinnings of the newly developing profession of occupational therapy (Hocking, 2007), also demonstrated an awareness of the importance of the relationship of the person with the environment.

Largely ignored for many years in occupational therapy, it is now also seen that the experience of some occupations may not always promote health or flourishing. While it was recognised that 'too much' of one occupation might not always be positive (e.g. muscle strain from excessive exercising), the view that some occupations in and of themselves may be actively detrimental is much more recent. For example we are seeing discussion of a dark side to occupation (Twinley, 2013), of addiction as an occupation (Wasmuth et al, 2014) and of violent occupations (Motimele & Ramugondo, 2014). This rediscovery is significant – earlier occupational therapy training programmes included education in psychoanalytic theories and group dynamics, which, based in the ideas of Freud, Winnicott and Klein admitted and explored destructive and annihilating impulses which were held to be an element of the development of human personality, and always present in the individual. However, since the 1990s these ideas, which in any case appear to have been specific to Western cultures, have lost credibility in clinical practices.

At the same time, there has developed a much greater focus on social occupation and collective processes related to the development of communities and meso level structures (Kantartzis & Molineux, 2017; Ramagundo & Kronenberg, 2015; Adams & Casteleijn, 2014). The power of collective occupation both to shape individual experience but also to shape the nature of the social world is evident throughout history. It is generally understood that the human species has always operated as communal groups with skills in social cooperation (Fukuyama, 2012). Primarily formed around kinship groups, despite the emergence of the state as an overarching structure, occupation continues to be largely undertaken within groups such as the classroom, the work place, the sports or arts club, the neighbourhood. Such collectives are maintained both through the ongoing day to day occupation but also through the collective experience of emotions (e.g. in rituals and sports events) (Von Scheve & Ismer, 2013), and though the power of collective action (e.g. organisation of a street party or a demonstration) (Dupree, 2015; Moore et al, 2015).

While such collective occupations are understood to be important in processes of social change facilitating social inclusion (see Frank, chapter 8), also acknowledged is their hegemonic practices that create and maintain disabling or exclusionary conditions for certain individuals and groups (Angell, 2014).

However, beyond this meso level of collective occupation a more critical turn in the social sciences in general, and the development of occupational science focusing on all aspects of the occupation of everyday life, has raised awareness of the influence of societal structures on the possibilities for occupation of individuals and groups (e.g.

Whiteford & Hocking, 2012; Laliberte Rudman, 2010; Townsend, 1997). A critical perspective informed the disability movement from the 1970's and their demand for the consideration of disabling societies, both in regards to the physical environment and societal norms and values influencing all aspects of daily life. Feminist theory and critical race theory supported understandings of the gendered nature of work and leisure as well as the ongoing influences of colonialism on society's structures and opportunities.

These influences together with the ongoing link between occupation and health and the increasing awareness of health inequalities based on the social determinants of health, has led to the development of an (occupational-) rights based discourse (WFOT, 2006), reflecting WHO positions on health as a human right (Office of the United Nations High Commissioner for Human Rights, 2008). The right to occupation, is particularly focused on occupation that enables participation, meaning, balance, and choice and control, which are identified as characteristics particularly linked to and supportive of health (Stadnyk et al, 2011). Concepts such as occupational deprivation, occupational alienation, occupational imbalance, occupational marginalisation (Wilcock & Hocking, 2015; Wilcock & Townsend, 2000; Whiteford, 2000) as well as occupational apartheid (Kronenberg & Pollard, 2005) express conditions of occupational injustice where opportunities for health-promoting occupation are denied by societal structures. These particular characteristics may be challenged, for example, occupational therapy, occupational science and their related concepts can be viewed as the products of colonialism, and the existence of occupational therapy may be viewed as a means of working on social problems and human rights concerns which are the outcomes of capitalism, and their universality has yet to be established (Guajardo & Mondaca, 2016). Nonetheless, they support an awareness of the importance of what people do, their occupation, to the possibilities of individuals, groups and communities to develop their potential and experience health and well-being.

The impact of historical and political events and processes in shaping what occupations are possible and how they are perceived by particular communities is illustrated in Cloete, Konstabel and Duncan's discussion of alcohol use in a South African township (chapter 13). Whether taking primarily an individual or a structural perspective, what is evident in these and many other chapters, is that the ongoing occupational process of living a life, is situated within and as part of the background knowledge 'a tightly woven fabric of interlaced and transversing understandings' (Polkinghorne, 2000, p.461), within which we 'feel' our way through daily occupation. Giddens (1984, p. 4) commented on the practical, shared knowledge, that does not usually enter discourse and which is 'inherent in the capability to 'go on' within the routines of social life'. This practical, shared knowledge, predominantly pre-discursive knowledge, leading to particular ways of doing, discussed by Bourdieu (1977) as habitus and by Dewey (1922/2007) as habits, arises in the different layers and interchanges of the cultures with which we live. What we do is formed through the conditions, social structures and culture in which we are born and live, as discussed, for example, in the work of Bourdieu on social, cultural and symbolic capital.

The impact of tacit, shared, beliefs and understandings, cultural narratives shaping occupation is evident. Touyin et al. discuss cultural attitudes shaping the occupations of people born with impaired vision in Malaysia (volume 3, chapter 3), and Laliberte Rudman et al discuss the facilitators and barriers encountered by Indigenous youth in London, Ontario, Canada as they attempt to move forward to post-secondary education (volume 3, chapter 11). Throughout the chapters of this book cultural shadings and interpretations are evident, actively illustrating their shaping of our everyday lives.

Occupation and health

A further perspective that runs through this discussion of social inclusion and occupation is their relationship with health. Occupational therapy was founded on the understanding that there was an integral relationship between occupation and health. This was not, and is not, a view of health as a normative state from which illness causes deviation, discussed within the boundaries of pathology (Alter, 1999) and with a focus on the individual as the location and cause of ill-health (Ogden, 2002), although at times occupational therapy practice has identified with such a bio-medical view of health. However, contemporary discussions of occupation and health reflect an approach to health from the position of human flourishing, the promotion of capabilities, and human development.

These approaches recognise that health is not only, or even primarily, a case of individual genetics and body functioning, and that there are fundamental requirements for health in terms of societal and environmental conditions (WHO, 1986). From the publication of the Ottawa Charter (WHO, 1986) to the 9th Global Conference held in Shanghai, China in 2016 (WHO, 2016), the WHO has made a sustained effort to support health through the identification of pre-requisites such as peace, sustainable resources and a stable eco-system, as well as shelter, education, food and income together with social justice and equity. That health is intricately linked to the social conditions of our daily lives was clearly outlined in the WHO report of the Commission on the Social Determinants of Health (2008). Although these refer primarily to the social determinants of disease and premature mortality (Venkatapuram, 2011), an understanding of health beyond an absence of disease and illness is evident in WHO documents, such as the Ottawa Charter (WHO, 1986, p. 1) that refers to health as a 'resource for everyday living'. This also reflects a newly introduced definition of health, supporting the importance of resilience and self-management, as: 'Health as the ability to adapt and to self manage, in the face of social, physical and emotional challenges' (Huber et al., 2016 p.1).

The recognition that health includes the ability to satisfy needs, achieve aspirations and adapt to the environment, not only of the individual but also of groups, is reflected in the increasing body of work with an expanded view of health that looks at the conditions of possibility for human development and flourishing. For the past 20 years understandings of development have moved beyond an economic foundation to recognise that people are the 'real wealth of a nation' with the basic objective of development to 'enable people to enjoy long, healthy and creative lives' (United Nations Development Programme, 1990, p. 9). The work of Max-Neef (1991) in South America, on Human Scale Development with a strong focus on human needs and local development, recognises the convergence of politics, economics and health. The conditions for human development include the satisfaction of fundamental human needs, increasing self-reliance and organic connections of people with nature and technology. Max-Neef supported the need for critical reflection on how we live together in our local communities and our social participation, to rediscover the components of the social fabric that support human development. We can see this vision of human potential expressed in David's chapter on creating the conditions to support the development of children born in some of the poorest areas of the Philippines, together with the importance of the engagement of families and the wider community in the process (volume 2, chapter 11).

The combined importance of individual abilities with the material and social preconditions also is at the core of the Human Development Approach, also known as the Capability Approach developed by Amartya Sen and Martha Nussbaum (Nussbaum, 2011, 2007; Sen, 1999). Although varying somewhat in their approaches they speak to the notion of human flourishing, the expansion of the real freedoms that people enjoy and to the importance of these for quality of life and well-being. Their concept of freedoms for each person to do and to be, reflects core concepts of occupation and the importance of the opportunities available to each of us.

Some of our chapters build upon these theoretical underpinnings to support the work the authors are undertaking around occupation-based social inclusion (see Simo, volume 2, chapter 8, and Perriera & Whiteford, chapter 9). Their resonance with understandings of the importance of occupation as the expression of and vehicle for a life worth living is strong, while authors in this book also emphasis the iterative relationship between what people do and the worlds so built. The chapter by Layton, Buchanan and Wilson (volume 3, chapter 12) clearly demonstrates (and challenges) the particular shaping of people with disability's possibility for engagement in the occupation of research, constructed by even the most well-meaning of researchers.

Venkatapuram (2011) with his theory of health justice clearly brings together the possibility to do and to be with theories of health. Together with the various theories noted earlier we can see considerable support for a concept of health considerably more complex than that of a normative concept from which illness and disease deviate. Health is not an end product but is the process that permits people to do and to be, a notion of unlimited and unbounded potential (Alter, 1999). Linked to much of the discussion in the chapters of this book, we also see the importance of moving away from a subjective evaluation of well-being that may well be influenced by the conditions of possibility with which the individual is living (Venkatapuram, 2011).

The particular capabilities that may be required can be defined in various ways, but both the needs described by Max-Neef (1991) and the capabilities identified by Nussbaum (2011), include not only those related to survival (life, bodily health and bodily integrity are named capabilities, subsistence and protection are named needs), but also discuss the importance of relationships, reason, understanding, creation, imagination and play, together with the importance of freedom and dignity. In this understanding of health as an overarching capability to do and to be, a strong compatibility with understandings of occupation is evident. Occupation here is linked to a positive and dynamic view of health, situated in everyday life and focusing on people's potential not only as individuals but as communities and populations.

A central element in this expanded understanding of human flourishing is the importance of the environment. The importance of the social to health has been thoroughly explored in theories of social capital, where extensive social networks are understood to provide access to a wide range of social and practical resources fundamental to health (Putnam, 2001). The impact of social inequality on health has also been investigated, and the importance of psychosocial determinants such as agency, control, dignity, and stress identified (Wilkinson & Pickett, 2010). However, not only the social aspects but the environment as a whole is seen as an integral part of the possibility for development and growth. Such contingency of person and context is reflected in the work of health ecologists who see that 'everything connects to everything' (Daysh, 1999, p. xvi) and describe the inter-relationship, interdependence and interplay of health and environment (Honari, 1999). This view of the person-in-the- environment-as-a-whole is also important in the transactional perspective of occupation proposed by Cutchin and Dickie (2012) based on the work of John Dewey. These ideas of the importance of the environment to support health and well-being underpin the development of Age Friendly Cities which aim to 'facilitate and support active ageing through adapting urban environments' (Zur and Rudman, 2013 p.371).

Here we can also see the importance of collective approaches. If health is not only the responsibility of the 'sick' individual, but like occupation is enabled and supported by the total environment in which one is situated, approaches that support the development of the whole community or positive change in the circumstances of the collective, are obviously advantageous in many circumstances. This may include raising consciousness of the situation, not only for those who are in greatest need, but for all those who are part of the situation, in order that the situation as a whole may change to facilitate new opportunities for health-promoting occupation.

Understandings of health are undergoing considerable revision and development at the present time, both in the increasing emphasis on health as a human right by the WHO (2002, 2011) and in the conceptualisation of health as a meta-capability to do and be things that reflect a life of dignity, influenced not only by biological and individual lifestyle factors but also by social and environmental factors (Venkatapuram, 2011).

Occupation, which is related to what we need, want and are able to do during the course of our daily lives, is thus seen to be a core expression of and a supporter of health (or poor health). As already stated occupational therapy was founded on the belief in a link between occupation and health (Wilcock, 2006, 1993), and the naming of the profession was based on such observations (Law et al, 1998). More recently, Wilcock (2007) has suggested that natural health and occupation may be one and the same.

While much of this discussion is based on professional and academic discourse, exploration of health as understood by people as they go about their everyday lives reflect notions of health as lived in daily life. An early and influential study exploring how people understood health within their daily lives was that of Herzlich (2004) in the 1960s in a Parisian suburb. Here people linked health not only with illness and but also with their way of life; where city life in particular was seen to not only exacerbate illness but also potentially to cause it. The experienced constraints of city life, including having no choice in the work one did and having to conform to time schedules, were major concerns, and reflect the importance of choice and control identified in studies of occupation and health (Law et al., 1998). In addition, people expressed the wish to be able to live in a more balanced manner, and this concern with balance, equilibrium and harmony has been found in a number of studies of people's health beliefs (Blaxter, 2004; Bury, 2005), while the notion of balance has been a reoccurring theme throughout the history of health, literature and philosophy (Helman, 2007). The complexity and multidimensionality of people's understandings of health was evident in these and later studies (e.g. Blaxter, 2004), where not only was the absence of illness frequently noted, but also vitality and good physical functioning, good social relationships, functioning (being able to do things), and mental well-being. A number of these studies also revealed the importance of social determinants to experiences of health as non-manual workers from higher social classes focused more on feelings of well-being, life without constraints, being in control and personal unfolding, while manual workers more on being able to work and avoiding excess (D'Houtard & Field, 1986, cited Blaxter, 2004, p. 50; Freund et al, 2003). People understood health along multiple dimensions and adapted these understandings to changing circumstances and contexts. Therefore, it appears that people incorporate their health beliefs into their way of life over time (Bury, 2005), with health being understood, experienced and worked on within the context of their daily lives.

An overarching theme is that health and everyday living are connected; people, their specific contexts and what they do, can be seen, using Dewey & Bentley's (1949) terminology, to be in a transactional relationship that is fundamental to health. As discussed, health is not a static and stable normative concept but is unbounded and potentially ever extending. It incorporates notions of people's flourishing, the ongoing satisfaction of needs and the development of their potentials, but these relate to the context both in regards to the possibilities and restraints on people's activities but also in that health incorporates notions of harmony, equilibrium and balance with the environment as a whole. Finally, and linking with the idea of a tacit knowledge that supports the usual, is the notion that people work at their health and that it is understood and experienced throughout day to day living.

Therefore health cannot be reduced to a diagnostic category, an individual story of illness or the progress of a condition, but is a rich narrative. It is a story not only of preventative measures and choices but of living in daily life within the pre-narrative action (Ricoeur, 1984) of the culture, health as lived; ill-health as lived and supported by the conditions of one's life. Within that we understand occupation as having 'moments' which constitute our narrative understanding of experiences of change or of life stages. Good moments (or bad moments) can sustain progress over time positively or negatively, e.g. Diggles drawing on his earlier art training (chapter 4).

The importance of the ongoing iterative relationship between social inclusion, health and its social determinants, and occupation, has strong implications for those wishing to take action on these issues. For example while focusing initially on the traditional foci of occupational therapy practice, i.e. the individual's physical and mental difficulties, the chapters by Cloete et al, (chapter 13), and Gupta et al, (Volume 3 chapter 2) then move the lens outwards to explore the multiple social, historical, political and cultural conditions in which these difficulties emerge, and their resulting long term impact on occupational opportunities and health. They strongly suggest the need not only for new ways of working with individuals and local community groups, but also the need to address the structures and systems, as well as cultural values, beliefs and traditions, that are limiting opportunities for health promoting occupation.

References

Adams, F., & Casteleijn, D. (2014) New insights in collective participation: A South African perspective. *South African Journal of Occupational Therapy, 44*, 1, 81-87

Alter, J. (1999) Heaps of health, metaphysical fitness: Ayurveda and the ontology of good health in medical anthropology. *Current Anthropology, 40*(S1, Special Issue Culture—A Second Chance?), S43-S66

Angell, A. M. (2014) Occupation-centered analysis of social difference: Contributions to a socially responsive occupational science. *Journal of Occupational Science,* 21, 104-116

Aristotle (n.d.) *Nicomacean Ethics. Book VI.* [Accesssed 6 July 2015 at http://classics.mit.edu/Aristotle/nicomachaen.6.vi.html]

Blaxter, M. (2004) *Health.* Cambridge: Polity

Bourdieu, P. (1972/1977) *Outline of a theory of practice* (R. Nice, Trans.). Cambridge: Cambridge University Press

Bury, M. (2005) *Health and illness.* Cambridge: Polity

Commission on the Social Determinants of Health (2008) *Closing the gap in a generation.* WHO. [Accessed 15 January 2015 at http://www.who.int/social_determinants/thecommission/finalreport/en/]

De Certeau, M., Giard, L. & Mayol, P. (1998) *The Practice of Everyday Life. Vol 2: Living and Cooking (trans. T. Tomasik).* Minneapolis: University of Minneapolis Press

Dewey. J. (1922/2007) *Human nature and conduct: An introduction to social psychology.* New York: Cosimo

Dewey, J. (1958) Experience and nature (2nd ed). New York: Dover

Dewey, J., & Bentley, A. (1949) *Knowing and the known.* Boston: Beacon Press

Diamond, J. (1999) *Guns, germs and steel. The fates of human societies.* New York: W.W. Norton & Co

Dos Santos, V. & Gallasi, A.D. (Eds.) (2014) *Questoes Contemporeanas da Terapia Ocupacional na America do Sul.* Curitaba, Brazil: Editions CRV

Dupree, N. (2015) My world, my experiences with Occupy Wall Street and how we can go further. in P. Block, D. Kasnitz, A. Nikishida & N. Pollard (Eds.) *Occupying disability: Critical approaches to community, justice and decolonizing disability.* New York: Springer (pp.225-234)

Freund, P., McGuire, M. & Podhurst, L. (2003). *Health, illness, and the social body. A critical sociology* (4th ed.) Upper Saddle Hall, NJ: Prentice Hall

Fukuyama, F. (2012) *The origins of political order.* London: Profile books

Giddens, A. (1984) *The constitution of society.* Cambridge: Polity Press

Guajardo, A. and Mondaca, M. (2016) Human rights, occupational therapy and the centrality of social practices. in D. Sakellariou, N. Pollard (Eds.) *Occupational therapies without borders: Integrating justice with practice.* Edinburgh: Elsevier (pp.102-108)

Helman, C. (2007) *Culture, health and illness.* (5th Edition). London: Hodder Arnold

Herzlich, C. (2004) The individual, the way of life and the genesis of illness. in M. Bury & J. Gabe (Eds.) *The sociology of health and illness: A reader.* London: Routledge (pp. 27-35).

Huber, M., van Vliet, M., Giezenberg, M., Winkens, B., Heerkens, Y., Dagnelie, P.C. and Knottnerus, J.A. (2016) Towards a 'patient-centred' operationalisation of the new dynamic concept of health: A mixed methods study. *BMJ Open* e010091. doi:10.1136/bmjopen-2015-010091

Hocking, C. (2007) The romance of occupational therapy. in J. Creek and A. Lawson-Porter (Eds.) *Contemporary Issues in Occupational Therapy. Reasoning and reflection.* Chichester:

Wiley (pp. 23-40)

Honneth, A. (2001) Recognition or redistribution? Changing perspectives on the moral order of society, *Theory, Culture & Society*, 18, 43–55

Kantartzis, S. and Molineux, M. (2017) Collective occupation in public spaces and the construction of the social fabric. *Canadian Journal of Occupational Therapy*, 84, 3, 168-177

Kantartzis, S and Molineux, M. (2011). The influence of western society's construction of a healthy daily life on the conceptualisation of occupation. *Journal of Occupational Science,* 18, 1, 62-80

Kronenberg, F. and Pollard, N. (2005) Overcoming occupational apartheid. in F Kronenberg, S. Simo Algado and N. Pollard (Eds.) *Occupational therapy without borders: Learning from the spirit of survivors.* Edinburgh: Elsevier/Churchill Livingstone (pp.58-86)

Laliberte Rudman, D. (2010) Occupational dialogue: Occupational possibilities. *Journal of Occupational Science,* 17, 55-59

Law, M., Steinwender, S. and Leclair, L. (1998) Occupation, health and well-being. *Canadian Journal of Occupational Therapy*, 65, 2, 81-91

Max-Neef, M. (1991). *Human scale development. Conception, application and further reflections.* New York: The Apex Press

Mirriam-Webster, 2016. Occupation. [Accessed 25 March 25 2016 at http://www.merriam-webster.com/dictionary/occupation]

Moore, L.F., Gray-Garcia, L. and Thrower, E.M. (2015) Black and blue: Policing disability & poverty beyond Occupy. in P. Block, D. Kasnitz, A. Nikishida and N. Pollard (Eds.) *Occupying disability: Critical approaches to community, justice and decolonizing disability.* New York: Springer (pp. 295-217)

Motimele, M. R. and Ramugondo, E. (2014) Violence and healing: Exploring the power of collective occupations. *International Journal of Criminology and Sociology,* 3, 388-401.

Nussbaum, M. (2007) Human rights and human capabilities. *Harvard Human Rights Journal 20 (Twentieth anniversary reflections)*, 21-24

Nussbaum, M. (2011) *Creating capabilities. The human development approach.* Cambridge MA: Harvard University Press

Office of the United Nations High Commissioner for Human Rights (2008) *The right to health. Fact Sheet no. 31.* Geneva: WHO

Ogden, J. (2002) *Health and the construction of the individual.* Hove: Routledge

Oldenburg, R. (1999) *The great good place.* Cambridge, MA: Da Capo Press

Polkinghorne, D. (2000) Psychological inquiry and the pragmatic and hermeneutic traditions. *Theory and Psychology.* 10, 4, 453-479

Reflection Group on the 2030 Agenda for Sustainable Development (2016) *Spotlight on Sustainable Development*, Report. [Accessed 20 November 2016 at www.reflectiongroup.org/sites/default/files/contentpix/spotlight/pdfs/Agenda2030_engl_160708_WEB.pdf]

Robinson, K., Kennedy, N. and Harmon, D. (2012) Happiness: A review of evidence relevant to occupational science, *Journal of Occupational. Science*, 19, 2, 150-164

Ricoeur, P. (1984) *Time and narrative. Volume 1* (K. McLaughlin & D. Pellauer, Trans. Vol. 1). Chicago: University of Chicago

Ryff, C. D., & Singer, B. H. (2008). Know thyself and become what you are: A eudaimonic approach to psychological well-being. *Journal of Happiness Studies,* 9,1, 13-39.

Sen, A. (1999) *Development as freedom.* Oxford: Oxford University Press

Stadnyk, R., Townsend, E. And Wilcock, A. A. (2011) Occupational justice. in C. Christiansen and E. Townsend (Eds.) *Introduction To Occupation: The art and science of living.* Upper Saddle

River, NJ: Pearson (pp. 329-358)

Townsend, E. (1997) Occupation: Potential for personal and social transformation. *Journal of Occupational Science,* 4,1,18-26

Turner, V. and Bruner, E. (1986) *The Anthropology of Experience.* Illinois: Illini Books

Twinley, R. (2013) The dark side of occupation: A concept for consideration. *Australian Occupational Therapy Journal,* 60, 4, 301-303

UNESCO (2016) *Social transformation.* [Accessed 17 August 2016 at http://www.unesco.org/new/en/social-and-human-sciences/themes/international-migration/glossary/social-transformation/]

United Nations Development Programme. (1990) *Human development report 1990.* New York: United Nations Development Programme

Von Scheve, C. and Ismer, S. (2013) Towards a theory of collective emotion. *Emotion Review, 5,* 406-413

Venkatapuram, S. (2011) *Health Justice.* Cambridge: Polity

Vertovec, S. (2007). Super-diversity and its implications, *Ethnic and Racial Studies,* 30, 6, 1024-1054

Wasmuth, S., Crabtree, J. and Scott, P. (2014). Exploring addiction-as-occupation. *British Journal of Occupational Therapy,* 77, 12, 605-613

Whiteford, G. (2000) Occupational deprivation: Global challenge in the new Millenium. *British Journal of Occupational Therapy,* 64, 5, 200-210

Whiteford, G. and Hocking, C. (2012) *Occupational Science. Society, inclusion, participation.* Oxford: Wiley-Blackwell

Wilcock, A. (2006) *An Occupational Perspective Of Health.* Thorofare: Slack Incorporated

Wilcock, A. and Hocking, C. (2015) *An Occupational Perspective Of health* (3rd ed.). Thorofare: Slack Incorporated

Wilcock, A. and Townsend, E. (2000) Occupational therapy interaction dialogue: Occupational justice. *Journal of Occupational Science,* 72, 2, 84-86

World Health Organization. (1986) *Ottawa Charter For Health Promotion.* Paper presented at the First International Conference on Health Promotion, Ottawa, Canada

World Health Organisation. (2002) *Questions And Answers On Health And Human Rights.* Geneva: World Health Organisation

World Health Organisation. (2011) *Impact Of Economic Crises On Mental Health.* Copenhagen: WHO Regional Office Europe

World Health Organisation (2016) WHO Global Health Promotion Conferences. [Accessed 15 March 2016 at http://www.who.int/healthpromotion/conferences/en/]

World Federation of Occupational Therapists. (2006) *Position statement on Human Rights*: World Federation of Occupational Therapists

Zango Martin, I., Flores Martos, J., Moruno Millares, P. and Björklund, A. (2015) Occupational therapy culture seen through the multifocal lens of fieldwork in diverse rural areas. *Scandinavian Journal of Occupational Therapy,* 22, 82-94

Zur, B. & Rudman, D. (2013) WHO Age Friendly Cities: Enacting societal transformation through enabling occupation. *Journal of Occupational Science.* 20, 4, 370-381

Chapter 3
Occupation-based approaches for social inclusion

Nick Pollard, Sarah Kantartzis, Hanneke van Bruggen

The previous chapter focused on occupation, that is, anything a person does. And as we stated in the manifesto which forms the preface for this book:

> 'The significance of doing is often overlooked because it is so fundamental to human existence. All our human stories are accounts of things we have done, to become who we are, and the expression of our belonging in a world with others'.

So, in some ways we are restating one of the core themes of human cultures recorded over and over since the beginnings of oral expression. What we also highlighted in the previous chapter is the way in which what we are able to do is shaped not only, nor even primarily, by our own choices but by the context in which we live. As we will see more fully in this chapter, social inclusion involves changes in the occupations or the nature of the occupation that people undertake. Change may be about the space in which occupation takes place, about the people who are in that space and their relationships, or about the occupation that takes place. It is also important to change our understanding, to raise to consciousness, our contexts, the situations and structures, our collective and individual occupations, which support our own and others occupation and thereby social inclusion. This chapter begins with a brief historical outline of occupation-based practice working for social change, primarily from within occupational therapy literature and from the English language perspective of the editors. The following section provides an introduction to some of the theoretical concepts that are underpinning current practice, before looking at what the various contributions to this book reveal in some detail about these positions and processes.

A historical overview of occupation-based social inclusion

Recognition of the influence of society in shaping the possibilities of occupation for people has been part of the philosophy of the profession of occupational therapy since its foundation. The perceived negative impact of industrialisation and of the resulting unhealthy patterns of living resulted in programmes that supported a healthy use of time and engagement in activities that were perceived to have a purpose by the person undertaking them (Meyer, 1922). However, throughout much of the 20th century the importance of occupation itself as promoting health and well being, together with critique of the nature of the changing social world, was largely lost, at least within the profession of occupational therapy. Activity (rarely meaningful occupation) became a means rather than an aim of therapy (McLaughlin Gray, 1998), and as such focused primarily on the remediation of bodily impairments.

From the 1960s within occupational therapy greater importance began to be given to the living of everyday life, to life roles, and to living in the community (Reilly, 1971). During the same period the civil rights movement in the USA was active to achieve equal rights and to end discrimination, while the disability movement emphasised living with impairments and the disabling nature of society. At the same time from a theoretical position Lyotard (1979) challenged universal, institutionalised forms of knowledge, instead supporting the importance of contextualised and local ways of knowing. These movements opened the way for a shift from a medicalised, reductionist understanding of health, to developing understandings of health as located in the everyday circumstances of peoples' lives, created in their day to day processes of living within specific contexts, and primarily to be understood through narrative ways of knowing (Bruner, 1986).

While these changes were occurring in the USA and Western Europe, influencing many English-speaking countries, in South America occupational therapy was already engaged with the social world, working with disadvantaged groups and communities. Barros, Ghihardi and Lopez (2005) trace the development of social occupational therapy in Brazil to the critical realisation of the late 1970s and the early 1980s, particularly in relation to the work occurring around psychiatric hospitals influenced by the Italian psychiatrist Franco Basaglia and the democratic psychiatry movement. They describe how the emerging field of social occupational therapy was defined around forms of exclusion, either in Goffman's (1961) total institution of the psychiatric asylum, or in the forms of social exclusions which occur in society through experiences of disability or unemployment. In social occupational therapy intervention the occupational therapist was recognised as a social and political agent for change who would employ activity as a means for building socialisation and interrelationships for inclusion. Their actions, organised and developed with people and social groups, would take place in communities and in the territories or geographical spaces of everyday life. The territorial concept was an important aspect of the development of Brazilian social occupational therapy as a focus for deinstitutionalisation, the freeing up of space for interaction – space which is limited if it exists at all in the total institution. It allowed therapists to recognise that their work might take them beyond the confines of the hospital, and to critically view how social conditions might also produce total institutions through the experiences associated with intergenerational poverty of the exclusions around disability.

However, due to the hegemony of English language publications and professional discourse concepts such as social occupational therapy were unable to have significant impact on developments in the profession in English speaking countries at the time; developments in Northern America, Australasia and the UK were occurring almost in isolation from the majority of the world. While the concept of social occupational therapy was being implemented in some Latin American countries, the discipline of occupational science was being generated in the USA. As occupational science took form in the late 1980s it gave impetus to developing knowledge and understanding of occupation for all people. The conceptualisation of people as occupational beings was developed (Clark et al, 1991) and scholarship around occupation flourished from a range of perspectives (Zemke & Clark, 1996) (although still primarily from English speaking countries). In her 1993 Canadian Association of Occupational Therapists Muriel Driver lectureship, Townsend discussed *Occupational therapy's social vision* (Townsend, 1993). A shift was underway from a narrow focus on the occupation of the person to expanding to consider the occupation of groups and communities, and from the treatment of ill-health to incorporate the importance of health promotion.

The introduction of the challenge of occupation for social justice (Townsend, 1997) was followed by the development of the concept of occupational justice, first introduced by Wilcock in 1998. A series of workshops and publications followed (e.g. Townsend & Wilcock, 2004; Wilcock & Townsend, 2000). Ideas around the potential of occupation for social change spread. Watson and Swartz (2004) wrote from South Africa of *Transformation through occupation.* A stream of occupational therapy publications began to deal with the issues of service learning and emergent role practice, community based rehabilitation and community development, seeking to include international perspectives and to explore an expanded field of practice for the profession (Sakellariou & Pollard, 2016; dos Santos & Gallasi, 2014; Pollard & Sakellariou, 2012; Kronenberg et al, 2011; Thew et al, 2011; Pollard et al, 2008; Lorenzo et al, 2006; Kronenberg et al, 2005; Whiteford & Wright St Clair, 2005).

In 1989 a series of radical political changes occurred in Europe, associated with the liberalisation of the Eastern Bloc's authoritarian systems and the erosion of political power in the pro-Soviet governments in nearby Poland and Hungary. After several weeks of civil unrest, the East German government announced the fall of the Berlin Wall on 9 November 1989. The enlargement of Europe since 1989 has been an important issue in the European occupational therapy world. Although it is difficult to speak about the development of occupational therapy in *the* Eastern European Countries, because of their different history, culture and language, there is a commonality that all countries are transitional states. Prior to 1989, these states formed part of the communist bloc and the former Soviet Union, and shared considerable similarities in health and social care systems within a common ideology. The historical changes in the socioeconomic system in ex-communist European countries greatly affected the quality of life of their populations. A European survey (Böhnke, 2004) provided evidence that an absolute majority of the people in transition countries view social injustice as the main driver of social exclusion processes. Within this context, between 2003 and 2007 ENOTHE (European Network for Occupational Therapy in Higher Education) applied successfully for grants from the European Commission to undertake several projects with the aim to facilitate the participation of disadvantaged groups in Eastern and Central European countries and to contribute to social and educational reform. This needed to be achieved by developing occupational therapy education and practice in collaboration with all stakeholders. Occupational therapy developed in several of these countries, such as Bulgaria, Armenia and Georgia, as a more social oriented and public health profession directed towards occupational justice and inclusion. Articles in the Georgian Journal of Occupational Therapy such as *Supporting inclusive employment for persons with learning disabilities in Georgia*

(Kapanadze, 2010), *Experience of daily occupations of internally displaced women in collective living centers* (Tavartkiladze, 2010) *Developing an assessment procedure for a transition program of youth with learning disabilities* (Loria, 2010), *Studying 'Street Youth' occupational needs through photo-voice* (Skhirtladze, 2010) and *Enabling teachers' active participation in the inclusion development process in a Georgian mainstream School* (Tsuladze, 2010) demonstrate the tendency of the occupational therapist to work on occupation-based community development. Moreover, various articles by Todorova and Mincheva (between 2005 and 2012) on the occupational therapy approach for inclusion of children with disabilities in mainstream schools in Rousse (for example, Todorova & Mincheva, 2005) and the chapter 'Occupational therapy for social inclusion of people with disabilities' by Todorova (2008) make clear from which angle the profession developed in Bulgaria. Occupational therapists in several of the Eastern European countries work in the social sector as well as in policy making positions around inclusion.

Through all this, as well as the continuing development and influence of occupational science, the challenges associated with daily life and of living in and with the social world came to be integrated in much of occupational therapy practice and seen as an important aim of many processes of intervention. Promoting participation was, and is, seen as particularly important. Influenced by the ICF (International Classification of Functioning, Disability and Health) of the WHO (WHO, 2016) and the history of a close relationship with the medical profession, this has been primarily a focus on the enablement of the individual to participate in society.

However, the power of existing structures were challenged, and the discussions of occupational justice have led to considerations of structural change. An early document described one of the theoretical foundations of occupational justice as:

> 'Enabling of social inclusion is a justice-orientated, client-centred practice, to create diverse opportunities and resources for people to participate in culturally defined, health-building occupations' (Townsend & Wilcock, 2004, p. 76).

In developing their discussion of occupational justice Townsend and Wilcock (2004, p. 80) proposed four occupational rights including 'The right to develop through participation in occupation for health and social inclusion', while proposing that occupational deprivation occurs when people are restricted from this right. Situations of occupational deprivation are important when occupation is understood to be part of human nature, and essential to fulfilling our needs and our wants (Wilcock, 1993). Situations which deprive us of the possibility to engage in occupation, and particularly occupation which has purpose and meaning and with which we engage in the social world, are increasingly seen as important points for intervention. Situations which may cause such deprivation may be physical, social, attitudinal, discriminatory, professional, institutional, racial, legislative, and/ or political (Whiteford, 2000).

As a result of consideration of situations of deprivation leading to exclusion from or limited access to occupation, practice has developed in the areas of advocacy and the promotion of occupation for disadvantaged groups, for example, with disabled women victims of domestic violence (Smith & Hilton, 2008), in prison services (Muñoz et al, 2016; Eggers et al, 2006) with the homeless (Thomas et al, 2011) and with refugees (Mayne et al, 2016; Whiteford, 2005). The international voluntary group OOFRAS (Occupational Opportunities for Refugees and Asylum Seekers) was established to support occupational therapists working with refugees and asylum seekers, recognising the importance of enabling their engagement in occupation and access to services and the development of 'occupationally-just communities' (OOFRAS, 2016, n.p.).

Work towards social inclusion has also been important for those working in mental health community practice, where stigma around mental illness is seen to be an important exclusionary factor, particularly in relation to employment. A number of articles discussing mental health and social inclusion (e.g. Dowling & Hitchens, 2008; Hutchinson, 2008) describe social inclusion as the aim of services, while service users engage in a range of occupations in the local environment (e.g. sports, arts and educational opportunities) and vocational opportunities are developed, to achieve this aim. However, while there is an implicit assumption that community-based practice is linked to social inclusion, it may largely focus on enabling the individual to join main-stream society. One of the motivators leading to the development of this book was the limited detail in the discussion of social inclusion as a process.

The complexity of the processes involved may be seen in Bryant et al's (2004, p.282) research that identified the 'living in a greenhouse' experience for those attending mental health services in the community - protected from society (a safe place) but highly visible. Kantartzis et al (2012) present the difficulties of finding employment which provides a good enough fit between the skills of the person and their management of their mental illness, within the limited flexibility of employment and benefits systems. Stewart and Park (volume 3, chapter 9) discuss occupational ghettoisation, when people with experience of mental illness become included in occupations that are perceived by professionals to be appropriate for people with their experiences and difficulties, effectively excluding them from a broader range of opportunities.

The importance of broad perspectives incorporating the multiple, transacting elements of the situation when working towards social inclusion, becomes evident. For example, while occupational therapists have worked for many years to support the development of the physical accessibility of environments to promote social inclusion, a study by Morrison and Burgman (2009) in an Australian school, noted that accessibility of the physical environment did not enable the social participation of children with physical disabilities. The development of friendships to support being valued, accepted and supported was not as well acknowledged, and the authors recommended that all those people involved in the situation – teachers and peers, as well as the students themselves – needed to be part of the process.

Looking beyond health services aiming to support those with specific conditions, there are a number of programmes which are working with institutions, organisations and/or communities to facilitate their change to become more inclusive. For example, in the UK the National Social Inclusion Programme (NSIP) has developed a project: Mental Health, Social Inclusion and the Arts. The programme has been developed with art galleries and museums, aiming to make these places more inclusive, particularly for people with experience of mental illness (Mitchel, 2008) (see also Guarini and Wicks, chapter 15). Other programmes are promoting the needs of particular groups in our communities. For example, Alzheimer Scotland (2016, n.p.) is working with the development of *Dementia Friendly Communities* which they describe as:

> '...made up of the whole community - shop assistants, public service workers, faith groups, businesses, police, fire and ambulance staff, bus drivers, school pupils, clubs and societies, and community leaders - people who are committed to working together and helping people with dementia to remain a part of their community and not become apart from it.'

Government policy is also directed at promoting certain occupations for all. For example, the Scottish Government (2013) has developed a *Play Strategy* which recognises the importance and works to improve the play experience of all children including those disadvantaged or with a disability. Play strategies are not only focussed on children, but on their households, parents and carers who may, for example, perceive that local environments, other children and adults may pose a threat to the well being of their children and discourage them from developing the independence and self discovery that goes with using community play-spaces (McKendrick et al, 2014).

Theory and approaches to occupation-based social inclusion

As understandings of social inclusion, participation and the impact of societal factors on the possibilities of groups of people expanded, occupation as an important element in the processes of change for groups and communities as a whole came to be considered. However the complexity of these processes has required new skills and tools for change, underpinned by existing and developing theoretical approaches.

As has been discussed, community-based approaches may be physically located *in* the community but may not be *with* the community. This may result in the ineffectiveness noted also in early development projects where *experts* (often from alternative cultural locations) decided what changes were required, and implemented projects without sufficient local negotiation for sustainable change. The consequences are socially damaging, because communities develop lowered expectations from involvement in any project, anticipating that skills, means and resources will not be handed over to them when the work is concluded (Kapasi, 2006). They will have been the subjects of a project but not participants in any achievement, not the owners of positive outcomes, nor will there be any palpable change. Contemporary approaches that aim to achieve sustainable development include campaigning (see Galvaan, chapter 7), partnership working (Tennyson, 2011), community mapping (see Cloete et al, chapter 13), capacity building (Sen, 2001; Baser & Morgan, 2008), and co-production (Scottish Co-production Network, 2016). In addition, different ways of thinking/ and professional reasoning, such as strategical reasoning (van Bruggen, 2016) development reasoning (Duncan, 2016) and political reasoning (Pollard & Sakellariou, 2012) are needed when social inclusion is the purpose of community development.

Participatory approaches are a cornerstone of the Participatory Occupational Justice

Framework (POJF) developed by Whiteford and Townsend (2011 and Whiteford et al, 2016) to guide the development of processes aiming for occupational justice. The POJF is based within a critical paradigm, as many chapters within this book. Such a perspective challenges existing social structures and systems that shape occupational possibilities for groups and populations, and through collaboration works towards action for social change. Important elements of these processes are seen to be critical reflexivity and the importance of raising consciousness of occupational injustices (Whiteford & Townsend, 2011).

Participatory Action Research (PAR) is used to understand the root/causes of the disadvantage and then take action to influence policies through the dissemination of their findings to policymakers and stakeholders (see Piskur et al, volume 3, chapter 13, and Simo, volume 2, chapter 8). PAR promotes leadership skills and emphasizes the abilities of the specific group/ community to be experts on issues of importance to them, and to work on social change.

Critical reflexivity is seen to be important for professionals in understanding how their knowledge is generated and produced, recognising the complex and contextualised nature of knowledge production and, importantly, how that influences their practice (Kinsella & Whiteford, 2009). Many chapters in this book demonstrate the importance of questioning what is known and what is considered possible, before finding ways of moving forward to be part of change processes. Critical reflexivity also facilitates consideration of existing power structures within which services have been traditionally based and which influence the relationships between service users and 'therapists'. The questioning of the use of traditional terminology (such as client, intervention, therapy and therapist) is part of this process which includes changing existing perceptions and positions, challenging ideas about who the experts are, who can be an expert and the basis for what each person brings and can do in a context.

As Godoy, Cordeiro, and Soares set out in chapter 5, occupational therapists need to reflect on their own position in the social system to which they belong, for example, their own place in the labour system of capitalist society. Occupational therapists are also engaged in the process of capitalist production and in the reproduction of social relations which are part of the structures in which illnesses are produced. An example would be injuries or stress arising from poor working conditions, or illnesses associated with poverty and poor living conditions. When people are subjected to inequalities through economically determined policies, it can be argued that this is a form of exclusion; the critical discussion of the needs identified by excluded people can be a means of generating an emancipatory approach to occupational therapy. People can develop a critical understanding and demonstrate an expertise which challenges the status quo which would perpetuate their position. Galvaan in chapter 7 points to the use of critical race theory in relation to occupation-based community development approaches, in which South African domestic workers recognise the structural factors which determine their occupational engagement in a society still marked by the legacy of apartheid and, using Photovoice as a medium, explore their capabilities and potential for activism.

A further important element in enabling change through occupation is based on the work of Freire (1970/1996), in particular the concept of conscientization – developing consciousness of the structural conditions within which we are living in order to bring about change. Conscientization in occupation-based approaches is frequently linked to action – exploration of current situations and needs through participatory approaches (see Shant & van Bruggen, volume 2, chapter 6) and methods such as photovoice (see Galvaan, chapter 7, and Rudman et al, volume 3, chapter 11), or which offer multiple means of data gathering to capture the complex and multifaceted nature of occupation, especially where language may be an issue (Huot & Rudman, 2015).

Galvaan and Peters' (2013) *Occupation-Based Community Development Framework* (see chapter 7) describes doing as being both the means and ends of the process, where with communities:

> 'doing is both the means and ends of actions that are aimed at bringing about changes in human connection and occupational engagement. ObCD involves long-term discursive processes where discourse and practices in and of everyday life are challenged. In the processes of facilitating ObCD, existing power relationships, structural inequalities, and entrenched mindsets are challenged. The ends are focused on actualizing more liberated forms of occupational engagement,' (Galvaan & Peters, 2013, n.p.)

Important to all these approaches is an emphasis on working with groups and communities, working with collectives of people, rather than with the individual. Frank and Muriithi (2015) particularly focus on the power of collective action in their theory of Occupational Reconstruction. They discuss social movements arising from an awareness of deficit or injustice and a collective desire for social transformation. Their theory combines a number of constructs, including the individual embodied experience, the power of collective action, and the narrative of change over time (see also Frank, chapter 8). Such theoretical developments are beginning to provide further tools that may be used to guide those working with processes of social change through occupation.

A further approach aiming specifically at tackling the poverty of many disadvantaged and excluded people is the development of social enterprises. This structure, by which any profits are re-invested in the business, has become a primary form of employment in many countries for people traditionally excluded from the work place. The development of such enterprise requires skills of entrepreneurship, including management, finance and marketing (see Simo, volume 2, chapter 8).

However, at the core of any inclusionary process are the relationships between people, and the experience of living in the world with others. Here theories of recognition, particularly those of Axel Honneth and Nancy Fraser (e.g. Honneth & Fraser, 2003) which discuss both inter subjective and institutional recognition, encourage work towards social inclusion to consider the equal dignity of all, ethical and justice implications, how to ensure the full status of all involved, as each person can experience these. Incorporated in many of the chapters in this book, recognition is specifically addressed by Stewart and Park (volume 3, chapter 9) and Pereira and Whiteford (chapter 9).

Working towards occupation-based social inclusion is underpinned by a range of theoretical approaches which challenge many of the existing structures of services and systems, but it is also important to remember that these are works in progress. One of the elements of working in communities is that everything is context dependent.

There are aspects which can be transferred from other experiences, but there will always be some components that have to be developed around the combinations of local interests and social actors in the setting. Often groups will have been established spontaneously around local needs, and as those needs will have been identified in relation to a particular community there may not be a connection to similar projects and similar needs elsewhere. There is a sense of having to reinvent the wheel, but this is also a reinvention, or an innovation of theory and practice. It is the authors' experience that in the heat of the process, with the immediacy of demands and the creative flow occurring as people develop their organisation the opportunity to record and to evaluate what is happening is often forgotten. Some of the chapters which follow may seem quite descriptive, but projects and schemes in different places have different needs and come from different stages of development. In these organic processes it is unwise to assume that knowledge which has not been written down is less valuable, or that what seems everyday is unimportant. Many of the ideas developed by small groups are revolutionary and can be very significant, because they are the low cost, easily implemented and realised practical approaches through which social inclusion can be enacted. They are tangible things in the community that people can begin to work around, such as Morishima and Diago's use of vacant urban spaces to develop local resources (volume 2, chapter 12), or the development of an adult literacy facility described by Fransen-Jaïbi and her colleagues (chapter 6).

Exploring approaches to occupation-based social inclusion

It is now possible to look with a little more detail at some of the ways in which occupation-based social inclusion may be approached. It is evident that occupation is a concept that spans across micro, meso and macro levels of society, while the possibilities for occupation for people and groups are shaped at and interwoven within all three levels. As we have seen, discussions of social inclusion may also consider an individually based level of analysis (micro), a socially based (meso) and structurally-based (macro) level (Cohen, 2013) and therefore in considering the occupation-based social inclusion all levels need to be considered.

Working to explore the nature and process of social inclusion, the ELSiTO European Learning Partnership (www.elsitio.net) identified the importance of not only the objective but also the subjective experience of inclusion (Kantartzis et al, 2012). They noted the importance of *feeling* included and noted the importance of awareness of small, everyday moments of doing, both with and without other people. Although social inclusion is usually conceptualised in relation to the social world, it is useful to recognise the importance of the individual and personal experience that both underpins but also influences that experience. Throughout the chapters small glimpses into everyday lives and the importance of even small acts for each person, become evident. Hayama (volume 2, chapter 7) describes the significance of making a meal of Japanese style pasta and how 'the occupation of cooking pasta started reconstructing my body and mind'. Over a longer period of time Ferguson, Jardine and Firth (chapter 10) discuss how placing occupation at the core of people's lives in the therapeutic process, enabled significant change in the life of one person. Diggles, writing the first of the personal narratives to be presented in this book (chapter 4), illustrates the power of the occupation of photography over a period of time in supporting the artist's well-being. While in all these chapters the contexts of the individual's lives are evident, central is the person's subjective engagement in occupation as part of the ongoing narrative of constructing a life, linking with memories and influencing future actions. These examples also illustrate the largely tacit, non-discursive level of such occupational experiences, habitual patterns of doing (Dewey, 1958) involving embodied memories and sensory experiences, inextricably part of one's context. This links to an experiential level of 'feeling included', not necessarily with other people, but a powerful feeling of being an inextricable part of one's world, a feeling that 'I fit'.

However, as noted by the United Nations Department of Social and Economic Affairs (UNDESA, 2009) an important element in working towards social inclusion is access to social interaction and the idea of being visible – to be noticed and to be recognised. Most occupation is essentially social, occurring with others, enabling the creation of networks of shared experiences, knowledge and skill, a sense of belonging with others through doing together, and being part of the social fabric or the social world. Sunderland, Wilson et al (chapter 12) discuss the ongoing importance of being part of a Bloke's Shed, a deceptively simple community-based occupation, which the authors unravel to reveal the complexity of doing and relationships involved.

It is also useful to note that this is social inclusion through occupation with people that share similarities between them – retired men in this case. An ongoing discussion is the degree to which opportunities for social inclusion refer only to those occupations in which all the diverse members of a community might participate. The Bloke's Shed is an example of a more limited membership. Discussions in ElSiTO between members revealed a desire for multiple opportunities - in the community and with the community with no fixed recipes; a variety of experiences, opportunities, and types of activities are required (Kantartzis, 2011). Clift and Morrison's (2011) example of the experience of singing in a choir for mental health service users, which offered emotional and social benefits, demonstrates that social inclusion occurs in many places and groups. When the importance of belonging, recognition and social relationships are considered, facilitating social inclusion becomes a process of finding the numerous ways that this occurs across the process of daily living.

In the descriptions of these occupations we can see elements of Nussbaum's (2011) description of the capability of affiliation: opportunities to be able to live with and toward others, to recognize and show concern for other human beings, to engage in various forms of social interaction and to be able to imagine the situation of another. The power of uncovering common histories of occupations in bringing together people with otherwise almost irreconcilable differences, is demonstrated in the case study of Columbian farmers in the discussion of participatory citizenship in chapter 6 in this volume by Fransen-Jaïbi et al. People who otherwise are *unrecognisable* become *visible* through stories of common experiences in occupation, powerful because they are strongly embedded in the personal history of each. At the same time each person becomes stronger through the process of building social connections, able to influence both their own health and the health of others (Hortulanus, 2006).

As well as the power of occupation to enable subjective experiences and to bring people together in processes of recognition and visibility, collective processes of occupation would also seem to incorporate a power for change. Schillar et al (volume 2, chapter 3) illustrate the power of employing collective occupation in a neighbourhood to promote inclusion. Simo's chapter (volume 2, chapter 8) explores collective working in schools with pupils and parents through occupation promoting inclusion, health and well-being. Frank (chapter 8) discusses the work of contemporary artist Vik Muniz with trash workers, known as *catadores,* in Rio de Janiero, Brazil. All illustrate the power of people coming together through occupation and the power of that process towards change, change in how the self is perceived, in how people perceive each other, and how the group or community as a whole recognises its agency.

Sunderland, Wilson et al's chapter (chapter 12), also illustrates the importance of spaces and places for inclusion. The physical layout of the shed enables the men to work and chat together, it is a safe and familiar place. Particularly in discussions of mental health recovery, the importance is noted of personal and social niches (Wilken, 2010) that need to be created, safe spots necessary for health. Risks can be taken in this safe environment and creative discoveries take place. Creating such safe spots is important for re-participation into the community, people need places where they can fit in with the whole, and where development can arise within a sense of freedom (Kal, 2011 cited Ammaraal et al, 2013, p.74). The Greek ELSiTO group (volume 2, chapter 1) argue that such spaces are places of inclusion, and finding and maintaining them is important for all people.

Awareness of the importance of space for all individuals' and communities' occupation is widely discussed in the literature. De Certeau, Giard and Mayol (1998) explore the conditions of possibility for urban life and particularly the social space of the neighbourhood. They describe the *practice* of living in a particular space which emerges in the relationship between concrete (buildings and objects), ideological and traditional elements. Oldenburg (1999) identifies the importance of 'third places' different to work and home, where public life is created and maintained. Bars, cafés, hair salons and bookstores are sites of occupation, where diverse people can come together and chat, joke and argue. The river bank, the well and the market place are also such locations. However, these may not always be inclusive places and raise questions about how we manage occupation in our social worlds. Pubs in the UK traditionally excluded women and children from certain areas designated for male drinking, while contemporary bars exclude social groups through pricing and dress code policies (Haydon, 1994). Attitudes to mental illness and physical disability limit access to public places for many. However, these are not always straightforward issues, as the members' of the Taieri Bloke's Shed reveal in their discussions of female membership (Sunderland, Wilson et al, chapter 12 in this volume). However, the possibility of collective occupation bringing diverse people together in new ways and the spaces for this is evident in discussion by Schillar et al. of urban gardening, and the importance of green spaces and nature in our cities (volume 2, chapter 3).

Occupation at the macro level of education and employment, part of national structures and systems, are discussed by other authors, particularly in relation to particular populations at risk of, or experiencing, limits to their inclusion. These broad categories of occupation – work, education, leisure – emerge from national legislative structures, interact with the local and social, and ultimately inform each individual person's possibility for inclusion in their particular context. Laliberte Rudman and colleagues (volume 3, chapter 11) focus on aspects of the higher educational systems in Canada and the challenges for indigenous youth. Funai (chapter 11) discusses the opportunities for employment available for those with chronic mental illness in the UK and describes the development of a social enterprise to facilitate employment opportunities. But it is significant that this is a social enterprise formed around arts-based activities, so that it is a fragile structure operating on the periphery of what might be considered business, the occupation of work. A number of chapters (Layton et al, volume 3, chapter 12, and Piskur et al, volume 3, chapter 13) illustrate the subtle elements of macro structures and their influence on occupation, in discussing the role of 'the researched' in traditional research projects. As in many other systems, people with disability have been traditionally prescribed the role of passive participant (or even subject), a role which prescribes specific and bounded occupations that they may perform. These positions have been maintained through the systems of the research structure including research review boards and publishing criteria.

Possibilities for inclusion and the nature of such inclusion through occupation are also influenced by the provision of health and social services. Murray's chapter (volume 3, chapter 4) is an indictment of the way in which people with learning difficulties were treated in the UK, demonstrating the historical oppression of people considered unable to live in society, and their story as they have emerged from such provision to services which support each as an individual. These services provide a different spatial and social context within which each person is able to begin to thrive, while the ongoing threat due to economic cutbacks and political will is evident. David (volume 2, chapter 11) demonstrates the importance of service provision in providing opportunities for education and employment for children with developmental difficulties living in deprived areas of the Philippines. However, the difficulties of changing service provision, even when structural processes are in place are also described (see Mlambo et al, volume 3, chapter 5).

The multiple levels influencing occupation range from, and intertwine, the micro level of the individual to the structural of state provision. Yoshikawa et al.'s narrative of ageing in Japan (volume 3, chapter 1) demonstrates the ongoing occupation of constructing a life that is satisfying across time and space, co-constituted by multiple elements from policies regulating the provision of services to a single moment of missed-communication between person and care staff. This raises further questions about how we can work together, to promote for the individual and the collective what we can do, and so be and become. This would seem to entail working with not only the conscious and the tangible conditions of our lives, but also working with the unforeseen outcomes of our own collective actions and macro processes.

Thus, we can see weaving throughout this book a central thread of how occupations may be engaged in as part of the process of raising to consciousness the processes of social inclusion, leading to change in those so engaged. For occupational therapy students a challenge, particularly in countries with long and well established professional structures, is to move beyond traditional perspectives of the client-therapist relationship, inherently unbalanced in its relationships of power, and to develop new ways of seeing and doing with others that support inclusive ways for people to be in the world together. Chapters by Karp and Block (volume 2, chapter 4), and Eyres et al (volume 2, chapter 2) describe processes of engaging students in occupation that aims to enable them to move beyond traditional relationships and views, to support their development reflections and reflexivity. The chapter written by the Greek ELSiTO group (volume 2, chapter 1) demonstrates a conscious process of learning to live and be together in new ways, through everyday occupation such as walks, games and meals. Here the power of 'normal' everyday occupations is used to create alternative dynamics to the traditional relationships of mental health service user and professional. We all eat meals, drink coffee and walk in the park, simultaneously managing and negotiating the tensions that inevitably arise in relationships between people engaged even in such 'simple' occupation.

Processes of conscientization based on the work of Freire are explicitly discussed in some chapters (Cloete et al, chapter 13; Fransen-Jaïbi et al, chapter 6) as an essential part of the processes enabling change in occupation, which although directed towards individuals, challenge internalised structural positions. Challenging the taken-for-granted positions that we all occupy is central to the chapters discussing research, and how the role of the 'researched' traditionally maintained positions of inequality and exclusion. The complexity of these processes of changing occupation, that is, changing the nature of our everyday lives, challenges notions of quick fixes through policy guidelines and statutory provision.

Finally, it is useful to reflect on the occupation of preparing this book as a process of inclusion. It is a powerful example of the complexities of working with multiple perspectives, languages and histories. Writing itself is perceived by many as an occupation of academics and of a literary establishment using a received idiom reflecting the dominance of the elite to whom it is a vehicle of daily expression. The experience of many people may be that writing is not for them and does not reflect their experience (Morley & Worpole, 2009). Even in a western country such as the UK, a significant proportion of the population may have reading or writing difficulties, with 5% of the adult population with a reading age of below 5-7 years, 16% with a reading age of below 11 years (Department for Business, Innovation and Skills, 2011). These people experience a profound and lifelong sense of exclusion, low self esteem, and often associated health issues (Marmot, 2013; Smart et al, 2011), and in some communities these issues may be concentrated to the extent that they may become a characteristic, as perhaps Cloete et al (chapter 13) and Mlambo et al (volume 3, chapter 5) describe. Yet many people managing their daily lives in a literate world with reading and writing difficulties demonstrate resilience and an ability to compensate - a key tenet of the radical adult literacy project developed by Pecket Learning Community (see Fransen-Jaïbi et al, chapter 6) was that 'a beginner writer is not a beginner thinker' (Smart, 2005). Conversely, the use of language, dialect and argot can be an affirming element of cultural identity as a form of resistance to oppression, as is evident in the promotion of many minority languages, and of occupational identity. In *Oliver Twist* Dickens gave an account of authentic cant as Oliver learned how to survive as a street child from Fagin and The Artful Dodger. Cant had evolved as the colourful language of the underclass to such an extent that during the 18th century courts had to employ translators (Linebaugh, 1991) so that those who were convicted could follow the process and those presiding understand both witnesses and defendants. Bonfim (2005) described how as a street child in Brazil he had to be adept at using the different forms of slang through which gangs of street children identified each other. These vast and rich aspects of language and occupation are just one of the areas of human experience which the literature of occupational therapy and occupational science has yet to recognise.

The international archipelago of occupational therapy communities is itself a diverse and multilingual community where writing in English compounds the exclusionary nature of the process which sustains the faultiness of history, the dissemination of Western ideas to the detriment of the epistemologies of other cultures. To take part people have to be able to express themselves sufficiently well in that colonial lingua franca or able to afford professional translators who can interpret their work. They are disempowered, just as if they were attempting to understand court procedures in 18th century England. There is a risk of being misheard, misinterpreted or misrepresented, if not ignored, because the challenge of translation is too great - but the risk has to be managed if an exchange of ideas is to begin.

From our network of colleagues we know that there are many people developing their ideas in other languages which will struggle to be heard in the Anglophone literature. Entire academic and professional literatures exist in other languages which are unknown, or very little explored in the Anglophone bloc, or to each other, addressing significant ideas and making important contributions to the development of occupational therapy. While we believe that including in our call a request for stories, cartoons, pictures and poems, this only partially enabled (new) voices to be heard. Another 'strategy' was to ask for writing teams of different disciplines and a mixture of professionals and people with experience of using services for the various chapters. Managed in various ways by our authors, this undoubtedly raised the known issues of the extra time always needed for shared working, as well as issues about how to write together collaboratively. Various examples were discussed by the Greek ELSiTO group (volume 2, chapter 1), and by Layton, Buchanan and Campbell (volume 3, chapter 12).

The need for the 'smoothing' of text by the editors reflects a conflict between homogeneity and diversity, perhaps at the core of social inclusionary processes. In previous editing practice Nick would have found this a highly contentious issue around authenticity of expression, where the right of the author not to have work interfered with editorially was sometimes vigorously defended in community publishing in the 1980s and 1990s. Spelling, grammar, and dialect were sometimes not to be corrected to a middle class received English usage where the linguistic characteristics of working class or ethnic identity were integral to the text and the author's expression (Morley & Worpole, 2009). As editors the decision for this book to be published in English places constraints and issues not only around the chapters' authors, but also on the reader, some of whom may be painstakingly decoding it through the medium of Google Translate into their own tongue. Using one language enables ideas to be shared across cultures, and promotes our understandings and our diversity. However, we must also question whether we have rendered content inauthentic and out of context. Although all editing was completed in consultation with authors, we recognise that the striving for understanding across languages and cultures is more than a momentary statement of agreement or comprise. We hope that the reader will engage with the chapters in this book in the spirit of ongoing exploration.

The book is organised in three volumes and seven sections. This first volume consists of three sections: introduction, theoretical views, and shifting perspectives. The second volume includes sections on learning inclusion and on projects, while the third volume is organised into two sections on the context of inclusion: working beyond individual perspectives, and participatory approaches and research. The three volumes together are not a hand book but rather an overview of where people are, capturing ideas of occupation-based strategies for inclusion. Powerful narratives from persons' experiences about managing life and local conditions introduce each section. The book includes perspectives from all continents, and from people with a variety of experiences. Authors include those with experience of using services and of working in services, of being researched and of researching, of learning and of teaching, people of all ages and using a number of different languages. Some authors are engaging with issues of social inclusion for many years, while others are only beginning such exploration. We consider that this book provides a tapestry of ideas and approaches, it indicates the complexity of the issues, and the difficulties of change.

References

Alzheimer Scotland (2016) *Dementia Friendly Communities* (on-line). [Accessed 15 September 2016 at http://www.alzscot.org/dementia_friendly_communities]

Ammeraal, M., Kantartzis, S., Burger, M. Bogeas, T. van der Molen, C. and Vercruysse, L. (2013) ELSiTO. A collaborative European initiative to foster social inclusion with persons experiencing mental illness. *Occupational Therapy International,* 20, 68–77

Barros, D.D., Ghirhardi, M.I.G. and Lopes, R.E. (2005) Social occupational therapy: a socio-historical perspective. in F. Kronenberg, S. Simo Algado and N. Pollard (Eds.) *Occupational Therapy without Borders: Learning from the spirit of survivors.* Edinburgh: Elsevier/Churchill Livingstone (pp. 140-151)

Baser, H. and Morgan, P. (2008) *Capacity, Change and Performance Study Report.* ECDPM Discussion Paper 59B. European Centre for Development Policy Management, Maastricht, the Netherlands

Böhnke, P. (2004) *Perceptions of Social integration and Exclusion in Enlarged Europe.* European Foundation for the Improvement of Living and Working Conditions, Dublin, Ireland

Bonfirm, V. (2005) Once a street child, now a citizen of the world. In F. Kronenberg, S. Simo Algado, and N. Pollard (Eds.) *Occupational Therapy without Borders - Learning from the spirit of survivors*, Edinburgh, Elsevier Science (pp. 19-30)

Bruner, J. (1986) *Actual Minds, Possible Worlds.* Cambridge, MA: Harvard University Press

Bryant, W., Craik, C. and McKay, E. (2004) Living in a glasshouse: Exploring occupational alienation. *Canadian Journal of Occupational Therapy*, 71, 5, 282-289

Clark, F., Parham, D., Carlson, M., Frank, G., Jackson, J., Pierce, D., et al. (1991) Occupational science: Academic innovation in the service of occupational therapy's future. *American Journal of Occupational Therapy,* 45, 4, 300-310

Clift, S. and Morrison, I. (2011) Group singing fosters mental health and wellbeing: findings from the East Kent 'singing for health' network project. *Mental Health and Social Inclusion* 15, 2, 88-97

Cohen, R. (2015) Reconsidering social inclusion/exclusion in social theory: Nine perspectives, three levels. *Mondi Migranti: Rivista di studi e ricerche sulle migrazioni internazionali* (Franco

Angelli), 1, 7–29

De Certeau, G., Giard, L. and Mayol, P. (1998) The Practice of Everyday Life. Volume 2: Living and cooking.(Trans. T. Tomansik). Minneapolis: University of Minnesota Press

Department for Business, Innovation and Skills (2011) *2011 Skills for Life Survey*. London: Author [Accessed 2 July 2019 at https://www.gov.uk/government/publications/2011-skills-for-life-survey]

Dewey, J. (1958) Experience and Nature. (2nd Ed.) New York: Dover

Dos Santos, V. and Gallasi, A.D. (Eds.) (2014) *Questoes Contempreanas da Terapia Ocupacional na America do Sul*. Curitaba, Brazis: Editias CRV

Dowling, H. and Hutchinson, A. (2008) Occupational therapy - its contribution to social inclusion and recovery. *A Life in the Day*. 12, 3, 11-14

Duncan, M. E. (2016) Development reasoning in community practice. in M.B. Cole and J. Creek (Eds.) *Global Perspectives in Professional Reasoning*, Slack, New Jersey (pp.203-237)

Eggers, M., Muñoz, J.P., Sciulli, J. and Crist, P.A.H. (2006) The community reintegration project: Occupational therapy at work in a county jail. *Occupational Therapy in Health Care*, 20, 1, 17-37

Frank, G. and Muriithi, B.A.K. (2015) Theorising social transformation in occupational science: The American Civil Rights Movement and South African struggle against apartheid as 'Occupational Reconstructions'. *South African Journal of Occupational Therapy*, 45, 1, 11-19

Fraser, N. and Honneth, A. (2003) Redistribution or Recognition? A political-philosophical exchange. New York: Verso

Freire, P. (1970/1996) *Pedagogy of the Oppressed*. London: Penguin Books

Galvaan, R. and Peters, L. (2013) *Occupation-Based Community Development Framework*. [Accessed 7 October 2016 at: https://vula.uct.ac.za/access/content/group/9c29ba04-b1ee-49b9-8c85-9a468b556ce2/OBCDF/index.html]

Goffman, E. (1961) *Asylums. Essays on the social situation of mental patients and other inmates*. New York: Garden City

Haydon, P. (1994) *The English Pub: A history*. London: Robert Hale

Hortulanus, R. (2006) Towards a new policy vision on social isolation. in R. Hortulanus, A. Machielse and L. Meeuwesen (Eds.) *Social Isolation in Modern Society*. Oxon: Routledge (pp.246-257)

Huot, S. and Rudman, D. L. (2015) Extending beyond qualitative interviewing to illuminate the tacit nature of everyday occupation occupational mapping and participatory occupation methods. *OTJR: Occupation, Participation and Health*, 35, 3, 142-150

Hutchinson, J. (2008) Promoting social inclusion for users of forensic services. *A Life in the Day*, 12, 3, 26-28

Kantartzis, S. (2011) *ELSiTO. Empowering learning for social inclusion through occupation*. Presentation at seminar Dialogue for Social Inclusion. Municipality of Irakleion, Attikis, Greece. 19th March 2011

Kantartzis, S., Ammeraal, M., Breedveld, S., Mattijs, L., Geert, Leonardos, Yiannis, Stefanos and Georgia. (2012) 'Doing' social inclusion with ELSiTO: Empowering learning for social inclusion through occupation. *Work*, 41, 447-454

Kapanadze, M. (2010) Supporting inclusive employment for persons with learning disabilities in Georgia: Facilitation of employees at the workplace. *The Georgian Journal of Occupational Therapy, 1*, 23-29

Kapasi, H. (2006) *Neighbourhood Play and Community Action*. York: Joseph Rowntree Foundation

Kinsella, A. and Whiteford, G. (2009) Knowledge generation and utilisation in occupational therapy: Towards epistemic reflexivity. *Australian Occupational Therapy Journal*, 56, 249–258

Kronenberg, F., Simo Algado, S. and Pollard, N. (Eds.) (2005) *Occupational Therapy without Borders - Learning from the spirit of survivors*, Edinburgh, Elsevier Science

Kronenberg, F., Pollard, N. and Sakellariou, D. (Eds.) (2011) *Occupational Therapies without Borders: Towards an ecology of occupation-based practices (Volume 2).* Edinburgh: Elsevier Science

Linebaugh, P. (1991) *The London Hanged: Crime and civil society in the eighteenth century.* Harmondsworth: Penguin

Lorenzo, T., Duncan, M., Buchanan, H. and Alsop, A. (2006) *Practice and Service Learning in Occupational Therapy: Enhancing potential in context.* Chichester: J Wiley and Sons

Loria, T. (2010) Developing an assessment procedure for a transition program of youth with learning disabilities in Georgia. *The Georgian Journal of Occupational Therapy, 1,* 30-34

Lyotard, J. F. (1979/ 1984) *The Post-Modern Condition: A report on knowledge* (Trans. G.Bennington, B. Massumi). Manchester: Manchester University Press

McKendrick, J., Horton, J., Kraftl, P. and Else, P. (2014) Bursting the bubble or opening the door? Appraising the impact of austerity on playwork and playwork practitioners in the UK. *Journal of Playwork Practice*, 1, 61-69

McLaughlin Gray, J. (1998) Putting occupation into practice: Occupation as ends, occupation as means. *American Journal of Occupational Therapy,* 52, 354-364

Marmot, M. (2013) *Health inequalities in the EU.* [Accessed 5 July 2016 at http://ec.europa.eu/health/social_determinants/docs/healthinequalitiesineu_2013_en.pdf]

Mayne, J., Lowrie, D. and Wilson, J. (2016) Occupational experiences of refugees and asylum seekers resettling in Australia a narrative review. *OTJR: Occupation, Participation and Health*, 36, 4, 204-215

Meyer, A. (1922/1977) The philosophy of occupation therapy. Reprinted from the Archives of Occupational Therapy, Volume 1, pp. 1-10, 1922. *American Journal of Occupational Therapy*, 31, 10, 639-42.

Mitchell, R. (2008) Policy and action. *A Life in the Day.* 12, 3, 36-37

Morley, D. and Worpole, K. (2009) *Republic of Letters* (2nd edition). Philadelphia/Syracuse: New City Communities Press/Syracuse University Press

Morrison, R. and Burgman, I. (2009) Friendship experiences among children with disabilities who attend Australian mainstream schools. *Canadian Journal of Occupational Therapy,* 76, 3, 145-152

Muñoz, J. P., Moreton, E. M. and Sitterly, A. M. (2016) The scope of practice of occupational therapy in US criminal justice settings. *Occupational Therapy International*, 23, 3, 241-54

Nussbaum, M. (2011) *Creating capabilities. The human development approach.* Cambridge MA: Harvard University Press

OOFRAS (2016) *Occupational Opportunities For Refugees and Asylum Seekers Inc.* (Web page). [Accessed 30 November 2016 at http://www.oofras.com/]

Pollard, N. and Sakellariou, D. (Eds.) (2012) *Politics of Occupation-Centred Practice.* Oxford, Wiley

Pollard, N., Sakellariou, D. and Kronenberg, F. (Eds.) (2008) *A Political Practice of Occupational Therapy*, Edinburgh: Elsevier Science

Reilly, M. (1971) The modernization of occupational therapy. *American Journal of Occupational Therapy,* 25, 143-6

Sakellariou, D. and Pollard, N. (Eds.) (2016) *Occupational Therapies without Borders: Integrating justice with practice, 2ed.* Edinburgh: Elsevier Science

Scottish Co-production Network (2016) *What is co-production?* [Accessed 10 July 2016 at http://www.coproductionscotland.org.uk/about/what-is-co-production/]

Scottish Government (2013) *Play Strategy*. [Accessed 15 September 2016 at http://www.gov.scot/Resource/0042/00425722.pdf]

Sen, A. K. (2001) *Development for Freedom*. Oxford: Oxford University Press

Skhirtladze, N. (2010) Studying 'Street Youth' occupational needs through photovoice. *The Georgian Journal of Occupational Therapy*, 1, 35-39

Smart, P. (2005) A beginner writer is not a beginner thinker. in F. Kronenberg, S. Simo Algado, and N. Pollard, (Eds.) *Occupational Therapy without Borders*. Oxford: Elsevier/ Churchill Livingstone (pp. 46-53)

Smart, P., Frost, G., Nugent, P. and Pollard, N. (2011) Pecket Learning Community. in F. Kronenberg, N. Pollard and D. Sakellariou (Eds.) *Occupational Therapies without Borders: Towards an ecology of occupation-based practices* (Volume 2). Edinburgh: Elsevier Science (pp. 19-26)

Smith, D. and Hilton, C. (2008) An occupational justice perspective of domestic violence against women with disabilities. *Journal of Occupational Science*, 15, 3, 166-172

Tavartkiladze, T. (2010) Experience of daily occupations of internally displaced women in collective living centres. *The Georgian Journal of Occupational Therapy*, 1, 15-23

Taylor, C., Appiah, K., Habermas, J., Rockefeller, S., Walzer, M. and Wolf, S. (1994) *Multiculturalism: Examining the politics of recognition*, Princeton: Princeton University Press

Tennyson, R. (2011) *The Partnering Toolbook*. [Accessed 15 November 2015 at http://thepartneringinitiative.org/publications/toolbook-series/the-partnering-toolbook/]

Thew, M., Edwards, M., Baptiste, S. and Molineux, M. (Eds.) (2011) *Role Emerging Occupational Therapy: Maximising occupation focused practice*. Oxford: Wiley-Blackwell

Thomas, Y., Gray, M. and McGinty, S. (2011). A systematic review of occupational therapy interventions with homeless people. *Occupational Therapy in Health Care*, *25*, 1, 38-53

Todorova, L. and Mincheva, P. (2005) An occupational therapy approach for inclusion of children with disabilities in mainstream schools in Rousse. *Journal of the Network for Prevention of Child Maltreatment 'Today's Children Are Tomorrow's Parents'*, 16, 32–39

Todorova, L. (2008) Occupational therapy for social inclusion of people with disabilities. in I. Topouzov (Ed.) *Occupational Therapy – 2nd part*. Sofia: RIK 'Simel' (pp. 278-302)

Tsuladze, M. (2010) Enabling teachers' active participation in the inclusion development process in a Georgian mainstream school. *The Georgian Journal of Occupational Therapy, 1*, 39-45

Townsend, E.A. (1993) Occupational therapy's social vision, Muriel Driver Memorial lecture 1993. *Canadian Journal of Occupational Therapy*, 60, 174-184

Townsend, E. A. (1997) Occupation: Potential for personal and social transformation. *Journal of Occupational Science*, 4, 1, 297-300

Townsend, E. and Wilcock, A. (2004) Occupational justice and client-centred practice. A dialogue in progress. *Canadian Journal of Occupational Therapy*, 71, 2, 84-86

United Nations Department of Social and Economic Affairs (UNDESA) (2009) Creating an Inclusive Society: Practical strategies to promote social integration. [Accessed 2 December 2016. http://www.un.org/esa/socdev/egms/docs/2009/Ghana/inclusive-society.pdf]

Van Bruggen, H. (2016) Strategic thinking and reasoning in occupational therapy. in M.B. Cole and J. Creek (Eds.) *Global Perspectives in Professional Reasoning*, Thorofare, NJ: Slack (pp. 25-43)

Watson, R. and Swartz, L. (2004). *Transformation Through Occupation.* London: Whurr Publishers

Whiteford, G. (2000) Occupational deprivation: Global challenge in the new Millenium. *British Journal of Occupational Therapy,* 64, 5, 200-210

Whiteford, G. (2005) Understanding the occupational deprivation of refugees: A case study from Kosovo. *The Canadian Journal of Occupational Therapy,* 72, 2, 124-130

Whiteford, G. and Townsend, E. (2011) Participatory Occupational Justice Framework (POJF 2010): Enabling occupational participation and inclusion. in F. Kronenberg, N. Pollard, N. and D. Sakellariou (Eds.) *Occupational Therapies Without Borders: Volume 2.* Edinburgh: Elsevier (pp. 65-84)

Whiteford, G., Townsend, E., Bryanton, E., Wicks, A. and Pereira, R. (2016) The Participatory Occupational Justice Framework: Salience across contexts. in D. Sakellariou and N. Pollard (Eds.) *Occupational Therapies without Borders: Integrating justice with practice, 2ed.* Edinburgh: Elsevier Science (pp. 163-174)

Whiteford, G. and Wright-St.Clair, V. (2005) *Occupation and Practice in Context.* Sydney: Elsevier/ Churchill Livingstone

Wilken, J.P. (2010) *Recovering Care. A contribution to a theory and practice of good care.* Amsterdam: SWP Publishers

Wilcock. A. (1998) *An Occupational Perspective of Health.* Thorofare, NJ: Slack Inc

Wilcock, A. and Townsend, E. (2000) Occupational terminology: Interactive dialogue. *Journal of Occupational Science,* 7, 2, 84-86

World Health Organisation (WHO) (2016) *International Classification of Functioning, Disability and Health (ICF).* [Accessed 12 November 2016 at http://www.who.int/classifications/icf/en/]

Zemke, R. and Clark, F. (1996) *Occupational Science: The evolving discipline.* Philadelphia: F.A. Davis Company

Section 2
Theoretical views

This section explores theoretical approaches to underpin occupation based approaches to social inclusion and outlines some research approaches. The chapters draw on ideas which until recently may have been unfamiliar territory for many occupational therapists.

The section begins with Diggles' account of developing personal photography based arts projects following a period of depression. Diggles falls back on his previous artistic training and discipline to produce a virtual gallery of photographs illustrating aspects of daily life, surroundings, and commentary. This chapter reflectively illustrates the important tacit and complex processes which precede the development of more formal theoretical approaches to occupation, in this case, artmaking (Huot, and Laliberte Rudman, 2015; Jarvis, 2007).

Godoy, Cordiero and Soares consider an emancipatory, Labour based approach to occupation allows it to be considered in its historical context rather than as simply a biomedical or health-disease process. Based in the work of the Hungarian Marxist philosopher Lukács, focusing on occupation as Labour enables questions such as social class, theory of consumption and production and the social conditions of capitalism to be critically considered as components of the experience of occupation, offering a holistic view of the production of illness and health through work relations and related living conditions, and even of occupational therapy itself as a part of the complex system which is engaged in reproducing itself. Godoy, Cordiero and Soares propose ways in which occupational therapy can be reimagined as a step in enabling social transformation, facilitating people in developing a critical consciousness about the structural conditions which produce ill health and their ability to resist them.

Fransen-Jaïbi, Viana-Moldes, Pollard and Kantartzis concern themselves with the relationship between occupation and concepts of citizenship. Using the ideas of Freire and Arendt, and UNESCO's approaches to education they set out a connection which is based in participation, illustrated by two case studies, one from the north and one from the southern hemisphere. To be able to participate, to be enabled to function as a citizen is central to most of the key occupations people enjoy interactively, whether in public or private spaces, and on which ideas of the self, of an identity which is shared with others can be based. Concepts of citizenship are not presented as universal, but related to different contexts; nonetheless citizenship can be a driver for transformative approaches using occupation.

Drawing on occupational science, Galvaan also considers social inclusion from a southern hemisphere perspective, looking at the experiences of participants in three occupation based community development research projects. Tools such as photovoice and critical race theory enable participants to elicit their everyday experiences as a step towards negotiating structural changes.

Finally Pereira and Whiteford review the application of theoretical constructs such as occupational justice to the experiences of marginalised people. Using a case study as an illustration to voice an experience based on one woman's unemployment, depression and other chronic health conditions, they interrogate theoretical concepts from some of the perspectives she offers. Using Honneth's theory of recognition Pereira and Whiteford's chapter drills through a complex set of interactions between systemic structures and actors within these systems to set out some foundations for generating the opportunities for participation and occupation based social inclusion. They conclude with a number of framing 'points of action' for sustainable social inclusion.

References

Huot, S. and Laliberte Rudman, D. (2015) Extending beyond qualitative interviewing to illuminate the tacit nature of everyday occupation: Occupational mapping and participatory occupation methods. *OTJR: Occupation, Participation and Health*, *35*, 3, 142-150

Jarvis, M. (2007) Articulating the tacit dimension in artmaking, *Journal of Visual Art Practice*, 6, 3, 201-213

Chapter 4
Getting back my ability
Tim Diggles

I had worked professionally for over 30 years in the arts in the UK, across many forms and in many fields. My work consisted of organising; finding funding; training and sharing skills; bringing people and organisations together; working with groups on things like strategic planning, constitutions and fund-raising; representation at conferences and meetings; recording and documenting. I worked in formal and informal settings. However it never included my own art practice for which I spent many years training and which is steeped in my soul.

In 2007 I was dismissed from my job for Unprofessional Conduct, due to a financial issue. Looking back I realise that I had 'burnt-out', and that over a period I made major errors of judgement both professionally and privately. I had not realised that for around two years I had had medium level depression. The signs were there; I didn't recognise them or seek help for them. I have never used this as an excuse for something I should and could have prevented. There were a number of possible triggers; my marriage had broken down; I had a major operation removing the bowel because of ulcerative colitis and a stoma fitted; my mother died. I was not allowing myself time to recuperate, and didn't take as much time off as I should, such as holidays. I became subsumed by work and felt constantly behind in what I was doing. I was finding the need to multi-task very difficult without realising it, and giving inordinate amounts of time to aspects of the post which could and should have been dealt with by a person trained in the specific role.

After losing my job I went into a deeper depression and for a period found even attending very straightforward meetings or attending things like a writers' group were impossible. I had anti-depression tablets, went to some group and one-to-one therapy. I found the tablets almost more debilitating because they stopped my creative abilities. During the following year I had to sell my home and get rid of my car; as well as deal with the 'shock' of not working and big drop in income. I understand why there were those who after losing their jobs continued setting off to work and wander round all day. Looking back it was probably a form of grief.

I was sent to Crown Court because I had bought a lot of 'sleepers' with the vague aim of having the means available to commit suicide, I didn't actually attempt it, but following a car accident, was accused of planning to sell them. I was found not guilty of selling but guilty of possession (I did not use the plans for suicide or depression as defence), which was correct and The Crown Prosecution Service were told in no certain terms by the judge they had wasted their time. I was given a one year suspended sentence.

When my depression levels had begun to even out, I started monitoring my levels of anxiety and depression through the forms the doctors and therapists were using to measure them - GAD-7 (Generalised Anxiety Disorder Questionnaire), and PHQ-9 (Patient Health Questionnaire for screening depression). When I got a second hand computer, I set these up as an Excel spread-sheet and was able to monitor myself. Over time I have been able to see patterns emerging when things are good and bad. I found that when I had had long conversations or visits with friends, done some creative work, my levels improved. During periods with no contact and lack of creative work things went worse.

So I instigated a self-motivated plan of action. I began by re-writing some poetry and two novels, as I had lost most of my writing when I left a usb stick at a library (and stupidly had no print versions); this meant I had both to plan out the work, remember what was important in my writing, do the work. I attended a couple of writers' groups, one of which has been most useful. I gave myself art based tasks, mainly with photography, and did some voluntary work such as at the local junior school looking at famous paintings and sharing some of my skills in fundraising. The photography increased greatly.

The computer, as well as giving me a new-found creative focus, linked me to people through social media and I have been able to find old friends as well as develop new friendships. Loneliness is a great issue for me, but social media helps greatly. By keeping close accounts of my personal finances I have been able to get my financial anxieties under control, which can be on the macro level of working out how much gas and electricity I was using per day on the pay meters so I would never run out (which can be very depressing). Or on a longer term planning how much I will need for things I may need. I have used the account set up on my computer for seven years and it has helped make me feel more in charge of my life, at least in those terms.

In general I have maintained a steady level of improvement mentally, periods of depression are now much fewer, perhaps twice a year, and more usually aligned to my physical health. I have a major operation coming up in early 2016 so am trying to plan for the possibility of becoming depressed again. This sets up regular contacts with friends and them knowing to phone or visit me regularly during recuperation. My main symptom now seems to be periods when I make every excuse not to attend things which I know help me, such as the very good writers' group I attend. Throughout my life I have suffered periods of lethargy and I am never sure if this is part of my depression, it appears to get worse at periods when I am under some form of stress. I am still finding ways of dealing with these periods. I cannot, and have not looked into why, perhaps I have suffered from levels of depression all my life, 1950's-60's childhoods were not exactly open to such ideas.

I receive Employment Support Allowance (ESA) and following a couple of extensive medicals examinations, have been told that my condition means I should not work. I regularly physically breakdown. The ESA means with good planning I have just about enough to survive on, I receive housing benefit which covers the rent on my flat.

Four years ago I came to the realisation that although I was statistically amongst the poorest people in the UK, I am time rich. I knew that this time could be used to develop my creative abilities. Compared to most of my artist friends I am able to give as much time as I need to my art. For a few years I had already concentrated on writing which was going fairly well, having had a couple of poems published and working on a couple of ambitious novels. I was lucky that the best writers' group I have come across was formed in Stoke-on-Trent at just the right time. It offers good and challenging critique, something I needed.

I have been taking photographs since 1970, so it was natural to take them as I went for walks or visited places and people. In 2012 as part of my plans I gave myself a project to write a blog (timdiggles.wordpress.com) and take at least one photograph a day for a year to use in it. As well as increasing my visual explorations, the blog developed in other ways and I have used it to publish some of my writing and interview people. It also gave me contacts around the world who I discuss things with and now have well over 1,000 followers. As I continue working my 'practice' has improved, I can see a progression in my work as an artist-photographer. My 'eye' had begun to 'return', seeing images and finding my visual 'voice' again. I have been studying photographers and technique I hadn't previously and see that what I am doing is getting positive feedback. Through some previous contacts I became a member of a local photographers' collective. This meant attending committee meetings and using skills I have in organisation and planning. I have been the lead in writing a new Constitution as the Collective becomes a more formal organisation and was elected their first Chair.

Most of my photographs are taken within a half mile radius of where I live due to not owning transport and my 'disabilities' makes walking further painful and exhausting, or within the confines of my one bedroomed flat. However, the limitations this imposes means I concentrate on compositional, light and time elements. I have been working on a number of projects and had an exhibition in early 2015 at Burslem School of Art called *Half Mile*.

My *Streets Project* is covering all the streets/roads/lanes/footpaths within half-a-mile of my flat, 142 of them. At each I concentrate sometimes for a few hours on the environment, buildings, road markings, nature, and human interventions. I am about a quarter-way through this. I wear a reflective jacket not just for safety (as I am often in the road photographing) but also to blend in, some people think I am from the council! I can see that it is about placing myself, which is important to me, knowing where I am.

Still Life was a photographic diary using the formality of a still life against a constant grey background. This lasted through 2014, with 52 images altogether. Each Friday I placed together objects representing things that I wrote down representing each day, then created and 'published' the photograph on my blog. These are best seen as a whole rather than individually.

Flat Life came from a long poem I was trying to write which would cover the whole of one day, dealing with the silences, light, corners, and loneliness of living alone. All the photographs were taken within the confines of my one-bedroomed flat, at all times of the day and night. I found in writing about these I couldn't find the words, but images such as the hands of a clock, edges of doors, corners of room, light falling through windows, captured what I was trying to write about. The project is now completed and has 200 photographs in the series.

I have also taken a lot of images of nature, landscapes, doors and gates in what I term a 'frontalist' style. I hope to find more exhibition outlets.

Looking at my work it does not include people. In a small group show we had in 2014 I felt my work looked 'cold' against the others. This does however reflect my personality, and I was pleased about that. However in 2015 I began a series of self-portraits called *Tim as...*, where I have recreated photographs of people in my front room portraying people such as Dylan Thomas, Christine Keeler, Matisse and Ben Nicholson. This adds a new element to my work and has stretched my abilities, which is what I want. This has also led me to make some portraits of people I know and is certainly an area I want to explore further.

I think I can now say that despite the financial difficulties and those of transport and illness, the discipline and rigour of working on quite large arts based projects has revived a self-confidence in my own work that I have not felt since the mid 1970's. I realise that maybe had I not dismissed my work at that time because of political belief and my abilities to organise and share came to the fore, my work as an artist may have flourished. However I was good at what I did and have many people who have thanked me for helping them develop their art and careers.

I can see that the committee and organisational work is also helping me. I do not see art as a therapy, it is not particularly a pleasure for me, and for most of my life it has been central to my thinking and living. However, without undertaking the work I do I am not sure where I would be, so it is therapeutic in that sense.

I am lucky in the quality of art education I undertook firstly at Leek School of Art then at Cardiff College of Art. It gave me the ability to work on my own and self-motivate; the eyes to see and create what I see envision; the discipline to take on and complete large projects.

Looking at this I can see that this is a very personal way of working. For 30 years my work life was one of supporting and encouraging others to create and be involved in the arts, sharing my skills, whether those were in arts practice or the raising of funds, organising groups, making things happen for others. For the past few years I have been making things happen for me, which was perhaps needed.

A selection of my writing and the catalogue for *Half Mile* can be found on ISSUU, and my blog with links to photographs from all the projects mentioned above on *timdiggles.wordpress.com/*.

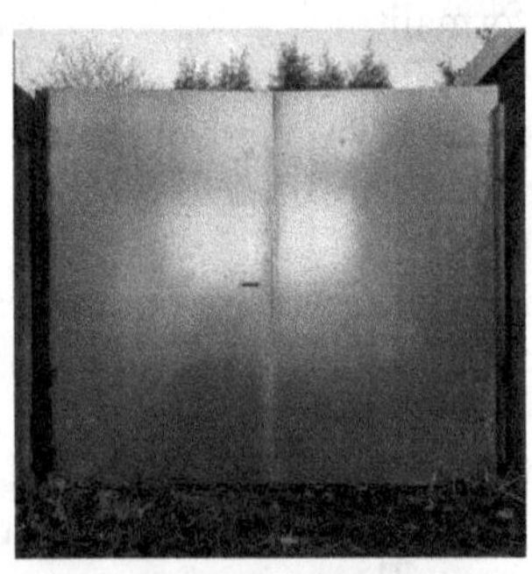

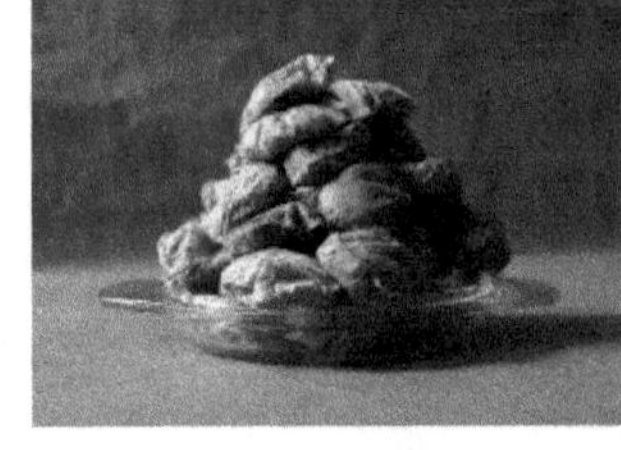

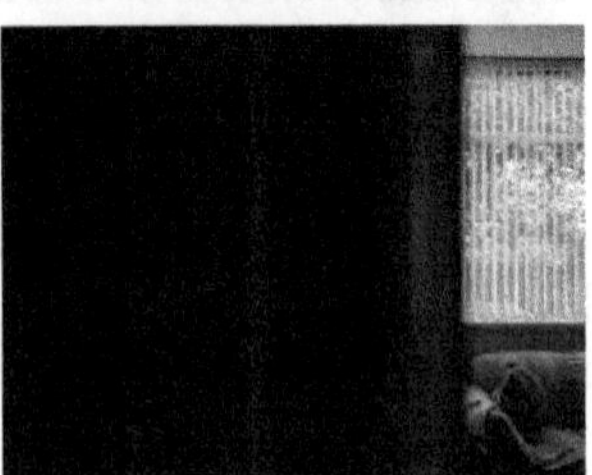

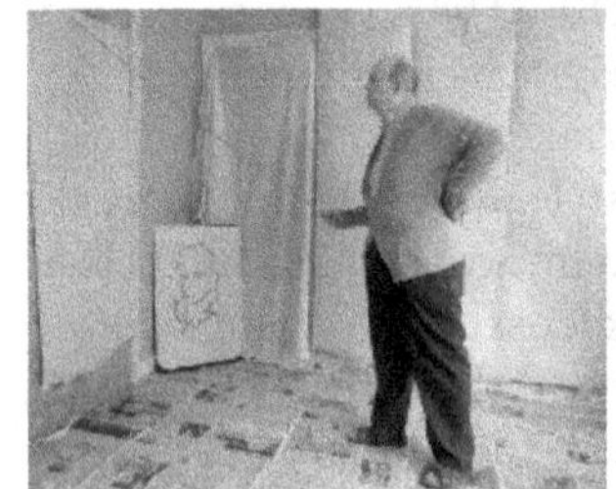

Chapter 5
Emancipatory occupation: Labour as the conceptual basis for occupation-based social practices

Aline Godoy, Luciana Cordeiro, Cassia Baldini Soares

This text presents a theoretical discussion about a critical epistemological foundation for occupation-based practices, from the discussion of occupational therapy and occupation as its object. We propose a definition of occupation under the concept of Labour - from Marx's theory of labour-processes (1982). Based on a Lukacsian[1] (Lessa, 2007) perspective on the centrality of Labour[2] in human existence, our intention is to present it as the basis for an emancipatory occupational therapy.

Occupational therapists are highly committed to occupation as the object of their practices. However, when asked about their theoretical basis, they usually speak of methods instead of epistemological foundations from which they work (Godoy, 2014; Hooper & Wood, 2002). In their practice descriptions it is not clear what humans and society concepts they defend and what transformation they propose for society. We intend, from the basis presented here, to strengthen the consciousness of practitioners to critically intervene on the social determination of health-disease processes through occupation-based practices, aiming for human emancipation.

In the first part of the chapter we present an overview of the theory of the social determination of the health-disease process (Borde et al, 2015; Rocha & David, 2015; Navarro, 2009), a structural element of the Collective Health field3 (Waitzkin et al, 2001) which is described by Laurell (1989) as the Latin American social medicine, locating Labour as a fundamental element of the health object of practices and therefore essential to its transformation. The second part of the chapter addresses the ontological place of Labour in the establishment of the social being and its transformation into alienated occupations in capitalist societies. Then, in the third part of the chapter we present occupational therapy as a social practice that historically developed from the capitalist social division of labour to respond to the needs of the mode of production in capitalism. Finally, in the fourth part, we present the emancipatory potentiality of social practices that no longer take alienated occupation as their object, but focus on Labour (as emancipatory occupation) aiming for the meaningful creative participation of assisted populations (and professionals) through their lifespan, as much as in the transformation of social determination of illness.

Labour as a fundamental element of the social determination of the health-disease process

Social medicine and critical epidemiology are critical paradigm disciplines that renewed the social determination of health-disease process theory in the late 1970s in Latin America by proposing 'an alternative model of objectivity' (Breilh, 2008, p.746). This theory explains the simultaneous presence of social and biological features in a disease process that can be analysed both by social and biological methodologies.

The Collective Health field of knowledge and practices conceives the health-disease process as a reverberation of the social reproduction (Rocha & David, 2015; Laurell, 1982). It sets out that there is an interdependence between society and nature: 'man determines himself and nature simultaneously and [...] health becomes the particular manner a man behaves as a social being according to his daily life conditions' (Nogueira, 2009, p.405).

Assuming that the health-disease process simultaneously presents social and biological features, the collective health-disease process determines the basic features on which the individual biological variation occurs. Supported by the Marxist concept of social reproduction, critical epidemiology's object is established in relation to work, life and health because social classes are characterised by the manner in which their members work and live. This means that epidemiology changes accordingly to the historical moment and the place the social class occupies in the social reproduction process (Laurell 1991; Laurell, 1982).

Therefore, social reproduction is a theoretical category which is essential for the social determination of health-disease process theory as it explains the hierarchical model of determination; '... the epidemiological profile of a social class indicates how the social class participates in the production process and the consumption process' (Soares et al, 2014, p.133). This means that the manner in which people work (including working conditions, daily use of techniques and instruments, earnings, autonomy on working processes, for example); and the manner in which people consume (access to food, education, leisure, clothing, and other commodities that respond to their needs) – their epidemiological profile - are determined by the production process of the society people live in.

Accordingly the conditions of work amongst different social classes and therefore the manner in which people work should be considered when studying the health-disease process of a social class or class fraction. This is because in capitalist societies debility and strengthening are produced differently in each social class (Laurell, 2008; Laurell, 1991).

We next present the concept of Labour as a central ontological category of social being, as that which makes us humans making and shaping the world (Marx, 1982). This concept differs from capitalist alienated labour over which workers have no control. Our aim is to propose a theoretical discussion about the basis for occupation as the object of social practices.

Labour[I] as a central ontological category of social being and the capitalist labour

Lukács (1980) responds to what seems to be the main question regarding the ontology of social being: why is Labour the central category to the establishment of the social being? What distinguishes Labour from other categories such as cooperation and language regarding the establishment of the social being? His response reveals that all other categories have operating ways developed in an already constituted social being, but Labour is in an intermediate situation between humankind and nature, marking the path from the purely organic and biological to the social being.

Labour-processes are generated to satisfy human needs. Humans are beings with needs and capacities. Both needs and capacities are susceptible to changes and development. Needs are everything that humans must have satisfied in order for them to continue to exist. When the satisfaction of these needs depend on the transformation of nature, it is achieved through the use of capacities during what are called Labour-processes. Needs and capacities are dimensions of one and the same thing. Humans only need what they actually identify in nature or in the material reality as something that could answer to their wants - this identification is called objectification, and it includes the possibility of achieving and consuming it through their capacities (Mendes Gonçalves, 1992).

During Labour-processes people transform materials from nature into products and this only happens if the human being has consciousness about the viability of their transformation. Consciousness is part of the transformation process and allows people to envision the necessary action. Consciousness therefore plays a decisive role in the materialist distinction between another animal and a human - the social being (Lukács, 1969). In other words, human consciousness organises the conduct of individuals during the Labour-process, which produces: a) a product; and b) knowledge about its production. The resulting knowledge of a specific Labour-process may serve to inform further Labour-processes and so on. Thus, consciousness comes to be more and more complex through Labour (Lukács, 1969).

The agents of the Labour-process produce themselves as members of the human race, since there is a progression of overcoming their natural instincts, toward conscious self-control of their behaviour (Lukács, 1980). Although Labour can be conceptualised in a universal manner as inherent to Humanity, the Labour-process changes accordingly to the modes of production and the forms of organization that are created to sustain the production process. Labour then, is a condition of human existence, that mediates the relations between humans and nature, and therefore a condition for human life itself. (Marx, 1976, p. 133 cited by Lukács, 1980).

It now becomes important to distinguish Labour (as the central human praxis) from labour (under capitalism). In capitalist societies, the worker is under the control of the capitalist who is the owner of his work (Viana, 2009). The capitalist wants the labour-process to be done properly and the means of production to be adequately applied, saving working tools and not wasting materials, spending only the money essential to execution of work. The final product is the capitalists' property, not the workers'. The capitalist pays for the daily value of the labour-force and incorporates the work done into the price of the product, which also belongs to the capitalist

(Marx, 1982). Workers do not receive the value they produce, only a part of it. To increase profit, the capitalist needs to control the labour-process, especially the time used for production, since more value is produced with the same investment if the worker works more, in less time.

At the beginning of 20th century a rationalisation of capitalistic interests called Taylorism or Fordism was applied in order to generate more profit. It was extremely efficient as it organized work along guidelines dividing labour between makers and performers and fragmenting the duties of each worker to improve managerial control over the labour process. Under Taylorism, workers do not control their rhythm of work, do not need to understand the ultimate purpose of their activities, and work individually, disconnected from other people around them during the labour-process. For the worker the only purpose from the labour-process is the wage.

Besides the labour-processes mechanism, it is also important to understand how the distribution of what is produced affects the organization of labour in capitalism. As the capitalist class craves increased profit, the working class struggles to sell their labour-force for better wages in the hope of increasing their access to consumable goods.

The decline in profitability during the crisis that triggered World War II led to a new round of expansion of capital, which according to Viana (2009) may best be called the *full accumulation regime*. After World War II, the Taylorist organization of labour was reformulated and a new model, Toyotism, added new forms of work intensification for the improvement of profit generation. Toyotism proposes the following elements: teamwork, which enhances productivity; the just-in-time strategy, which is used to respond quickly to demands; flexibility in working contracts, which aims to free capital from juridical and legal barriers; and polyvalence, which determines how workers perform various functions and operate different machines rather than working at one task only. It includes also appeals to the emotional involvement of the workers in their production, through the exploitation of the worker's subjectivity (Antunes, 2009), through team building and work based social events to generate a company identity, for example.

All over the world one can witness increasing unemployment in different fields of activity, under the name of *flexible labour practices*, an euphemism for the deliberate policy of labour force fragmentation and precarious jobs relations. Although this practice dogged industrial development through the late 18th and 19th centuries, it became central to contemporaneous capitalism, in which the production of commodities is not continuous, but is in response to demand, under just-in-time methods. Therefore, hiring permanent workers is not profitable, and workers are called only when necessary (during the Christmas season, for example) (Durant, 2003). This is followed by a significant reduction in the standards of living, even in that fraction of the working population that is necessary to the operational demands of the production system (Viana, 2009; Mészáros, 2002).

As the capitalist mode of production invades all areas of social life, the Toyotist rationality is also applied to organised waged labor in the service sector, which is also dominated by profit making. Service sector profit is obtained from the difference between what buyers pay for services and employees receive for doing them (Viana, 2009).

Besides Toyotism, neoliberalism is an ideological model of society that was triggered to support the full accumulation regime, aiming to reduce capital expenditure by undermining the social rights acquired by working class struggles, such as those expressed in labour laws (Viana, 2009).

Since individuals fit into the productive machinery of the capital system as mere instruments of the general mechanism, human qualities are considered as obstacles to effectiveness. Correspondingly, the same criteria are applied in the evaluation of both human performance and that of a railway locomotive (Mészáros, 2002), when workers are expected to produce as efficiently as possible for the least investment. This cost-benefit logic does not account for all human specific needs, desires, opinions, values, since workers are only considered as the components of a bigger process.

Capitalism adopts authoritarian measures to overcome the difficulties in the management of working conditions, which are increasingly harsh to social and economic life. Some examples are forms of control over the rhythm of work that consider physiological needs as obstacles, limiting rest intervals to the minimum, and the demand for results despite the lack of conditions for achieving them. These measures are created to support the most aggressive postures of capital with respect to its labour-force, with the threat of the law and, where necessary, with the use of force (Mészáros, 2002). The threat of unemployment, for example, pressures workers to bear long unpaid hours of work, situations of institutional violence (as racism, sexism, and xenophobism), moral harassment (like being treated in a hostile manner that affects ones' dignity, physical or psychological well-being), among other forms of exploitation and oppression.

Undoubtedly one can see that the capitalist idea of labour is highly negative with regard to creativity and freedom, as opposed to the positive value of Labour implicit in the ontology of social being (Antunes 2009). The possibility of full human realization is stolen from the worker through alienated labour.

Occupational therapy: Occupation as an element of social division of labour and emancipation possibilities

In the USA and some other western capitalist countries after World War II, the tension and disputes between the interests of corporate owners (efficiency in production and profit), and the interests of workers (for labour rights) resulted in increased access to health and social care services, since these responses to the social needs of the working class also generated profit for dominant social classes (Viana, 2006; Navarro, 1982). From the late 1940s the United Nations Organization (UN), International Labour Organization (ILO) and United Nations Educational, Scientific and Cultural Organization (UNESCO), together with local governments became responsible for the dissemination and implementation of rehabilitation policies. Consequently in many countries protectionist laws were created for people with mental illnesses and disabilities, which proposed the establishment of special programs for these populations (De Carlo & Bartalotti, 2001). The creation and development of occupational therapy at this time bore a close relationship to the capitalistic needs of maintaining the workforce. The world wars were determinants for the expansion of health and rehabilitation professions both to meet the needs of disabled soldiers and for the consequent development of medical practices. This context was responsible for the expansion of work for a number of health and social care professions, including occupational therapists, stimulating the development of specific technical knowledge around the world.

Marxist literature posits that occupational therapy was a product of the complex relations among the social production of illness, the mediations of the State and the permanent class struggle (Soares, 1991). In capitalist societies the social reproduction and maintenance of existence for the majority of individuals and groups depends on selling alienated labour-forces (labour performed without understanding the whole process of production, and from which workers do not receive the total value they produce) and consuming goods. It means that there is a whole apparatus such as public health systems, public education systems, and social services systems whose function is to maintain life under capitalism and its excludent mechanisms of reproduction.

Cordoba (2012) states that the constitution of occupational therapy was based on liberal positivist thoughts. These thoughts explain health problems by focusing on dysfunctional individuals and their manifestation in occupations as the expression of these dysfunctions. Thus, occupation was made the object of occupational therapy practices and it can be simultaneously understood as both the instrument and product of practices of which the ultimate purpose is to fit the person or group to the requirements of the labour market and a concept of social usefulness (Hooper & Wood, 2002; Ambrosi & Schwatz, 1995a; 1995b). Nevertheless, it is possible to identify several experiences of social practices that show other possibilities for addressing needs, developing the ability to determine and create individuals' and groups' own history, and to change the course of events around them and transform their own lives through occupation (Van Bruggen, 2011; Kronenberg et al, 2005; Watson and Swartz, 2004; Medeiros, 2003; Galheigo, 2003).

Emancipatory practices should promote a comprehension of reality, of the real origin of social and health problems (Soares, 2007). Understanding that people cannot individually avoid the social determination of illness may enable them not only to develop the individual abilities to face problems but also the possibility for their political engagement toward wider social transformation.

An example of emancipatory practice was developed in a supervision process with the workers of a psychosocial mental health centre for drug users (Cordeiro et al, 2014). The whole team (psychologists, occupational therapist, nurses, physicians, social workers and others) participated in the supervision process, the aim of which was:

1 to evaluate whether the practices developed in the centre were addressing the health needs presented by the assisted population, as proposed by Trapé, Soares and Dalmaso (2012);
2 to transform practices through reflection about the healthcare production process and the team's Labour-process.

It was expected that the workers were capable of exposing and challenging the reality contradictions in the structural (capitalism), particular (health sector), and individual (psychosocial centre and its patients) dimensions. The supervision was taken as an emancipatory education process, meaning it intended to overcome the technical issues and establish a political dimension of the practices, so the workers were able to dominate the elements of their labour process (Saviani, 2003).

Another example was a workshop with community health workers (CHW) that intended to promote reflection and understanding about the drug consumption phenomena (Cordeiro et al, 2013). By being encouraged to describe their labour-process and conceptions of drugs and drug consumption, the CHW realised that their practices were expected to control drug users' behaviours and habits instead of transforming health needs. Therefore, they realised they were mere instruments (i.e. the workforce) of the healthcare team chain. They also realised that they were the weakest part of the health production process. The workshop allowed them to explain part of their lack of enthusiasm about their work, to develop meaningful practices oriented to the social determination of health, and become active individuals able to shape their practices, intentionally.

Occupational therapists and occupational scientists affirm that humans are occupational beings, and that

> 'people´s engagement in occupations that they themselves find meaningful and useful in their given environment, is as fundamental to experiencing health and wellbeing as eating, drinking, and being loved.' (Kronenberg & Pollard, 2005, p. 62).

According to this, meaningful human activity is a result of a complex relationship between awareness and practice/experience in the world. This is a manifestation of the dialectics of the series of activities we will describe as a series of labour-processes that humans assume daily, from preparing breakfast to building a house, as Lukács would call, a complex of complexes (Tertulian, 1990).

Emancipatory occupation: Labour as the conceptual basis for occupation-based social practices

> 'If meaningful occupation is related to a sense of social belonging, then both the nature of the society to which individuals are obligated and the basis on which membership is determined are problems for occupational therapists' (Kronenberg et al, 2005, p. 57).

Epistemological and theoretical groundings locate practices in relation to the social structure and allow practitioners to clearly establish the basis from which they work. From Marxism, we assume that to achieve critical social practices it is not enough to make social inclusion through fitting people to social structure - but it is necessary and obligatory to engage them in critical and inquiring reflection about the determination of the deprivation and marginalization (social determination of disease-health processes) and the human potentiality of overcoming this structure (through Labour).

Humans change reality accordingly to their needs. Beyond their biological needs they are capable of intentionally transcending those needs through creativity, establishing new needs when desiring things that require instruments that have not yet been invented (Paro, 2001), motivating new inventions and the creation of culture.

By this process humans are able to create their own history through collective Labour as it englobes the social historical construction of technology and culture.

An important explanation is necessary at this point, since there is a complexity in understanding the production of needs. Needs are individual and occur in each person. Nevertheless, as needs are socially produced dialectically accordingly to how humans live in each social group, it is not possible to determine a unique general list of social needs to be satisfied when aiming for social inclusion. The identification of social needs by social inclusion initiatives often does not take this fact into account. If these initiatives are not composed by the people in need themselves, there is a huge risk that the needs addressed are not those of the people they intend to support.

When discussing the importance of challenging occupational apartheid Kronenberg and Pollard (2005) present an important discussion that took place on World Federation of Occupational Therapists debate around the first position paper on community-based rehabilitation, in 2004. This international document was built by members of rich countries and poor countries, and there was a dispute about the use of terms which some considered to be 'too politically charged': occupational apartheid, occupational deprivation and occupational justice. The terms were held important and were kept in the document mainly because without them the document would have represented 'a colonialist position which did not recognize the situations of those countries and communities with fewer health resources' (Kronenberg et al, 2005, p. 68). What the dominant classes consider as important needs must not be taken generically, as the needs of individuals and groups in suffering. For this reason the individual and collective aspects of health-disease process must be taken dialectically into consideration when developing emancipatory practices.

Humans produce their history in the process of social reproduction through Labour, which satisfies needs and also creates new ones. In this process, as part of the human widening of their appropriation of the relations with nature, despite the functionality of these needs (eating, wearing clothes, building a house), some other special needs may and must be produced. Those special needs cannot be satisfied by including people within the existing socio-historical structure that generates them: beyond the quantitative satisfaction of several new needs, those special needs are those of qualitative diversification of the humans (such as the need not only to sleep, but to sleep comfortably, thus inventing a mattress; or the need not only to move from a place to another but to move faster, thus inventing cars; or even the need not only to accept a precarious job that pays the bills, but to be recognized and be capable of operating meaningful transformations that respond to human needs instead of capitalism's needs). Those special needs are defined as radical needs which demand a transcendent movement to overcome current structures (Mendes Gonçalves, 1992). This means: radical needs are those not only of merely fitting within an existing oppressive structure, but of overcoming it and creating new forms of social relations of production.

Radical needs express the confluence between the conscientious creative self-determination of humans through Labour and the social determination of their conditions. Labour is the intentional transformation of nature by humans to satisfy their needs. Needs are produced in humans through their relations with nature, with other humans and with the products of labour-processes. From this perspective,

Labour is a structural element of determination of humans relations to themselves, to the objects of the world and to other humans. Wilcock (1999) and Wilcock and Jakobsen (2001) connect Marx's theory to the concept of occupation, and, as occupational scientists, postulate that humans are occupational beings.

We propose to understand occupation as Labour, to deepen the discussion about the mechanisms of occupation in order to provide instruments for developing emancipatory practices. Emancipation is understood as the consciousness one has of oneself in relation to the whole social structure, associated to the possibilities of interfering in oneself and collectively in the structure. With the term occupation defined as Labour, occupation will be qualified as emancipatory occupation, that is, as a form of affirmation of the specificity of this concept in opposition to capitalist occupation.

Occupation-based professions which are essentially concerned with the social production of needs (those restricted to social reproduction and those of overcoming of the social structures) will not take capitalist occupation as object, but will be concerned with emancipatory occupation instead. Emancipatory occupation, as Cordoba (2012) explains the practices of a critical occupational therapy, will be an expression of collective occupations, practices, historically produced social relations, materialised through the lives of each individual and through the characteristics of each social group.

Social reproduction through Labour is composed of both the individuals' reproduction and the reproduction of a social totality. Besides the material products of the labour-processes, complex relations are also created such as language, laws, philosophy, and religion, for example; and these complex relations produce human history in a social development through time (Tertulian, 1990).

One of the outcomes expected from emancipatory occupation based practices is a conscious understanding of active and creative participation in the political, social, cultural structures that determine one's living and working conditions. And from this awareness, the possibility to produce broader needs, other labour-processes, other occupations, different from the previous ones, in an emancipated human dialectical production of individual and social history.

Examples of emancipatory occupation

From the Collective Health perspective the aim of social practices is human emancipation (Soares, 2007). To propose occupational therapy as a social practice committed to human emancipation, it is necessary to deliver practices that respond to real and broad needs; that respond to the conflicts produced by the contradictions of the social system; and that build the strength necessary for a radical social transformation (Medeiros, 2003). Next we present some practices performed by occupational therapists that take emancipatory occupation as an object.

In a psychosocial mental health care center for drug users, an occupational therapist together with a social worker coordinate a group for women. In the group, they discuss themes brought by the participants about their living situations. Analysing those situations, they realise how much they feel imprisoned by their daily activities.

Together, they create noticeboard displays of news about sexist situations, the roles of women in their society, reflecting on the meaning of their daily choices, and other identity possibilities through experiencing a better knowledge about the social determination of their conditions. From a new perspective, it is expected that what they choose in reality to fit their needs will be different from the limited previous ones (e.g. consuming drugs) (Godoy, 2014).

In an income-generation group for people in highly vulnerability situations, another occupational therapist also developed emancipatory practices. During the production process of keychains and book covers the participants realised that it took more time to produce keychains than book covers, but the price did not follow the same logic: the commodity that was easier to make was more expensive in the market. They discussed profit and how commodities are valued in capitalism. With the support of the occupational therapist, the social mechanisms of the determination of their poverty became clearer to them. The conscious and reflexive participation in the activity created complex relations which allowed the women to widen their ability to understand and value their own Labour (Godoy, 2014). This understanding helped them to overcome the idea of individual responsibility for their conditions, thus the importance of perceiving the potential for collective work for transformation. It is expected that from this experience they will be stronger to resist oppression in labour-processes (mainly subjective violence such as moral harassment), since they know they are not individually responsible for their labour conditions or the results of production process, and since they have the experience of collective strengthening through critical reflection.

While assisting workers with musculoskeletal injuries in an occupational therapy rehabilitation service, it was also possible to identify with them not only which movements, but also which working and living conditions determine their condition. The lack of rest between tasks; the pressure to work quickly; the restriction of movement to only a small repetitive part of a whole production process - were associated with harmful body postures due to long hours spent in overcrowded commuting to work and home; poor nutrition due to lack of accessible healthy food near the job or time to prepare a lunch box; and lack of exercise due to exhaustion from work and shortage of time. All those elements contribute to the complex damage manifested in a musculoskeletal injury. This structural complexity of proposing a process of understanding illness together with the workers during the activity assessment is part of an emancipatory practice.

Conclusion

It is possible to produce the basis for truly transformative occupations which aim for the improvement of the social determination of health by deepening the discussion about emancipatory occupation mechanisms, its structural participation in social reproduction, and its potential of producing freedom for humans to create their own history.

From the discussion proposed in this chapter it is possible to affirm that the social dimension of practice should not be restricted to practices with people in the context of social needs and deprivation - these may be trying to include them into a structure that is based on exclusion. It is extremely important to define a basis from which every worker concerned about occupations will be able to address social change. From this grounding, even when an occupational therapist is exercising a hand muscle, this practice is consciously connected to social determination of health and the other social practices in the society.

To take emancipatory occupation as object of social practices means to promote discussions and experiences that may raise awareness about the existent contradictions in peoples' lives so they might reflect on labour's essentiality to promote strength (in a positive sense) and/or weakness (in a negative sense). Thus, they might reflect on labour participation in the social determination of health-disease processes; the mechanisms in which people engage through labour in this determination process - individually and collectively; and the recognition and transformation of their needs - from alienated needs to conscious and radical needs of social transformation.

The consciousness about the social determination of diseases creates the potential to develop new needs from other perspectives: the possibility to choose more efficiently what to change in the production of one's own life in order to offer better resistance to exploitation and oppression and to start to aim to transcend harmful structures. Inevitably, life conditions of an individual are the life conditions of a whole social group, with similar needs, thus the change must also consider collective action. Individual and/or collective creative action towards transforming reality, generated by needs produced through critical reflection about the social determinants of health-disease processes will be called emancipatory occupation.

Notes

1. Lukács worked from the beginning of the 1960s on a set of writings that became known as The Lukács' Ontology. His work is a milestone for contemporary thought. He wanted to demonstrate the possibility of human emancipation through overcoming exploitation by one person of another. During the capitalist period humans have been adjudged to be capitalist in essence. Investigations of the essential in human beings need to confront this false and ahistorical conception. According to Lukács the category of labour is the original form of the human action. Human and social praxis could not exist without labour (Lessa, 2007).
2. The term Labour (with a capital L) is used in this chapter as the concept from Marx's theory of Labour Process as the intentional and conscious transformation of nature by humans to respond to necessities. The terms labour (with small l) or work are used to identify employment and / or income generation in capitalism.
3. The field of Collective Health developed in Latin America in the late 20th century. Although the field is not characterized by a single influence, the common grounds are an interest in the social dimension of health, and having dialectical and historical materialism (Marxism) as an important epistemological foundation (Osmo & Schraiber, 2015). The authors of this chapter share the Marxist approach to this field of knowledge and practices (Soares et al, 2013).

Acknowledgements

Special thanks to Eurig Scandrett, who believed there was a contribution to occupation-based practices in our ideas, and presented us the possibility to write this chapter. Thanks also to Maria Giatsi Clausen and Elaine Ballantyne, who so willingly listened to the ideas and fondly offered supportive words when they began to take shape.

References

Ambrosi, E. and Schwartz, K. B. (1995a) The profession's image, 1917–1925, Part I: Occupational therapy as represented in the media. *The American Journal of Occupational Therapy*, 49, 7, 715-719

Ambrosi, E. and Schwartz, K. B. (1995b) The profession's image, 1917–1925, Part II: Occupational therapy as represented by the profession. *The American Journal of Occupational Therapy*, 49, 8, 828-832

Antunes, R. (2009) *Meanings of Labour: Essays about Labour affirmation and denial.* 2nd ed. São Paulo: Boitempo Editorial

Borde, E., Hernández Álvarez, M. and Porto, M.F.S. (2015) Critical analysis of social determinants of health approach from social medicine and latin-american collective health. [Uma análise crítica da abordagem dos determinantes sociais da saúde a partir da medicina social e saúde coletiva latino-americana]. *Saúde Debate*, 39, 106, 841-54

Breilh, J. (2008) Latin American critical ('Social') epidemiology: New settings for an old dream. *International Journal of Epidemiology*, 37, 4, 745-750. [Accessed 25 January 2016 at http://ije.oxfordjournals.org/content/37/4/745.full]

van Bruggen, H. (2011) Eastern European transition countries: Capacity development for social reform. in F. Kronenberg, N. Pollard, and D. Sakellariou (Eds.) *Occupational Therapy without Borders: Towards an ecology of occupation-based practices.* Vol, 2. Oxford: Elsevier Science (pp. 851-878)

Cordeiro, L., Soares, C.B. and Campos, C.M.S. (2013) Action research in the collective health perspective: Report of experience of a community health workers education program to face harmful use of drugs. *Saúde and Transformação Social*, 4, 2,106-16. [Accessed 25 January 2016 at http://incubadora.periodicos.ufsc.br/index.php/saudeetransformacao/article/view/2239]

Cordeiro, L., Godoy, A. and Soares, C.B. (2014) Supervision as educative process: Building a paradigm of Emancipatory Harm Reduction with a team from a CAPS -AD. *Caderno de Terapia Ocupacional da UFSCar, 2,* suppl esp, 153-159. [Accessed 25 January 2016 at http://dx.doi.org/10.4322/cto.2014.040]

Córdoba, A.G. (2012) Focus and praxis in occupational therapy: Reflections of a critical occupational therapy perspective. *Terapia ocupacional Galícia (A Coaruña) 5, 18-29.* [Accessed 28 April 2015 at http://www.revistatog.com/mono/num5/prologo.pdf]

De Carlo, M.M.R.P. and Bartalotti, C.C. (2001) Occupational therapy paths. in M.M.R.P. De Carlo and C.C. Bartalotti (Org.) *Occupational Therapy in Brazil. Foundings and perspectives.* São Paulo: Plexus (pp. 19-40)

Durant, J.P. (2003) The refounding of Labour in tensioned flow. *Revista Tempo Social*, 15, 1, 139-158. [Accessed 25 January 2016 at http://www.scielo.br/pdf/ts/v15n1/v15n1a08.pdf]

Galheigo, S. (2003) The social: Going forth and back in an occupational therapy action field . in E. M. M. Pádua and L. V. Magalhães (Eds.) *Occupational Therapy: Theory and practice.* Campinas: Papirus (pp.29-48)

Godoy, A. (2014). *Occupational Therapist Practices In CAPS AD.* Master Thesis, Nursing School, University of São Paulo, São Paulo. [Accessed 13 November 2015 at http://www.teses.usp.br/teses/disponiveis/7/7141/tde-17042015-110935/]

Hooper, B. and Wood, W. (2002) Pragmatism and Structuralism in occupational therapy: The long conversation. *The American Journal of Occupational Therapy*, 56, 1, 40-50

Kronenberg, F. and Pollard, N. (2005) Overcoming occupational apartheid. A preliminary exploration of the political nature of occupational therapy. in F. Kronenberg, S. Simó-Algado, N. Pollard, (Eds.). *Occupational Therapy without Borders. Learning from the spirit of survivors.* Oxford: Elseviers Science (pp. 58-86)

Kronenberg, F., Simó-Algado, S. and Pollard, N. (2005) (Eds.) *Occupational Therapy without Borders. Learning from the spirit of survivors.* Oxford: Elsevier/Churchill Livingstone

Laurell, A.C. (1982) Health-disease as a social process. *Revista Latinoamericana de Salud*, 2, 7-25. [Accessed 28 April 2015 at https://fopspr.files.wordpress.com/2009/01/saudedoenca.pdf]

Laurell, A.C. (1989) Social analysis of Collective Health in Latin America. *Social Science Medicine*, 28, 11, 1183-91

Laurell, A.C. (1991) Labour and health: Knowledge status. in: S. Franco (Ed.) *Social Medicine Debates.* Quito: Organización Panemericana de La Salud (pp. 249-339)

Laurell, A.C. (2008) Advancing towards the past: Neoliberalism social policy. in A.C. Laurell (Ed.) *State And Social Policies In Neoliberalism.* São Paulo: Cortez (pp. 151-178)

Lessa S. (2007) *Understanding Lukács Ontology.* [Accessed 2 July 2019 at https://www.researchgate.net/publication/255644683_Lukacs_Ontologia_e_Historicidade1]

Lukács, G. (1969) *Ontological Basis of Thought and Man Activity.* [Accessed 28 April 2015 at http://www.giovannialves.org/Bases_Luk%E1cs.pdf]

Lukács, G. (1980) *The Ontology of Social Being Vol 3: Labour.* London: Merlin Press

Marx, K. (1976) *Capital.* Vol 1, Harmondsworth: Penguin. [Accessed 28 April 2015 at https://www.marxists.org/archive/marx/works/1867-c1/ch16.htm.s/d]

Marx, K. (1982) *Capital.* Vol 1. São Paulo: Difel

Medeiros, M.H.R. (2003) *Occupational Therapy: An epistemological and social focus.* São Paulo: Hucitec, EdUFSCar

Mendes Gonçalves, R.B. (1992) *Health Practices: Work processes and needs.* Centro de Formação dos Trabalhadores em Saúde da Secretaria Municipal da Saúde. São Paulo: Secretaria Municipal da Saúde

Mészáros, I. (2002) *Beyond Capital.* São Paulo: Boitempo

Navarro, V. (1982) The Labour process and health: A historical materialist interpretation. *International Journal of Health Services.* 12, 1, 25

Navarro, V. (2009) What we mean by social determinants of health. *International Journal of Health Services,* 39, 3, 423-41

Nogueira, R.P. (2009) Social determinants, determination and determinism. *Saúde em Debate*, 33, 83, 397-406. [Accessed 25 January 2016 at http://www.cebes.org.br/media/File/Determinacao.pdf]

Osmo, A. and Schraiber, L.B. (2015) The field of Collective Health: Definitions and debates on its constitution. *Saúde and Sociedade,* 24, 1, 201-214. [Accessed 07 November 2015 at http://www.scielo.br/pdf/sausoc/v24s1/en_0104-1290-sausoc-24-s1-00205.pdf]

Paro, V. H. (2001) *Writings about Education*. São Paulo: Xamã

Rocha, P.R. and David, H.M.S.L. (2015) Determination or determinants? A debate based on the Theory on the Social Production of Health. *Revista da Escola de Enfermagem da USP*, 49, 1, 129-135. [Accessed 11 November 2015 at https://dx.doi.org/10.1590/S0080-623420150000100017]

Saviani, D. (2003) *Historical-Critical Pedagogy*. Campinas: Autores Associados

Soares, L. (1991) *Occupational Therapy: Capital or Labour logic?* São Paulo: Hucitec

Soares, C.B. (2007) *Contemporary Drugs Consumption and Youth: Object construction in collective health perspective*. Lecturer dissertation, Nursing School, University of São Paulo, São Paulo. [Accessed 25 Jan 2016 at http://abramd.org/wp-content/uploads/2014/06/2007_Tese_Consumo_de_drogas_e_Juventude.pdf]

Soares, C.B., Campos, C.M.S. and Yonekura, T. (2013) Marxism as a theoretical and methodological framework in Collective Health: Implications for systematic review and synthesis of evidence. *Revista da Escola de Enfermagem da USP, 47, 6, 1403-1409.* [Accessed 23 January 2016 at http://www.scielo.br/scielo.php?script=sci_arttextandpid=S0080-62342013000601403andlng=en. http://dx.doi.org/10.1590/S0080-623420130000600022]

Soares, C.B., Trapé, C. A., Yonekura, T. and Sivalli Campos, C. (2014) Marxismo, trabalho e classes sociais: Epidemiologia crítica como instrumento da saúde coletiva (Marxism, Labour and social class: Critical epidemiology as a collective health instrument). in J. R. Carvalheiro, L. Sterman and M. Derbli (eds.). *O Social Na Epidemiologia: Um legado de Cecilia Donnangelo (The Social Epidemiology: A legacy of Cecilia Donnangelo)*. São Paulo: Instituto de Saúde

Trapé, C.A., Soares, C.B. and Dalmaso, A.S.W. (2012) The labour of health comunitary worker: Educational dimension of supervision. São Paulo. *Sociedade em debate*, 119-138

Tertulian, N. (1990) A presentation of Lukács social being ontology. *Crítica Marxista - eletronic journal*. [Accessed 28 April 2015 at http://www.ifch.unicamp.br/criticamarxista/arquivos_biblioteca/3_Tertulian.pdf]

Viana, N. (2006) Public policies constitution. *Revista. Plurais*. 1, 4, 94 – 112. [Accessed 28 April 2015 at http://www.nee.ueg.br/seer/index.php/revistaplurais/article/viewFile/69/96]

Viana, N. (2009) *Capitalism in the Integral Acumultaion Era*. Aparecida: Idéias e Letras

Waitzkin, H., Iriart, C., Estrada, A. and Lamadrid, S. (2001) Social medicine then and now: Lessons from Latin America. *American Journal of Public Health*, 91, 10, 1592–1601

Watson, R. and Swartz, L. (2004). *Transformation Through Occupation*. London and Philadelphia: Whurr Publishers

Wilcock, A. (1999) Reflections on doing, being and becoming. *Australian Journal of Occupational Therapy*, 46, 1, 1-11

Wilcock, A.A. and Jakobsen, K. (2001) Occupational terminology interactive dialogue. *Journal of Occupational Science*, 8, 3, 25-31

Chapter 6
Reflections on occupation transforming citizenship

Hetty Fransen-Jaïbi, Inés Viana-Moldes, Nick Pollard, Sarah Kantartzis

Introduction

Issues of citizenship and rights are central to contemporary academic, political and social debate. The potential of occupation to transform citizenship and rights needs to be highlighted both in the wider debate on citizenship in society and within occupational therapy and occupational science. The possession of rights is no guarantee that people effectively have the opportunity or access to exercise them and be full and contributing citizens of their society. Furthermore, rights are essentially focused on the individual; the question remains how people can live together and to shape their common public life together. A citizenship-perspective extends the rights to the public realm, in other words to collective living and doing together (Fransen et al, 2015; 2013).

The authors of this chapter are members of the ENOTHE (European Network of Occupational Therapy in Higher Education) citizenship project group engaged with investigating citizenship in relation to occupation and the contribution of occupational therapy. This chapter deals with a citizenship perspective on occupation and an occupational perspective on citizenship in order to facilitate participation and social justice. Our aim is to address how occupation transforms citizenship, looking for potentialities, and to identify and reflect on what we see to be central issues. Firstly we will introduce the concept of citizenship and some of its various and conflicting interpretations. We will explain the notion of participatory citizenship as an occupational practice and relate this to situations of dis-citizenship. Two case-studies will be presented to allow the exploration and analysis of occupation transforming citizenship in context.

We take a socio-political perspective as a guiding framework mainly drawn on the ideas of empowerment and social justice as expressed by Paulo Freire (Brett, 2007; McCowan, 2006; Freire, 1985; 1968), on Arendt's conception of citizenship and the public sphere and political agency and identity (Hann, 2013, Beltran, 2009; Tubb, 2006; Arendt, 1961; 1958) and on the work of UNESCO on education for citizenship (UNESCO, 2014).

The idea of citizenship

Citizenship and how it is defined and approached

The notions of being a citizen and of citizenship express ideas about how people live together and how we all take care of and are responsible for our shared world. The relationship between the citizen and the state as well as the nature of citizenship has changed over time. These relationships have different meanings depending on their underpinning social, cultural, historical and political contexts.

The word citizen is derived from the Latin for city (Painter, 2005). It means literally: (1) inhabitant of a city, (2) a member of a state (Oxford English Dictionary, 2004). In the middle ages it referred almost exclusively to the inhabitant of a town. The 19th and early 20th century in particular was a period of political struggles over political and social rights - over what citizenship meant and who could be a citizen. Citizenship includes important concepts of the rights and responsibilities of the individual in relationship to the state, which are historically situated within the theories developed in 19th century Northern Europe and America. These ideas of citizenship remain significant today (Hoskins et al, 2012).

Models of citizenship

Citizenship takes many different forms. Ensuring effective practices and policies to promote citizenship for all people demands a clear recognition of the differences in understanding of the concepts and their variations. Most of the literature on citizenship distinguishes four main and competing models of citizenship, which are presented in Table 1:

These models of citizenship result from different historical, cultural, economic, political and social developments. They identify what it means to be a citizen and how the role, principles and focus of the citizen depends on the underlying ideology. In this sense, it is important to highlight that more than one of these models coexists simultaneously in society and social institutions (schools, health and social care, professional organisations, etc.). There are conflicting and changing ideas in the resulting dynamism amongst which people are living, articulating different discourses, roles and actions depending on each scenario.

In recent years the notion of active citizenship has developed. It is seen as a practice and not merely a passive legal status. The terminology of participatory citizenship or active citizenship has been introduced to highlight these active and action based dimensions of citizenship. As noted in its definition: participatory citizenship is 'participation in civil society, community and/or political life, characterised by mutual respect and nonviolence and in accordance with human rights and democracy' (Hoskins, 2006, p. 4).

Some examples are the urgent questions about the future of the earth and its sustainability, which put demands on 'planetary citizenship' (Padilha et al, 2011). These are about issues such as taking responsibility and care of our global world today and how to do this collectively in the face of threatening climate change as a product of human activity. Without collective action the earth will be impoverished and lose its natural cycle of renewal, because of overexploitation. Without collective action, the contemporary problems of humanity, such as migration, poverty and conflict will increase in an exponential way (UNESCO, 2014).

Citizenship Models	Liberal	Communitarian	Civic republican	Critical
Principles	Citizens' involvement in public life is minimal, and is primarily enacted through the vote.	Citizenship focuses on identity and feelings of belonging to a group, and the need to work towards the collective benefit of this group.	Citizens become the actors of positive laws for social change and the instruments to prevent corruption.	Citizens critique and improve society through social and political action based on the ideas of empowerment and social justice.
Focus	Atomized individuals.	Communities.	Emphasizes the need for citizens to act politically within the public sphere, and to be actively engaged within a political community as equal and free citizens.	More dynamic view on democracy that is grounded in critical and engaged citizens. Focus on equal participation in the power relations of democracy.
Citizens role	Citizens' conform to the rules. Volunteering.	More hierarchical and top-down decision making.	Equality in political participation. Learn civic competences.	Create change towards greater equality.

Table 1: Models of Citizenship: characteristics. Adapted from *Contextual Analysis Report. Participatory Citizenship in the European Union Institute of Education (*Hoskins et al, 2012).

Citizenship, inequalities and dis-citizenship

Citizenship is central to contemporary politics. It is one of the most important and controversial concepts in social and political debate, and a focus of education (UNESCO, 2014; Painter, 2005). However, citizenship is also a highly problematical concept. Having legal rights and obligations is insufficient to enable equal opportunities for all citizens and to guarantee that all citizens are able to exercise their rights. Although having equal rights is invaluable, inequalities are often a barrier to effectively practicing and realising full citizenship and enjoying the civil, political and social rights which go with this. This brings the concept of citizenship from the legal into the socio-political domain, revealing significant tensions: between homogeneity and diversity, belonging and inclusion and exclusion. There is also an emphasis in this legal discourse on the individual and their relationship with the state, ignoring citizenship as relationships between people, fellow citizens. As much as the collective living and doing together as citizens in communities may be positively recognised as places of cooperation and mutual recognition, they are also places of inevitable conflict, social control and exclusion (Ferreira et al, 2012).

This problem is seen in the definition of citizenship in terms of a Northern hemisphere perspective, which is culturally Western and shaped through socioeconomic privileges in relation to other parts of the world (Kabeer, 2002). An increasing awareness of the transcultural demographic composition of most states through globalisation and migration is challenging these 'old' concepts. Models of differentiated or transcultural citizenship are needed as alternatives or complements to local contextualised, national and universal conceptions of citizenship (Sousa dos Santos, 2012; Painter, 2005).

Furthermore, these old concepts of citizenship are not grounded in the lived experiences of people in most Southern or Eastern countries (Sousa dos Santos, 2012; Kabeer, 2002). They have been introduced as foreign elements in struggles for self-determination, or imposed by governments within old colonial borders, but never delivered or enacted, making their promises hollow words. They have not expressed the perceptions of so-called 'minorities' whose cultural and social geography may exist on other boundaries than those drawn up in the ages of empires. To claim that a Western definition of citizenship is universal is at least West-Eurocentric.

The use of words such as *integration* may be a denial of discrimination and a cover term for mechanisms of exclusion, producing stale forms of multiculturalism which deny differences and serve only dominant values (Gilroy, 2012). Even appointing people to a *minority*, particularly those minorities seen to be less-able, less-valuable, makes them different and belonging to *the others* (us-them) and indirectly expresses denial of human diversity.

As can be seen, citizenship involves more than an individual status; it is also a practice that locates individuals in the larger community (Devlin & Poitier, 2006). This suggests, that the inclusion or the exclusion of individuals from the status of citizenship is something which is as much arbitrated at the local contextual level as it might be ordained through the connections of power (not just through government but also through cultural, corporate, or other organised institutions, both legal and extra-legal in character). The consequences of such arbitration are experienced in terms of personal identity and belonging; access to and participation in resources and facilities; the experience of personhood and of freedom, that is, the components of agency in the social world. Many persons as well as whole groups experience exclusion at different levels. In an absence of recognition they are silenced, absent and invisible citizens (Sousa dos Santos, 2012) assigned to the status of 'dis-citizen', a form of citizenship-minus, a disabled citizenship. Dis-citizens experience exclusion from the co-creation of the collective history and social change.

Citizenship as an occupational practice

As an ongoing, contested process citizenship is expressed through occupation, which is shaped within the particular context and circumstances that arise through human relationships. Occupation is an essential part of inclusive societies and based on the participation in public life of people as citizens of their society (Galheigo, 2011). Socially excluded groups are not only denied access to the formal structures and activities of decision-making which govern the collective life of a society, but also their dependent status or their marginalisation may undermine their capacity to exercise voice and agency on their own behalf, to act like citizens (Kabeer, 2008). Perspectives of the multidimensional continuum of inclusion-exclusion are important for the contemporary debate around citizenship as an occupational practice.

Occupation transforming citizenship as an everyday life practice

We present two case-studies of citizenship as an everyday life practice that illustrate the power of occupation in transforming citizenship. The first (see Example 1), a narrative of displaced farmers, illustrates the power of former common occupations in bringing people together and enabling healing, shaping identities and new paths. The second (see Example 2) is about literacy and the creation of possibilities, a changing relationship to others, recognition and dignity.

Case study 1. Farmers in Columbia

Seated in the vacant room, Ana* knew she had witnessed tangible evidence of the true transformative power of occupation. As a Colombian citizen and occupational therapist, Ana had grown up and pursued her education in a country where a 60 year-civil war had gone from being at the forefront of all citizens' minds, to one that had taken permanent residence as a defining piece in the fabric of their lives. Possibly the longest-running internal conflict in the Western hemisphere (Centre for Justice and Accountability, n.d.), Colombia's armed conflict was rooted in political violence and a chronic persistence of social and economic inequalities, worsened by drug trafficking, corruption and abuse of power. In recent years, several collective efforts across the nation produced the disarmament of some guerrilla and paramilitary groups, as well as the public admission of government involvement in human right violations. However, the healing of a nation touches every life and peace must overcome in a few years what conflict has had decades to shape, namely citizenship and trust. With more than 5.7 million internally displaced people, occupational therapists in Colombia labour daily to see the power of occupation enable healing, shape identities and rediscover new paths.

Earlier that day, Ana had conducted a workshop for internally displaced peasants. As part of a public funded initiative that aims to provide victims of internal displacement with opportunities to engage in entrepreneurial initiatives, Anna had been instructed to lead the group in discovering options for alternative productive occupations. The day before Ana had conducted the workshop with catastrophic results. Having come from different parts of the country, typically identified as being influenced by specific guerrilla or paramilitary groups, participants had found it impossible to work in collaboration as the wounds inflicted to their families and heritage by each of the groups was associated with the places of origin of others in the room. But in her knowledge of occupation Ana found her greatest skill. This time she called for each person to participate in a workshop specifically for people who shared a particular occupation back home, such as farmers. Now, with all farmers who had lost the only land they had known to be theirs sitting in the room, their common occupation provided them with a means of connecting and empathising. They realised that regardless of their stories, they could all relate to the loss of an occupation that shaped their identity, and that common place was the platform upon which they stood to collaborate, imagine, create and move forward. That afternoon, having used her knowledge of how occupation shapes identity, Ana could see clearer than ever: that sometimes occupation is all we have in common; and there is room to heal in that common place (Liliana Alvarez Jamarillo, OT, PhD, Colombia)

*For confidentiality and privacy purposes, the name of the therapist has been changed.

Case 2: Pecket Learning Community, UK

Pecket learning community was a radical basic adult education college which was set up in 1985 by a group of adult learners working with an adult educator who decided to set up their own college. None of them had any fundraising experience or of running an organisation.

They wanted to do away with distinctions like tutor and student, and campaigned and fundraised to set up and run their own college. With the help of the adult educator they bought space in an old Co-operative shop in the village of Pecket Well, in West Yorkshire, UK. The college opened in March 1992, run by volunteer directors, two thirds of whom were people with direct experience of adult literacy difficulties. Other directors might come from a professional background but had to recognise that they were learners themselves, and the process adopted by Pecket towards all its adult learning programmes was of co-operative education. This was liberating: everyone could recognise that there would be things they did not understand, people had "to learn to be a learner".

Classes thus became workshops in which people worked on their struggles with writing, reading, numeracy or community skills. People learned in a non-hierarchical way and they learned to empower each other. This is very important when working with the multiple barriers and depleted confidence which adult learners often have. People can be quickly demoralised and never come back to the learning environment. In the co-operative education model which Pecket developed, the recognition of this issue was part of almost everyone's experience. Many of the members had at some time been afraid to enter classrooms, and one of the most important feature of the college was the tea urn, which was available all day if you needed a place of refuge. Workshops appointed special roles such as the 'word watcher' to ensure that no terms which were difficult were left unexplained, residential weekend courses appointed 'toffee twins' (who had drawn sweets with identical coloured tags wrapped in them) whose role was to offer each other support through the course. Many people learned basic computer skills on a computer in a plywood case – Pat Smart's famous 'wooden computer', which itself took the anxiety out of coping with new technology. Members of the college campaigned locally on literacy and disabled access issues.

Pecket learning community was not an occupational therapy programme, but it could be described as occupation based. Access to literacy and numeracy skills is fundamental to many aspects of everyday occupation. In the villages of West Yorkshire many people were isolated because they could not read bus timetables, experienced multiple exclusions, the biggest of which was that their needs had been abandoned in the educational process. Pecket's educational methods were about peers skill sharing, negotiating their learning about literacy and numeracy through activities which included running their own college (Hamilton et al, 2014; Smart et al, 2010; Smart, 2005).

Both cases present coinciding and relevant aspects when we consider occupation as empowering and transforming citizenship. Participatory processes are needed to ensure that all the stakeholders have the ability to access opportunities to express their voice and to participate in decision making, including decisions about the development of the process itself. Another key element, described in the cases, is the recognition that all the participants have knowledge. Respect for everyone, carried through negotiation and agreement on the methods and actions as well as the discussions of the dilemmas the groups encountered, raise awareness and critical consciousness of this process of individual and collective transformation, as a lived experience.

The role of occupation is the 'backbone' of the life process itself, through which one develops as a citizen, learning and doing citizenship. In both cases we see that the power of occupation is evident throughout the life cycle and that what has been developed in the past may serve in the present. In Case 1, the common occupation of farming and loss of land creates a sense of belonging which assists in re-focusing participants' lives. In Case 2, occupation is a common starting point from which the Pecket members start a process of emancipation, participation, co-empowerment and civic transformation. These stories of real events about individuals, situations and structures offer insight into *how* occupation can be connected to understandings of citizenship and used for exploratory analysis and discussion of four central issues of occupation transforming citizenship as an everyday life practice which we present in the next section.

Recognition and equal dignity

Both cases show us how engagement in occupation and collective occupation provides a scenario for exploring and living experiences of equity, social value and reciprocal recognition. But collective occupation can also reproduce the processes of exclusion, for example, through anti-social actions, and also through the effects of discriminatory practices which are operated through both institutions and the locally social (the local community) against minorities (Ramugondo & Kronenberg, 2013). These occur whether they are identified specifically, covertly, because they identify secondary characteristics such as geographical areas where people live rather than clear categories such as skin colour, or because the needs of minorities are not accounted for. Often the trajectories which are involved in these practices are not made explicit, but they emerge in individual narratives or collective protests representing experiences. Thus exploring equity, social value and multiple recognition as a living experience is an interesting and powerful process because it implies a redistribution of power, voices, roles, tasks and decision making in the process of building and doing together. Ana makes this possible with the Colombian farmers by finding a common experience of loss; the Pecket members achieve this by working out their own processes to enable each other to pursue an approach to education that works around the barriers they have experienced.

Recognition is a central concept in the work of Arendt. She notes that a starting point of becoming human is *to have the rights to have rights* and a key to rights as a whole. Social recognition as not just as a human, homo sapiens, but as a person with social value and social esteem comes with recognition (Hann, 2013). For Arendt the question is not to be or not to be, but *to belong or not to belong*. The Colombian case shows that legal citizenship does not go far enough when the state has little ability, or interest, in guaranteeing citizenship rights. The violence in some regions of Colombia dehumanises and disrupts the lives of those it affects. One of the most significant consequences has been the forced displacement of millions of people, which, for Colombian farmers makes human rights largely paper constructions with little possibility of realisation in the immediate future. Everything, including rights, depends on belonging – on being recognised as a member of a given political community and thus having access to the right to have rights (Tubb, 2006). The farmers' loss of their home means the loss of their socially constructed identity from where they were born and raised and where they have created a unique socially connected existence (Arendt, 1961). This loss of connections and relationships entails the loss of the relevance of speech, because there is nobody there to listen, and the loss of the importance of human relationships, because there is nobody there who cares.

The effectiveness of collective occupations in helping displaced refugees or victims of violence to construct new identities and navigate new ways of belonging is shown in research in occupational therapy (Motimele & Ramugondo, 2014). The power of collective occupations, alluding to social cohesion and a common good, for example mutual cooperation and support in order to develop and divide labour (Ramugondo & Kronenberg, 2013), has synergies with collective aspects of healing as a process that extends beyond the individual. The examples of the Pecket learning community and the Colombian farmers illustrate this synergy and the main role of occupation in this process.

Freire (1968) describes dehumanisation as processes resulting from an unjust order that engenders violence in oppressors, which in turn dehumanises the oppressed. Critical consciousness of this unjust order together with reflection on action is the collective process, transcending the individual, based in recognition and equality by which the transformation can take place (Freire, 1985). Freire's main thought is that human beings must move forwards increasing humanisation, and moving away from becoming mere *objects*, determined by other peoples' intentions and without real agency to becoming *subjects* of history (McCowan, 2006). This allows the will and the opportunity to act as citizens for a common interest and a common good. We note the parallels with Arendt's concepts of recognition and being a person.

A way of doing in the world with others

The cases described above make explicit the power of occupation as the core of social life itself. In the examples, occupation enables people to begin to transcend and transform issues of horror, hatred, discourses, ideologies and to work for strategies to confront their non-recognition and non-rights status. Thus, through their collective occupation and actions, individuals, relationships, common places, nature, culture and society are intertwined and reconnected in a new configuration or space, but now with more respect, dignity and recognition for others.

Thibeault (2002) discusses the vital role that occupation can play in the rebuilding of civic society following the extreme violence and disruption of civil war. Being intimately related to all aspects of daily life yet conceptually neutral, occupation 'becomes the instrument of mediation: offering a silent bridge between perpetuators and victims, it allows for a softer adaptation...' (Thibeault, 2002, p. 43), giving examples including not only mediation ceremonies but also the rebuilding of schools by communities together. This demonstrates concretely that the rebuilding of civic society is not only about physical reconstruction, but also about the transformation into active contributing citizens to society. Both cases presented illustrate the emergence and importance of this transformational process based in reciprocal recognition, sharing voices and doing together.

The cases demonstrate this power of shared, community or collective occupation. Arendt (1958) builds upon this concept of action in the common world through the coming together of people based on their equality and plurality, and the power that emerges from this to create and sustain the common or public world. The importance of this public world has been emphasised as the place where the previously un-noticed can act and be heard, have voice and visibility, claiming both space and an entry to political life (Beltran, 2009). At the same time the public world often operates as a meritocracy and makes minor assumptions about inclusion and equality which prevent those who are overlooked from participating. For example, non-attendance might be the result of inaccessibility rather than lack of interest. A combination of such exclusions can render the invisible more invisible, and promote greater inequality (Iqbal, 2013; Fraser & Honneth, 2003).

While collective occupation may take different forms, from the construction of social organisations to celebrations, requiring various skills, roles, tasks, etc, however the core principle is about the deep understanding of diversity as a natural potential and expression of mankind. Using this perspective, it is important to be aware of and work through our individual/group/societal/centrism, instead using that diversity to diffuse discrimination and human oppression in any of its expression (Sousa dos Santos, 2012). It is important to recognise how discrimination and oppression are also enacted through occupation at the collective level. Sometimes differences have become a core element of individual and community identity and the issues they bring can give a strong sense of purpose to a group, but the community is also the place where such relationships can be mediated.

Physical, social and virtual spaces in which to practice citizenship

Citizenship is practiced in occupations that take place in our communities: in urban/rural spaces, schools, work places, and in local associations and organisations. Again, in both examples the importance of citizenship being enacted in the real world, in time and space is evident. In Case 1 reconciling alienated people following civil war requires the coming together of people in places, regardless of their previous political positions. This may be regulated through policy but the coming together in space and time, allowing all to have their voice heard and to participate in decision making and in doing, is necessary for the development of a sense of belonging and that change may happen.

Places are also important sites of exclusion and discrimination, encouraging the increased visibility of some citizens and the 'disappearance' of others. In the second case we see how the people from the Pecket Learning Community had experienced difficulty in entering traditional learning environments and were demoralised. In addition, because of their literacy difficulties they were not fully able to participate in community life. They developed a co-operative form of education and the collective occupations within the classrooms or around the tea urn were important for empowering and providing a safe point from which to explore learning. They were sites for occupations of doing, being, becoming and belonging (Wilcock, 1998).

Spaces for participation and the expression of citizens' voices are rarely neutral. The fact that public spaces for participation exist, whether in law or social practice, does not mean that they will always be used equally by various actors for realising the rights of citizenship. Rather, each space is itself socially and politically located, with dynamics of participation varying across differing levels and arenas of citizen engagement, and across differing types of policy spaces (Di Massio, 2012; Painter, 2005; Fraser & Honneth, 2003). Many are regulated by local government – such as market spaces, or have become areas which are the focus of corporate styles or the regulation of social behaviour, like shopping malls (Dennis et al, 2010), sports events (Lera-López et al, 2012), the suppression of fairs (Cameron, 1998) or interior design of pubs (Haydon, 1994). The establishment and maintenance of much 'public' space, is today largely governed by institutional and/or the hegemonic order of the locally social world, which regulates the possibilities for voice and action within them. In this context, occupation in place may also change the meaning of these places. Places become receptacles for memories of the collective life developed within them, violence and horror as well as celebrations, reconciliation, and moments of change.

Of note is the virtual world as an emerging place for citizenship. Many social movements are utilising the increasingly participatory opportunities for communication and collaboration that the Internet offers. Citizens may participate through accessing information and participating in discussions, signing petitions, lobbying politicians and organising action (see Shant and van Bruggen, volume 2, chapter 6). In regions of the world where state institutions may restrict full access to information, the Internet is an increasingly important vehicle for communication and mobilisation particularly of the youth (Herrera, 2014).

Within this discussion we can see the relevance of Arendt's concept of the public sphere comprising two distinct but interrelated dimensions, both essential to the practice of citizenship. The first is the 'space of appearance', a space of political freedom and equality which comes into being whenever citizens act together. The second is the 'common world', a shared and public world of human artifacts, institutions and settings which separates us from nature and which provides a relatively permanent and durable context for our activities (Arendt, 1961). Here we can see the contribution of occupation to the places that are created through it, for example the importance of art, as human expressions occupying cultural spaces promoting democracy, tolerance, education, diversity, critic, ethics and aesthetics.

Participation in political life

'For the things we have to learn before we can do them, we learn by doing them' Aristotle

The spaces in the case-studies allow people to participate in the processes of creating and shaping together a common place for a common good. Although the cases describe quite specific populations and localities these issues of participation in community life can also be understood as an issue of participation in political life.

Political participation - by which we mean taking part in a range of activities such as discussion and speaking out about political matters, taking forms of action, contributing to the organisation of events, campaigns or political parties - is much more than merely casting a vote. It is valued and at the core of the democratic definition of citizenship and social justice offered in the ideas and work of Arendt and Freire or through UNESCO. Involvement and participation in decisions and actions is clearly important to transforming community, yet it is complex and has many different facets. Arnstein's ladder of citizen participation (Arnstein, 1969) is frequently referred to in analyses of citizen participation because of its clarity concerning the different forms of participation and their relation to power and empowerment as main organiser. This ladder of citizen participation sets a progression in terms of power and citizenship control through eight different levels, from the 'non-participation' of manipulation and therapy, through 'tokenistic' forms of participation to 'citizen's power' and ultimate level of citizen control. Arnstein made clear that participation without real opportunities and power to affect the outcomes of the process is empty and superficial, and maintains social injustice. The quality of the participative process and experiences needs to be considered (Ferreiro et al, 2012). Both cases presented consideration of the process itself, enacted and facilitated by the quality of the collective occupation that was at the core of the transformational change that took place.

From a 'democratic' perspective, simply being able to participate is a major achievement (a principle of the liberal citizenship model, see Table 1), but to the poor and disadvantaged lack of resources means that the participatory process must yield tangible benefits (Brett, 2007). This point of view is a depoliticisation of the idea of participation and citizenship, making it rather mechanistic. We argue that a more critical model of citizenship (see Table 1) is required, that moves towards recognising that participation and occupation need to be present in order to make transformation and full citizenship possible. A concern with the qualities of citizenship emphasises the importance of political participation because it permits the establishment of relations of civility, solidarity and tolerance among citizens.

We follow Arendt in her vision that reactivation of citizenship in the modern world depends on the recovery of a common, shared world and the creation of numerous spaces of appearance and occupation in which individuals can disclose their identities and establish relations of reciprocity and solidarity. This public interest has little to do with our private interests, since it concerns the world that lies beyond the self. It refers to the interests of a public world which we share and shape by coming together as citizens, and which we can pursue and enjoy only by going beyond our private self-interest. Political action and discourse are, in this respect, essential to the constitution of collective identities and the public world.

Freire also values universal political participation, seeing political participation in the terms of co-operation with others and which he sees as considerably threatened by the alienated individualism of neo-liberalism and the consumer society (McCowan, 2006). In his view the process of humanisation and the transformation of society is only possible by education and political participation in the context of the collective.

Reflective conclusions: Towards occupation in a transformative approach to participatory citizenship

Occupation and participation are vital for social justice in relation to the effective functioning of society, which demands the participation of all individuals in its processes, and makes them intrinsically political. The quality of these processes, their inter-relatedness and the synergy of all aspects and elements in making the transformational process happen, are foregrounded in our case-studies and in the main issues discussed in them. The emphasis in both case-studies is put on the learners' personal experience in the world as a starting point, from which real-life problems and contradictions are revealed and problematised through dialogue. The sense of being a subject and having the ability to intervene in the external public world, to be citizens, is embodied in the processes of conscientisation and empowerment of Freire and capture ideas of political agency and collective identity as exposed by Arendt. Both underscore the importance of praxis, reflection and action and with this enactment in occupation.

In our analysis we have mostly drawn on the work of Freire and Arendt for their transformative critical analysis. We have emphasised the importance of citizens as active inter-relating subjects participating in the public realm with a strong enactment in occupation. The significant issues discussed are intertwined and are related to understandings of occupation as belonging, being, doing and becoming (Wilcock, 2006). Recognition and equality (belonging and being), a way of doing in the world with others (being and doing), physical, social and virtual places in which to practice citizenship (doing and becoming) and participation in political life (becoming and belonging) are all grounded in occupation. Citizenship and rights have an impact on occupation in the sense of doing, being, becoming and belonging (Wilcock &

Hocking, 2015) and on occupation as a human right (Algado et al, 2016; Galheigo, 2011; WFOT, 2006). However, we stress the dialectical relationship where occupation also has the power to transform citizenship and rights.

Both Arendt and Freire were strongly influenced by their own life context and historical period. It is important to recognise that approaches, interpretation and focus vary within a critical sociopolitical perspective, placing in diverse configurations the most relevant issues regarding occupation and citizenship. Context is paramount and should be acknowledged, understood and explored. Pretending that there is one universal model of citizenship denies the very different historical construction of citizenship experiences. No one model can address them all and no one model can be prescriptive. For example, in countries where there are intensive conflicts or post-conflicts settings (Colombia, South Africa) citizenship approaches are often considered with regard to working towards peace and collective identity (Bloomfield et al, 2003) including the rethinking of collective being, collective awareness of the realities and the needs for transformation. In other contexts, for instance in Brazil, citizenship notions drive social occupational therapy (Malfitano et al, 2014). Although the word citizenship is absent, the concept underpins occupation in practice which shapes social cohesion, consciousness raising and social transformation (Malfitano et al, 2014; Lopes et al, 2008; Barros et al, 1999). In countries which are experiencing transitions in government regimes, such as in Eastern Europe, the Middle East or Tunisia, the citizen perspective has been considered as reinforcing principles of democratic participation and universal values (UNESCO, 2014). Regional integration policies, as in the European Union, or within countries, for better cooperation around societal issues, have emphasised the citizenship perspective for increasing tolerance and respect for diversity and encouraging people to be receptive to different cultures and the potential benefits of diversity (UNESCO, 2014; Tsaliki, 2007). These approaches involve a learning process which addresses both what and how people learn about themselves and others. They are concerned with how people learn to do things and interact socially and towards encouraging them to develop active and participatory roles. We have demonstrated through the cases and the discussion, how occupation has the potential to be catalytic in the transformative process, engaging people through a collective process.

This chapter aims to be orientated towards the future, with an open perspective simultaneously encompassing the movements of globalisation and the need for authentic sustainable local communities. However, a historical perspective is useful and an understanding of underlying causes is important for raising awareness about injustices as well as awareness of the complexities of the processes involved in moving towards more active and positive participation and citizen engagement. It enables us to establish a point from where the processes of belonging, being, doing, and becoming can move us towards active participation in the public realm, around the dynamics of 'how to empower the future' in a rapidly changing world with major challenges. It is challenging, but essential, to find a common place, where everyone is a participant, an ordinary and valuable person (farmers, students, teachers ....). These common places, where the dialectical process between occupation transforming citizenship and citizenship transforming occupation can be built, are places of occupation.

Acknowledgments

We wish to thank Liliana Alvarez Jamarillo and the Pecket Learning Community (www.pecket.org) for the case-stories.

References

Algado, S. S., Guajardo, A., Correa, F., Galheigo, S. and Garcia, S. (2016) *Terapias Ocupacionales desde el Sur: Derechos Humanos, CIudadanía y Participación* [Occupational therapies from the South: Human rights, citizenship, and participation]. Santiago, Chile: Editorial USACH

Arendt, H. (1958) *The Human Condition* (2nd Edition). Chicago: The University of Chicago Press

Arendt, H. (1961) *Between Past and Future: Eight exercises in political thought.* New York: The Viking Press

Arnstein, S. (1969) A ladder of citizen participation. *Journal of the American Institute of Planners,* 35, 4, 216-224

Barros, D., Ghirardi, M. and Lopes, R. (1999) Terapia ocupacional e sociedade. *Revista de Terapia Ocupacional da Universidade de São Paulo,* 10, 2/3, 69-74. [Accessed 5 March 2016 at http://doi.org/10.11606/issn.2238-6149.v13i3p95-103]

Beltrán, C. (2009) Going public: Hannah Arendt, immigrant action, and the space of appearance. *Political Theory,* 37, 5, 595-622

Bloomfield, D., Barnes, T. and Huyse, L. (2003) *Reconciliation After Violent Conflict: A handbook.* Stockholm: International Institute for Democracy and Electoral Assistance. [Accessed 29 February 2016 at http://www.un.org/en/peacebuilding/pbso/pdf/Reconciliation-After-Violent-Conflict-A-Handbook-Full-English-PDF.pdf]

Brett, P. (2007) *Endowing Participation with Meaning: Citizenship education, Paolo Freire and educating young people as change-maker.* [Accessed 8 January 2016 at http://www.citized.info/pdf/com marticles/Endowing%20Participation%20Peter%20Brett.pdf]

Cameron, D. (1998) *The English Fair.* Stroud: Alan Sutton

Dennis, C., Newman, A., Michon, R., Brakus, J. and Wright, L. (2010) The mediating effects of perception and emotion: Digital signage in mall atmospherics. *Journal of Retailing and Consumer Services,* 17, 3, 205-215

Devlin, R. and Pothier, D. (2006) Introduction: Towards a critical theory of dis-citizenship. in R. Devlin and D. Pothier (Eds.) *Critical Disability Theory. Essays in philosophy, politics, policy, and law.* Vancouver: UBC Press (pp. 141-175)

Ferreira, P., Coimbra, P. and Menezes, J. (2012) Diversity within diversity: Exploring connections, between community, participation and citizenship. *Journal of Social Science Education,* 11, 3, 118-132

Fransen, H., Kantartzis, S., Pollard, N. and Viana-Moldes, I. (2013) *Citizenship: Exploring the contribution of occupational therapy.* ENOTHE. [Accessed 14 June 2015 at http://www.enothe.eu/activities/.../CITIZENSHIP_STATEMENT_ENGLISH.pdf]

Fransen, H., Pollard, N., Kantartzis, S. and Viana-Moldes, I. (2015) Participatory citizenship: Critical perspectives on client-centred occupational therapy. *Scandinavian Journal of Occupational Therapy,* 22, 4, 260-266

Fraser, N. and Honneth, A. (2003) *Redistribution or Recognition?: A political-philosophical exchange.* (Translators: J. Golb, J. Ingram, and C. Wilke, Trans.). New York: Verso

Freire, P. (1968) *The Pedagogy of the Oppressed.* (Translator: M. Ramos). Harmondsworth: Penguin

Freire, P. (1985) *The Politics of Education: Culture, power and liberation* (Translator: D. Macedo). USA: Bergin and Garvey

Galheigo, S. (2011) What needs to be done? Occupational therapy responsibilities and challenges regarding human rights. *Australian Occupational Therapy Journal*, 58, 60-66

Gilroy, P. (2012) 'My Britain is fuck all' zombie multiculturalism and the race politics of citizenship. *Identities*, 19, 4, 380-397

Hann, M. (2013) *Recognising Recognition: Hannah Arendt on Human Rights.* Political Studies Association Annual Conference 2013. Cardiff. [Accessed 7 October 2016 at https://www.psa.ac.uk/sites/default/files/988_509.pdf]

Hamilton, M., Nugent, P., Pollard, N. and members of Pecket Learning Community Steering Group (2014) Learner voices at Pecket: Past and present. *Fine Print,* 37, 1, 15-20

Haydon. P. (1994) *The English Pub: A history.* London: Robert Hale

Herrera, L. (2014). *Wired Citizenship: Youth learning and activism in the Middle East.* New York: Routledge

Hoskins, B. (2006) *Draft Framework on Indicators for Active Citizenship.* Ispra: CRELL

Hoskins, B., Abs, H., Han, C., Kerr, D. and Veugelers. W. (2012) *Contextual Analysis Report. Participatory citizenship in the European Union.* Institution of Education. [Accessed 15 November 2015 at http://ec.europa.eu/citizenship/pdf/report_1_conextual_report.pdf]

Iqbal, K. (2013) *Dear Birmingham: A conversation with my hometown.* Bloomington, Indiana: Xlibris

Kabeer, N. (2002) *Citizenship and the Boundaries of the Acknowledged Community: Identity, affiliation and exclusion.* IDS working paper 171. Brighton: Institute of Development Studies; 2002. [Accessed 10 May 2015 at http://www.ids.ac.uk/files/dmfile/Wp171.pdf]

Kabeer, N. (2008) *Social Protection Strategies for an Inclusive Society: A citizen-centred approach.* Institute of Development Studies, Sussex UK. Note prepared for UN Expert Group Meeting On Promoting Social Integration, Helsinki 8-10 July 2008. [Accessed 10 May 2015 at http://www.un.org/esa/socdev/social/meetings/egm6_social_integration/documents/Social_protection_strategies_Naila_Kabeer.pdf]

Lera-López, F., Ollo-López, A. and Rapún-Gárate, M. (2012) Sports spectatorship in Spain: Attendance and consumption, *European Sport Management Quarterly*, 12:3, 265-289

Lopes, R., Adorno, R., Malfitano, A., Takeiti, B., Silva, C., and Borba, P. (2008). Poor youth, violence and citizenship. *Saude e Sociedade,* 17, 3, 63-76

McCowan, T. (2006) Approaching the political in citizenship education: The perspectives of Paulo Freire and Bernard Crick. *Educate*, 6, 1, 57-70

Malfitano, A., Lopes, R., Magalhães, L. and Townsend, E. (2014). Social occupational therapy: Conversations about a Brazilian experience. *Canadian Journal of Occupational Therapy,* 81, 5, 298-307

Motimele, M. and Ramugondo, E. (2014) Violence and healing: Exploring the power of collective occupations. *International Journal of Criminology and Sociology*, 3, 338-401

Oxford English Dictionary. (2004) Oxford: Oxford University Press

Padilha, P. R., Favarão, M.J., Morris, E., Marine, L. (2011) *Educação para a Cidadania Planetária: currículo intertransdisciplinar em Osasco. [Education for Planetary Citizenship: Intertransdisciplinar curriculum in Osasco].* São Paulo: Editora e Livraria Instituto Paulo Freire

Painter, J. (2005) *Urban Citizenship and Rights to the City.* Background paper to the Office of the Deputy of the Prime Minister. International Centre for Regional regeneration and

Development Studies. Durham University. UK

Ramugondo, E. and Kronenberg, F. (2013) Explaining collective occupations from a human relations perspective: Bridging the individual-collective dichotomy. *Journal of Occupational Science*, 20, 1, 1-14

Smart, P. (2005) A beginner writer is not a beginner thinker. in F. Kronenberg, S. Simo Algado, and N. Pollard (Eds.), *Occupational Therapy without Borders – Learning from the spirit of survivors.* Edinburgh, Churchill Livingstone/Elsevier Science. (pp. 46-53).

Smart, P., Frost, G., Nugent, P. and Pollard, N. 2010) Pecket learning community - where the stem of knowledge blossoms. in F. Kronenberg, N. Pollard and D. Sakellariou (Eds.) *Occupational Therapies without Borders* (Volume 2). Edinburgh, Elsevier Science (pp. 19-26)

Sousa dos Santos, B. (2012) Public sphere and epistemologies of the south. *Africa Development*, 37, 1, 43-67

Thibeault, R. (2002) Fostering healing through occupation: The case of the Canadian Inuit. *Journal of Occupational Science*, 9, 3, 153-158

Tsaliki, L. (2007) The construction of European identity and citizenship through cultural policy. *European studies*, 24, 157-182

Tubb, D. (2006) Statelessness and Colombia: Hannah Arendt and the failure of human rights. *Undercurrents*, 3, 2, 39-51

UNESCO (2014) *Global Citizenship Education: Preparing learners for the challenge of the twenty-first century.* Paris, France. [Accessed 12 December 2015 at http://unesdoc.unesco.org/images/0022/002277/227729E.pdf]

Wilcock, A. (1998) Reflections on doing, being and becoming. *Canadian Journal of Occupational Therapy*, 65, 5, 248-256

Wilcock, A. (2006) *An Occupational Perspective of Health, 2nd Edition.* Thorofare NJ: Slack Incorporated

Wilcock, A. and Hocking, C. (2015) *An Occupational Perspective of Health, 3rd Edition.* Thorofare NJ: Slack Incorporated

World Federation of Occupational Therapists (2006) *Position Statement on Human Rights.* [Accessed 12 December 2015 at http://www.wfot.org/Resourceentre.aspx]

Chapter 7
Facilitating inclusion through occupation-based community development

Roshan Galvaan

This chapter begins with a brief rationale for and overview of an Occupation-based Community Development framework. This framework guides practice through addressing social inequalities and promoting occupational justice. It provides insights into the key elements that inform developing an understanding of the needs of a marginalised group, as they emerge across the phases of the framework. An emphasis is placed on the adaptation of participatory methods, with photovoice explained to demonstrate application.

Introduction to an occupation-based community development framework

Many people experience social exclusion, reflected subtly or overtly in their daily experiences of participating in human occupations. Structural restrictions, such as social, economic, political, or cultural factors, may limit their access to opportunities for equitable participation in occupations. Nussbaum (2011) suggests that marginalisation and discrimination should be addressed to promote social justice through making opportunities more accessible. Viewing capabilities as opportunities, the Capability Approach recognises that core opportunities are required so that people are able to achieve functionings that enable them to live meaningful and dignified lives (Nussbaum, 2011). While the Capability Approach, as an economic and political theory supports occupational therapy's social justice pursuits, further theoretical direction is required for occupational therapy to address social and occupational injustices.

Acknowledging that occupational therapists have to formulate ways of practicing that embraces critical approaches to practice, Galvaan and Peters (2013) established the Occupation-based Community Development (ObCD) framework. ObCD as both a framework and particular approach to community development aims to generate long-term discursive processes, where the discourses and practices of everyday 'doing' are challenged (Galvaan & Peters, 2013). These discursive processes emerge across the four phases of the ObCD framework that is a theoretical framework that guides the occupational therapists reasoning and thinking through their practice decisions. The four phases are summarized in text box 1.

Text box 1: Phases of ObCD (Galvaan & Peters, 2013)

Phase I: Initiating a Campaign

As suggested by the name, this phase involves initiating a collaborative relationship with stakeholders in the community. The aim of this phase is to develop mutual understandings of how participation in occupations occurs in context, identifying instances where limitations are imposed or possibilities for authentic participation are limited. Together with community stakeholders, the challenges to participating in human occupation are explored and possibilities for taking action are articulated. A Campaign refers to actively organized, collaborative processes of pursuing change.

Phase II: Design

This phase extends on insights emerging through gaining mutual understanding during the Initiation phase by interpreting and applying occupational science concepts and constructs to develop and design a strategy to address the mutually identified needs. Actively and collaboratively developing strategies for change in ObCD involves participating in occupations, giving careful consideration to applying participatory methods and strategically accessing necessary and available resources available. Drawing on key processes of community development (Taylor et al, 1997) together with occupational science concepts and constructs, it assists therapists to collaboratively design campaigns that address identified needs, particularly in relation to occupational injustice.

Phase III: Implementation

Implementing the designed strategy occurs through building on the processes emerging from the participatory methods applied in the previous phases. This phase involves participation in occupations. Throughout this phase the collaborators reflect on, improvise or create new strategies, as is necessary to address the identified needs. This reflection occurs through ongoing application of the Action Learning cycle (Taylor et al, 1997).

Phase IV: Monitoring and Evaluation

Continuous critical reflection and improvisations during the previous phases means that monitoring occurs throughout the phases of the ObCD framework. Notwithstanding, this phase focuses on monitoring and evaluation of the intervention in terms of the extent to which the needs are being met, as reflected in shifts in participation. It allows for different interpretations of the needs to emerge across time and so informs the ongoing Development process. Evaluation of particular aspects of interventions implemented provides feedback to all involved on what works and areas that need refinement and change.

ObCD as a critical occupational therapy practice

ObCD is a form of critical occupational therapy that is informed by research and practice with communities (Galvaan, 2015, 2010; Galvaan, Peters & Gretschel, 2015; Peters, 2011). The critical approach to practice is aligned with the use of critical theories, such as critical race theory, postcolonial theory, critical disability theory, each aimed at transforming society. Such theories aim not only to describe or justify what is happening or being experienced, but offers a critique and explores possible conditions for change. These theories may also be applied to inform which marginalised groups are worked with as a priority in the face of resource constraints. The choice of selecting marginalised groups to work with may thus be a political and strategic decision that is informed by the social, economic and political landscape within communities. In so doing, the application of these theories promote questioning of how things are, together with re-imagining what may be or become in future, thus creating mindsets of possibilities.

ObCD addresses the conditions that limit participation in human occupation, emphasizing individual change together with policy and contextual changes in order to develop more equitable opportunities and privileges for marginalised groups to participate to their full potential and to exercise, without subjugation, control over what they do every day. Text box 1 illustrates how critical race theory is applied in research related to domestic work in South Africa. The insights gained into relationships provided a glimpse of the need to challenge hegemonies in order for domestic worker's work conditions to change. This shows the kind of reasoning that informs the practice that draws on the ObCD framework.

Text box 2: Use of critical race theory to frame domestic work

Domestic work is an undervalued form of work and domestic workers, as a group of workers, are known to be vulnerable (Fall et al, 2013). Thus domestic workers would typically be a group of people rendered vulnerable through societal structures, who occupational therapists could work with. In South Africa, the majority of domestic workers are Black women. While previous research explored the experiences of domestic workers engaging in occupations (Galvaan, 2011), it also highlighted the pivotal influence of employers on the domestic workers' experiences. The study described below, focused on the employers' experiences of employing a live-in domestic worker.

A phenomenological study was conducted to explore the experiences of employers of live-in domestic workers in the Cape Town metropolis, South Africa. Six employers were purposively selected and two interviews were conducted with each person. A thematic data analysis was completed between interviews, followed by two more levels of analysis (Galvaan et al, 2015).

A significant aspect emphasised in the theme and categories was the way that the relationship between the employers and domestic workers left the employers feeling weighed down (Galvaan et al, 2015). The employers experienced some tensions in how they were supported by their domestic workers; however, their access to domestic workers enabled them to participate with more choice. This participation was possible since employers were able to orchestrate the conditions of employment in ways that prioritised their occupational identities while showing sympathy towards the limitations in the domestic worker' occupational identities. The research showed that through the particular manner in which employers' accessed their own occupational rights, they placed their domestic workers in situations where they experienced occupational injustice. The employers recognised that although they depended on their domestic workers, they felt burdened by the relationship. For example, one participant's privilege is seen in her expression of admiration for domestic workers:

"Um, I think it's very sad, because I think it's very unfair or sad that these women are having to leave their children behind, often in the Eastern Cape with their mothers or indeed alone and come and work here to send money back. I think and I also sometimes think it's really sad that, that you know, like I felt with Thandi, gosh, what must it be like to have children who are 7 or 9 or whatever, who aren't with you and then you are looking after someone else's children. I mean life isn't a fair process, but I find that really a sad thing that it has to be like that for them. But you know, the thing I really admire about these women and I'll tell you something, my experience, my experiences, Xhosa women, really reliable, I mean I admire them cause they bite the bullet and say this is what we got to do to survive."

In the above quote, the employer's admiration for the domestic worker's resilience occurs against a background of sympathy. In referring to life not being fair, she acknowledges that she has not experienced this unfairness. However, she does not recognise how the history of colonization and apartheid, through migrant labour, contributed to the separation of black mothers from their children. The employer in this extract was a white female and the domestic worker, a black female and the employer was from a higher social class compared to the domestic worker. Intersectionality draws attention to the way that people hold multiple social identities and that these identities give them different power in social situations (Yuval-Davis, 2006). In this example, the employer does not consider that she may be experiencing privilege in contrast to the struggle faced by the domestic workers. This exchange could be considered in terms of white privilege. White privilege (Case, 2012) refers to the obvious and subtle extent of social, political, and economic advantage experienced by white individuals, as a systematic product of racial domination. Thus, while the employers used their dominant race and class positions, the domestic workers remained subjugated. Applying critical race theories allows for more nuanced understandings of power to emerge. The way in which structural and systemic racism affects everyday exchanges are revealed. This would assist in informing how occupational therapists may work to advance the rights of and enhance the possibilities with domestic workers. This description is also significant in relation to considering the way that relationships influences participation in occupations. The application of critical theories is not limited to the participants, but should extend its analysis to the therapists. In this regard, the therapists involved in ObCD processes should draw on these theories to self-critique and reflect on their interactions with all stakeholders. This means that therapists have to critically examine their privileges and work towards eliminating prejudices or discriminatory practices that may operate during the ObCD processes. In this way, change may equally occur for therapists and all stakeholders in the ObCD process. This involves identifying how power operates within everyday occupational engagement. Power is understood in terms of how people relate to each other and their contexts.

Human occupation in ObCD

In ObCD, the reference to *occupation-based* signals that occupation is both used as an analytic tool and as a basis for practice. As an analytic tool, occupational science concepts and constructs are interpreted together with occupational therapy concepts to guide occupational therapy practice. Occupational science concepts refer to abstractions about human occupation drawn from observations made of cases related to the performance or participation in human occupation. Occupational science constructs (Ramugondo, 2015) are developed by drawing on occupational science concepts together with relevant other abstractions to formulate theoretical interpretations of human occupation. Both occupational science concepts and constructs may inform theories and concepts in occupational therapy.

Text box 2 provides a brief description of the use of occupation as an analytic tool before presenting how occupation may be applied as a basis for practice. A key element of this analysis is an awareness of the politics of human occupation. An appreciation of the politics of human occupation, particularly during the initiation and design phases, guides the therapist away from a purely individual focus, towards considering how contextual factors contribute to the patterns of participation available. The politics of human occupation has been theorized within the occupational science constructs of occupational choice (Galvaan, 2015), occupational consciousness (Ramugondo, 2012), occupational possibilities (Rudman, 2010), collective occupations (Ramugondo and Kronenberg, 2013) and occupational justice (Whiteford & Townsend, 2011; Stadnyk, Townsend & Wilcock, 2010). The theoretical coherence between these constructs has been referred to as a cluster of constructs (Ramugondo, 2015). In the above example of domestic workers' employers, the power relationship between the employer and domestic workers, expressed through the occupations that the domestic worker has to perform, reflects some of the politics of human occupation in that the occupational choices available to domestic workers are limited by structural factors in their context, but that these same structural factors, such as the influence of a capitalist economy, also influence the employers' need for and experiences of having domestic workers.

Text box 3: The Mitchell's Plain Workgroup – Leigh Ann Richards, Liesl Peters and Roshan Galvaan

Mitchells Plain is an area located on the Cape Flats in Cape Town. High unemployment, low education levels, substance abuse, gangsterism and crime are typical challenges in this area. Marginalisation and limited participation are common experiences for people with disabilities living in this community. The recognition of the way in which people with disabilities are compromised here led to the development of the Mitchell's Plain Work Group, supported by the Cape Town Association for Persons with Physical Disabilities (APD). This group consisted of people with physical disabilities who live in Mitchell's Plain, are unemployed and who are dependent on a disability grant. The group was registered as a satellite workgroup of Cape Town APD and started to receive a subsidy toward their operating expenses, from the Department of Social Development on a monthly basis.

The initial purpose of the group was for the members to earn an extra income by making products to sell. The group met every day and consisted of nine members. When the group began, the Cape Town APD social worker was primarily responsible for the day-to-day operations of the group. This included recruiting members, registering them, purchasing stock and consumables, book-keeping and organising refreshments for the members. This led to a situation where the members in the group were totally reliant on the social worker and the attendance of the group was poor. The products manufactured by the group were not being sold which compromised the main goal of the group, that is, to generate an additional income for people with disabilities and their families. Income generation could be seen as the end occupation that members aimed to participate in. Members were unhappy and indicated that they desperately wanted to change their situation. The occupational therapist, who contributed to development processes within Cape Town APD, was approached to assist.

Through the application of an Occupation-based Community Development approach, the occupational therapist thought strategically about the way in which the group viewed themselves, their participation, and their potential to succeed. This involved recognising that there were limitations in the way they were positioned in relation to their work, particularly their agency. As a result she collaborated with members to construct a space that could be used to enable the members to view their participation differently and begin to reconstruct a more strategic action plan that would assist them to redirect the development of their group. Through this members began to identify and articulate their needs and reflect on the purpose of the workgroup in addressing these. Utilising discussions created the opportunity for them to critically examine their role in the direction and development of the workgroup, acknowledging how this interfaced with their needs. The occupational therapist used key questions informed by organsational development (Taylor, 2003) that assisted members to open up their own thinking to new possibilities while facing the shortcomings in their participation and the evident failure of the workgroup to meet their needs. Through this opportunity to think differently about the interface between themselves and their situations members began to recognise that they owned the power to (re)direct the group.

In order to harness this renewed sense of power the occupational therapist supported the group to consider the options at their disposal to move the group forward. This was done by encouraging members to re-evaluate the goals for their group and to develop an action plan for the future. Although this was a good strategy to support the development of new occupational choices the group found that acting on their identified goals was not as easy because of the way in which practical consciousness informed their usual occupational choices. For example, they had to re-think how they wanted to access the resources (including finances) that they needed. As a result the group faced challenges, but through continued support while they performed the occupations of the group, were able to own their power. They actively reflected with the occupational therapist on what their available options or possibilities for action were so that they could move towards meeting their needs. The outcome has been that the group is better established, as illustrated for example, in their success in negotiating a crafts contract with the City of Cape Town. Group members became completely responsible for managing their finances and have not been dependent on a social worker for the past few months.

This case example emphasises the importance of doing as a means to reflect and develop new ways of participating. Although the occupational therapist enabled the opportunity to critically reflect on their situation the workgroup had to act more consciously in making occupational choices in order to realise change. This proved difficult, although not insurmountable. Through strategic support in the form of challenging dominant occupational choices and liberating ways of thinking incisively, individuals and groups are able to carry their own agenda forward and realise their development. This particular case also highlights that when community members take responsibility and a partnering approach is promoted, the waste of resources and funding is prevented. If the roots for sustainable planning and learning are nurtured in this way, groups of people are able to carry forth their own goals with little professional support.

The interpretations made based on the analytic use of human occupation, informs the practical use thereof. Since ObCD aims to disrupt hegemonies that perpetuate social inequities, such as the power imbalance that exists between employers and domestic workers in South Africa, the continuous exploration of how participation in occupations maintains such hegemonies is needed. Analysing the patterns of occupational engagement seeks to reveal the ways in which hegemonic practices are perpetuated through entrenched assumptions and mindsets. Applying this within the design phase of ObCD, the facilitator has to consider which occupational science constructs and assumptions assist in conceptualising the issues that emerge during occupational engagement with stakeholders and assist in identifying possibilities for change. Practice thus involves facilitating processes that contest how people navigate the social, economic and political struggles associated with their occupations in context. A key mechanism through which this occurs is the application of occupation as means and as end is pertinent in the Design and Implementation phases of ObCD (Galvaan & Peters, 2013). Once a mutual understanding of the needs has been reached and a possibility for change in occupation has been identified, this change may be identified as the participation in occupation that is being aimed for as an end. Simultaneously, it may be possible to apply the use of occupation as a means whereby occupations are participated in, in real time so that efforts are made towards the intended changes in occupation. This perspective of focusing on occupations as means and end is distinct from the view of using occupations towards enhancing performance components (McLaughlin Gray, 1998). When considering occupation as an end, the goals of occupation-based community development are always focused on actualising more liberated forms of participation. In some instances, the occupations that are intended as the end, may be participated in as a means. In the above example, the group members were engaging in income generation toward the end of being able to participate in viable income-generating occupations. However, the focus of the facilitated process was not merely on income. Through ongoing processes of facilitating participation in occupations as means and end, change may be facilitated. Liberated forms of participation allow people to participate as their authentic selves without being compromised by or conforming to dominant hegemonies. Through designing and strategically selecting or constructing opportunities for participation in real world occupations, occupations are applied as means and ends.

Facilitating participation

Participation in processes of community development is understood as emerging from active political struggle through which identity and position are negotiated (Cornwall & Brock, 2005). Working with the influence of each person's multiple subject realities and across situations, ObCD aims to facilitate participation, acknowledging that such facilitation requires considering these multiple subject realities. Thus, participation and non-participation are not seen as opposites. Instead even non-participation may be viewed as a form of active engagement, that is - resistance. To this end, an occupational therapist has to gain an understanding into the active struggles reflected in people's participation. Since this understanding is deepened and changes as people participate in occupations and situations over time, the level and type of understanding evolves as participants engage. Occupational therapists have to remain alert to such changes. Thus, to practice community development, occupational therapists need to develop ways of gaining understanding that do not just focus singly on an individual or their environment, but explores both. This involves critical reflexivity to challenge the gaps between occupational therapy philosophy, ideas, theories and the practical realities of everyday practice (Whiteford & Pereira, 2012).

Participatory methods have been utilised in occupational therapy practice in community settings, with the aim of promoting emancipatory goals (Galheigo, 2011; Whiteford & Townsend, 2011). Through the application of such methods connections between people, with what they do and with what matters to them are facilitated. Participatory methods are applied as a way of engaging with people so that they can bring their authentic selves to bear on the development process. Photovoice is a particularly useful example of such a method which has been discussed as a method for occupational therapy research (Galvaan, 2010) and will be described further here.

Facilitating participation through photovoice methods

Photovoice methods are participatory-action research methods which draw on critical consciousness-raising and feminist theory (Wang et al, 2004) to facilitate participation. It allows people to define for themselves what is worth remembering. Thus, participants are able to define and select what they represent in their photos. By drawing on Freire's concept of education for critical consciousness, photography is used to apply the principle of reflecting with the community (Wang et al, 2004). Through a facilitated, self-generated process of producing photos, individuals or groups of people and communities can reveal the social and political realities affecting their lives. Thus, people are able to produce rich photographic images representing what they want to communicate as community activists. Occupational therapists have identified that photovoice methods hold value as a research method (Lal et al, 2012) while the use of photovoice applied as a distinct project through which participants are able to express themselves publically during community activism has not been documented. When applying photovoice within ObCD, the therapist should consider how to draw on the method in a way that will best facilitate participation and serve the emerging needs. It may thus be to adapt and apply elements of photovoice methods. The key elements of photovoice have been identified as 'Getting the picture'; 'Unpacking the picture' and 'Using the findings' (Galvaan, 2007).

Getting the picture

The process of producing the photos in a way that allows for the participant to exert their agency is deemed of utmost importance (International Visual Methodologies for Social Change Project, 2009). In ObCD, the application of photovoice is adapted to serve the unfolding development process. The facilitator has to consider whose perspective is being sought, recognising that there are sub-groups amongst participants. Thus the 'participants' in the focus group may be different stakeholders, rather than a single participant or group. To inform the negotiation about who is involved in the project, the therapist should critically reflect on what more needs to be understood and what may not have been said, collaboratively discussing this with all involved. This assists with identifying what needs further exploration that could be revealed through the photos.

It is essential to build a relationship of trust with participants before and while initiating the photovoice project, this allows for open discussions about any possible risks associated with capturing the images. These discussions have to identify what the potential risks are, for example risks to privacy or safety, and find ways of managing these. Practical consideration should be given to which cameras are accessible and the timing of taking the photos. A simple point-and-shoot disposable or inexpensive camera (Wang, 1999) can be used to capture the images. Cell phones with cameras, when accessible, are also an easy way to capture the desired images.

Discussions reflecting on actual images and practice sessions using the camera are essential to assist the participants with thinking about what they want to capture and how they may choose to frame it. It is suggested that clear production prompts be used to assist the participants in knowing what they are expected to do and to ensure that they capture what is intended for the project (Mitchell, 2008). An example of a prompt could be as simple as drawing a participant's attention to a comment that they may have made during an interview and checking if this is something that they could explore further through the images that they capture. It is advised that prompts are kept simple and focused (International Visual Methodologies for Social Change Project, 2009). The length of time allocated for the production of the photographs is negotiated between the therapist and participants. Previous researchers have allocated between forty-five minutes (Mitchell et al, 2005) to weeks (Ewald & Lightfoot, 2001a) depending on the subject and process being followed.

Unpacking the picture

Many participants in photovoice projects are novice, first-time photographers, but are able to produce rich data (Mitchell et al, 2007). Once the images have been captured, the facilitator collects the photos or copies of the images and prints these for discussion with the participants. Participants would view their collection of photographs and photo-elicitation interviews can be applied to explore the content of the photographs. Photo-elicitation interviews allows for seeing the context and for flow in the participants account. The quality of being able to capture action in a photograph is particularly important for the doing, action-orientation of occupation. During photo-elicitation interviews, the participants should be requested to share their experiences of capturing the images (Ewald & Lightfoot, 2001b). Aspects of this experience can be further probed and following from this elements related to participation in occupation can be further explored. Insights into tacit, explicit, individual and group knowledge about how occupations occur and what occupations may or may not be participated in are critically discussed. The occupational therapist should be concerned with both the content and context of the photograph and thus can investigate both of these during the photo-elicitation interview. This creates opportunities to explore how hegemonies, for example those associated with neo-liberal ideologies, where participation in occupations may be disproportionately influenced by market-driven identities and values, are challenged. In this way the process of unpacking the picture may feed into the way that the findings are used.

While engaging in these discussions, the facilitator should be aware of how personal and positional power influences participation.

Using the Findings

Through reflecting on the occupations captured in the images, mutual understanding of the way forward and the issues that should be addressed is reached. Insights gained into how occupations occur, factors that prevent participation from occurring and the way in which power is navigated during participation becomes apparent through unpacking the photos. These very issues may be the focus of the ongoing development process and inform the design of the occupations that are applied as means or end.

Adaptation of photovoice methods in ObCD

Although the application of photovoice methods may be applied as described above, the therapist may also apply aspects of the photovoice method. In the example in text box 4, Cornelius and Peters describe how the student therapists were able to create a code through capturing the images of participants engaging in daily occupations. This created a stimulus for critical discussions about possibilities for change. This provides one example of the utility of a participatory method within the ObCD process. It also alerts facilitators to the need to think about what aspects of the method is most relevant and how they may use themselves to contribute to the emerging understanding.

Text box 4: Nonzamo Seniors' Club
Christelle Cornellius and Liesl Peters

Ikamva Labantu (IL) (Ikamva.org.za) is a non-profit organisation dedicated to providing services to the most vulnerable people in South Africa's township communities. In response to the challenges facing seniors', as well as the lack of services and support for them in the township communities, Ikamva Labantu volunteers and community leaders began supporting and establishing community-based seniors' clubs during the era of apartheid. The organisation formally oversees seventeen seniors' clubs under the umbrella of its Senior Sector. The aim was to create a supportive environment for vulnerable older persons and to enable them to remain active in their communities for as long as possible through the provision of community-based care and support. Services provided by Ikamva Labantu aim at reducing vulnerability and increasing dignity. These services are based on the premise that older persons know what they need and that they can provide support to each other. It is with the support of Ikamva Labantu that they are able to organise themselves and access resources that enable their needs to be met. Ikamva Labantu's response is not about bringing the services to the people. Rather, it is about utilising the resources of the people to create more opportunities for them. One strategy applied in providing support is to develop leadership structures within the seniors' clubs that encourage club members to critically consider their preferences for self-governance.

Nomzamo is one of the Ikamva Labantu seniors' clubs and is situated in Langa. The club did not have a suitable venue in which to meet and had no cook or club assistant. Although Ikamva Labantu had assisted other seniors' clubs to attain such resources this provision was not always possible. Final year University of Cape Town occupational therapy students were placed at this club as part of their practice learning requirements. They were required to consider designing campaigns that focused on occupation-based community development. At the point of the intervention described below, Nonzamo club members did not draw on their authority to effectively run their club in the way that they were felt satisfied with. Initially they held the view that they were the subjects of change rather than the change agents. As a result the club members tended to wait for Ikamva Labantu to sort out their problems and members did not all participate in or take control of the day-to-day running of the club. There were few opportunities for participation in meaningful occupations available to them at Nonzamo Seniors' club, despite this being one of the central reasons for the club's existence. This framed the Initiation stage of the ObCD process.

Occupational therapy students recognised the need to consider how the club members wanted to view and enact their self-governance. In response, the occupational therapy students created opportunities for the club members to view themselves differently through a process of critical storytelling. Thus the occupational therapy students saw themselves as participating with the club members and storytelling involved multiple views of the club members' participation. This enabled the members to gain a different and deeper understanding of themselves as a collective (Taylor, 2003). This process involved an opportunity for club members to view their participation from the 'outside-in' through the use of photographs as codes. This adapted use of photovoice method involved the students taking photos of the club members engaging in daily tasks during the course of the week. All the documented occupations captured were then presented to the club members for critical reflection.

Club members were shocked to realise both what they were missing and what was beneficial about their current participation. For example, a particular photograph depicting club members engaged in the informal activity of reading the newspaper on a particular morning provided members with the insight to realise that some of their occupational choices could be shaped into more formal opportunities for participation, which would benefit all the club members. This was since some of the members had not realised that they could access or read the newspaper at the club, but upon reflection saw this as an opportunity to discuss current events. Through facilitating participation drawing on photovoice, agency was set in motion.

Thus the opportunity for critical storytelling, prompted by these photographs, was coupled with opportunities to dialogue (Senge, 2006) together as a club. This created the platform to engage with the outcomes of the storytelling process and to consider together what mechanisms they required to more effectively self-govern. They began to work collaboratively to put a more structured activity programme in place for themselves. The outcome was the development of an active and participatory approach to electing an executive committee, as well as a cooking committee. This has meant that all club members now contribute to the provision of their daily meals. Overall, the process resulted in group of seniors who are more active in their processes of change.

This case example has highlighted how the opportunity to view ones' participation in context can begin the process of changing how occupations are participated in. This together with the space to engage in critical dialogue enables groups to transform their mindsets. The process enabled the group to assume the power they had as a resource and utilise this to contribute as productive citizens.

In text box 4, the students and participants both contributed to developing the understanding. Each partner's contribution made it possible for the change to be set in motion. This equal, but different contributions offered by different stakeholders recognises the value that each person can contribute to the development process.

This section has highlighted facilitating participation and drawing on participatory methods such as photovoice as techniques that support occupation-based community development practice. In addition to participatory methods, facilitation techniques drawn from organisational development, such as Dialogue (Senge, 2006; Isaacs, 1999) and the Thinking environment (Kline, 1999) are applied in ObCD. Adaptation of these methods to suit the development process and enhance the use of occupation or achievement of participation in occupations informs the application and selection of methods.

Conclusion

This chapter has provided an overview of Occupation-based Community Development as a way of promoting occupational justice. It identified how practice may be designed, drawing from occupational science concepts and constructs. Particular focus is given to the influence of the politics of human occupation. This is extended into the way that occupations are used as a means and end and the adaptation of participatory methods to facilitate change. This provides a glimpse of how occupational therapists together with others could contribute to enabling access to real opportunities in people's lives in order to enhance the capabilities available and functionings that they are able to achieve. While this approach may have therapeutic qualities, it is not aiming to address impairments through applying therapeutic techniques. Instead it provides a way of facilitating change at the local and micro level, in people's everyday lives, while situating this in relation to the structural challenges that they have to negotiate.

Note

1 The word Intervention has been replaced with 'Campaign' as a more accurate reflection of the processes and action involved

References

Case, K.A. (2012) Decoding the privilege of whiteness: White women's reflections of anti-racist identity and ally behavior. *Journal of Social Issues,* 68, 1, 78-96

Cornwall, A. and Brock, K. (2005) What do buzzwords do for development policy? A critical look at 'participation', 'empowerment' and 'poverty reduction'. *Third World Quarterly,* 26, 7, 1043-1060

Ewald, W. and Lightfoot, A. (2001a) *I Wanna Take Me a Picture: Teaching photography and writing to children.* Boston: Centre for Documentary Studies in association with Beacon Press

Ewald, W. and Lightfoot, A. (2001b) Literacy through photography. in W. Ewald and A. Lightfoot (Eds.) *I Wanna Take Me a Picture.* Boston: Centre for Documentary Studies in association with Beacon Press

Fall, Y., D'Cunha, J., Lewis, N., De Freitas, N., Courteille, C., Koning, M. and Smenjaud, C. (2013) *Domestic Workers Count too: Implementing protections for domestic workers.* [Accessed 7 October 2016 at http://library.pcw.gov.ph/sites/default/files/documents/resources/domestic_worker_count_too.pdf]

Galheigo, S. M. (2011) What needs to be done? Occupational therapy responsibilities and challenges regarding human rights. *Australian Occupational Therapy Journal,* 58, 2, 60-66

Galvaan, R. (2007) Getting the picture: The process of participation. in N. de Lange, C. Mitchell, and J. Stuart (Eds.) *Putting People in the Picture: Visual methodologies for social change.* Rotterdam: Sense Publishers (pp. 153-161)

Galvaan, R. (2010) *A Critical Ethnography of Young Adolescents' Occupational Choices in a Community in Post-Apartheid South Africa.* (PhD thesis), Cape Town: University of Cape Town. [Accessed 7 October 2016 at https://core.ac.uk/display/29056866/tab/similar-list]

Galvaan, R. (2011) Domestic workers' narratives: Transforming occupational therapy practice. in F. Kronenberg, N. Pollard, and D. Sakellariou (Eds.) *Occupational Therapies without Borders – Volume II: Towards an ecology of occupation-based practices.* (2nd ed.) Philadelphia: Churchill Livingstone Elsevier (pp. 349-356)

Galvaan, R. (2015) The contextually situated nature of occupational choice: Marginalised young adolescents' experiences in South Africa. *Journal of Occupational Science,* 22, 1, 39-53

Galvaan, R. and Peters, L. (2013) *Occupation-based community development framework.* [Accessed 7 October 2016 at: https://vula.uct.ac.za/access/content/group/9c29ba04-b1ee-49b9-8c85-9a468b556ce2/OBCDF/index.html]

Galvaan, R., Peters, L., and Gretschel, P. (2015) Embracing an 'occupational' perspective to promoting learning in context. *South African Journal of Higher Education,* 29, 3

Galvaan, R., Peters, L., Smith, T., Brittain, M., Menagaldo, A., Rautenbach, N, and Wilson-Poe, A. (2015) Employer's experiences of having a live-in domestic worker: Insights into the relationship between privilege and occupational justice. *South African Journal of Occupational Therapy, 45,* 1, 41-46

International Visual Methodologies for Social Change Project. (2009) *Doing Photovoice.* [Accessed 7 October 2016 at http://www.ivmproject.ca/tools/photovoice.pdf]

Isaacs, W. (1999) *Dialogue: The art of thinking together.* New York: Doubleday

Kline, N. (1999) *Time to Think: Listening to ignite the human mind.* London: Octopus Books

Lal, S., Jarus, T. and Suto, M. (2012) A scoping review of Photovoice method: Implications for occupational therapy research. *Canadian Journal of Occupational Therapy,* 79, 3, 181-90

McLaughlin Gray, J. (1998) Putting occupation into practice: Occupation as ends, occupation as means. *American Journal of Occupational Therapy,* 52, 354-364

Mitchell, C. (2008) Getting the picture and changing the picture: Visual methodologies and educational research in South Africa. *South African Journal of Education,* 28, 365-383

Mitchell, C., De Lange, N., Stuart, J., Moletsane, R. and Buthelezi, T. (2007) Children's provocative images of stigma, vulnerability and violence in the age of AIDS: Re-visualisations of childhood. in N. De Lange, C. Mitchell and J. Stuart (Eds.) *Putting People in the Picture: Visual methodologies for social change.* Rotterdam: Sense Publishers (*pp.* 59–72)

Mitchell, C., Moletsane, R., Stuart, J., Buthelezi, T. and De Lange, N. (2005) Taking pictures/ taking action! Using photovoice techniques with children. *Children First,* 9, 60, 27-31

Nussbaum, M.C. (2011) *Creating Capabilities. The human development approach.* Cambridge, MA: The Belknap Press of Harvard University

Peters, L. (2011) *A Biographical Inquiry into the Occupational Participation of Men who Drop Out of School.* (MSc (OT) thesis), University of Cape Town, Cape Town. [Accessed 7 October 2016 at https://open.uct.ac.za/handle/11427/12249?show=full]

Ramugondo, E. (2015) Occupational consciousness. *Journal of Occupational Science,* 22, 8, 488-501

Ramugondo, E. and Kronenberg, F. (2013) Explaining collective occupations from a human-relations perspective: Bridging the individual-collective dichotomy. *Journal of Occupational Science.* 22, 1, 3-16

Ramugondo, E.L. (2012) Intergenerational play within family: The case for occupational consciousness. *Journal of Occupational Science,* 19, 4, 326-340

Rudman, D.L. (2010) Occupational possibilities. *Journal of Occupational Science,* 17, 1, 55-59

Senge, P. (2006) *The Fifth Discipline. The art and practice of the learning organisation.* London: Random House Business Books

Stadnyk, R., Townsend, E. and Wilcock, A. (2010) Occupational justice. in C.H. Christiansen and E. Townsend (Eds.) *Introduction to Occupation: The art and science of living (2nd ed.).* Upper Saddle River, NJ: Pearson Education (pp. 329-358)

Taylor, J. (2003) *Organisations and Development: Towards building a practice.* Cape Town: CDRA

Taylor, J., Kaplan, A. and Marais, D. (1997) *Action Learning for Development.* Cape Town: Juta

Wang, C. (1999) Photovoice: A participatory action research strategy applied to women's health. *Journal of Women's Health,* 8, 2, 85-192

Wang, C., Morrel-Samuels, S., Hutchison, P.M., Bell, L. and Pestronk, R.M. (2004) Flint photovoice: Community building among youths, adults and policymakers. *American Journal of Public Health,* 94, 6, 911-913

Whiteford, G.E. and Pereira, R. (2012) Occupation, social inclusion and participation. In G. E. Whiteford and C. Hocking (Eds.) *Occupational Science: Society, inclusion, participation.* London: Wiley-Blackwell (pp.117-136)

Whiteford, G. E. and Townsend, E. (2011) Participatory occupational justice framework: Enabling occupational participation and inclusion. in F. Kronenberg, N. Pollard, and D. Sakellariou (Eds.) *Occupational Therapy without Borders (Volume II): Towards an ecology of occupation-based practices.* Philadelphia: Churchill Livingstone Elsevier (pp. 65-84)

Yuval-Davis, N. (2006) Intersectionality and feminist politics. *European Journal of Women's Studies,* 13, 193-209

Chapter 8
Social transformation in theory and practice: Resources for radicals in participatory art, occupational therapy and social movements

Gelya Frank

Introduction

This chapter digs into foundations of 20th century social thought and action to reveal a panorama of radical practices in participatory art, social movements, and occupational therapy. The purpose is to provide resources for interventions that engage people in collective actions of varying scales, from neighborhoods to international publics. A sharp right turn in world politics – marked by Britain's withdrawal from the European Union and the 2016 presidential election in the United States – makes the need for such 'social occupational therapies' compelling. Beginning with the example of a high-profile participatory art project by Brazilian-born artist Vik Muniz, the chapter offers a framework called *occupational reconstruction* that is derived from the study of theories and practices used to engage, organize and mobilize people to transform everyday situations of marginalization and oppression.

More than ever before, the occupational therapy profession is concerned to enable marginalized, oppressed and excluded populations to participate more fully in social life (Whiteford 2011, 2000). While nothing less than 'transformation' is envisioned in this important critical agenda (Farias & Rudman, 2016), changes typically take place on the ground incrementally through everyday practices and policies (Renton & Van Bruggen, 2015; Galvaan, 2012). In the Global South, critical, alternative, indigenous and local epistemologies suggest new forms of occupational therapy practice in this social realm (Guajardo et al, 2015; Guajardo & Pollard, 2010; Smith, 2013). In Brazil, for example, a non-medicalized practice called 'social occupational therapy' targets opportunities and outcomes for vulnerable youth through workshops and coordination with other social services (Malfitano et al, 2014; Barros et al, 2011; Galheigo, 2010).

The *occupational reconstruction* framework is a nontraditional way of thinking and practicing occupationally to build cooperative participation and collective action (Ramugondo, 2015; Ramugondo & Kronenberg, 2015). While occupational therapy practice typically focuses on the ability of an individual to function and participate in society, occupational reconstruction focuses on group participation and social outcomes (Frank, 2012). Occupational reconstructions can be defined as hopeful *experiments that involve collective action to improve a problematic situation. Participation takes place through shared narratives about the situation and collaboration in highly focused occupations within a bounded event structure.* Key elements of the framework are:

1. *Collective Occupation*
   Occupational reconstructions involve shared actions with an articulated purpose
2. *Situations/Problem Solving*
   Occupational reconstructions are a kind of cooperative problem solving to make a problematic situation better
3. *Experience*
   Occupational reconstructions work because of experiences of 'doing.' Participation takes place through embodied action, with emotional and other felt dimensions
4. *Narrative Meanings/Event Structures*
   Occupational reconstructions involve narratives that coordinate individual and shared experience. They also depend on narratively structured events – with a beginning, middle and end – that focus attention and action
5. *Creative Possibilities*
   Occupational reconstructions open up spaces for doing, being, becoming and belonging – in other words, transformational growth and discoveries
6. *Intrinsic Motivation*
   Occupational reconstructions build intrinsic motivation – or desire. Participation is a function of freedom – voluntary, by choice
7. *Reflective Experimentation*
   Occupational reconstructions are hopeful experiments. Participation may produce changes in consciousness and circumstances, but require reflection and interpretation.

The occupational reconstruction framework can be used to understand and also guide participation in actions related to decolonization, civil rights, racial equality and social justice (Frank & Muriithi, 2015, also see Kronenberg et al, 2015; Motimele & Ramugondo, 2014). Occupational reconstructions also occur in situations that are less overtly confrontational, as in the example of 'Incredible Edible' Todmorden, a once-prosperous industrial town in the north of England. Bitter and critical of government inaction to improve their situation of joblessness, Todmorden's citizens took direct action and planted edible vegetables everywhere in public and private spaces. The result has been a thriving economy based on environmental tourism and teaching and development of sustainable technologies (J. Thompson, 2012).

Vik Muniz's 'Pictures of Trash' as occupation-based practice in participatory art

The documentary film *Waste Land,* addresses the social exclusion of trash workers, known as *catadores,* on the world's largest landfill located on the outskirts of Rio de Janiero (Walker, 2010). Readers are encouraged to view this 99-minute film on the Internet. With a crew of artists, Vik Muniz engaged several members of a *catadores* (trash pickers) union to participate in the participatory art project 'Pictures of Trash.' The artist recruited and hired the *catadores* to be interviewed and observed as they recycled garbage. Eventually, under the artist's direction, they turned recycled objects into works of art. Together, Muniz and his assistants worked with the trash pickers to produce a series of major art works that were meant to transform viewers' perspectives and relationships with waste and the people who work with it.

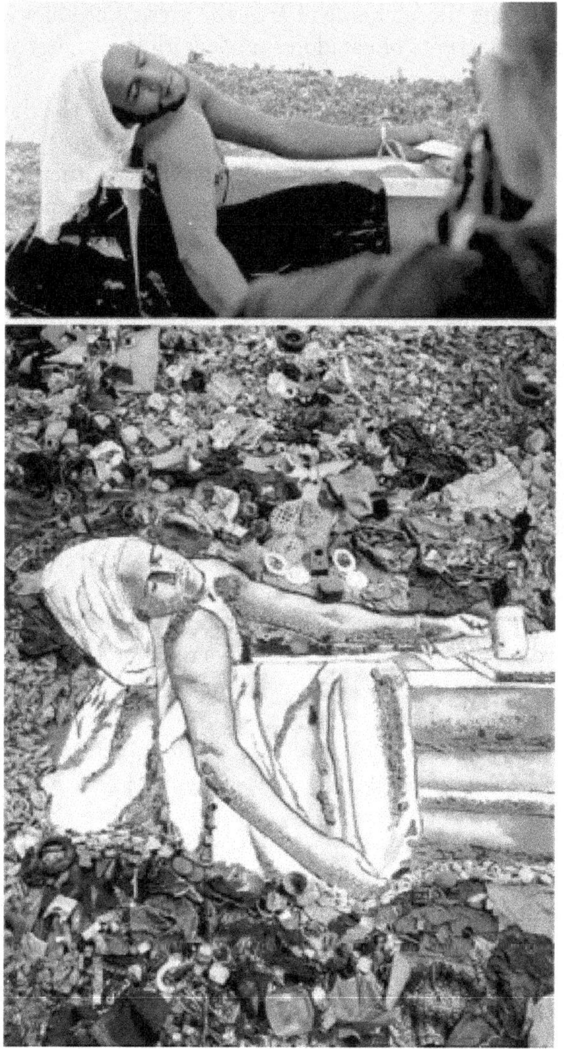

Figure 1. Artist Vik Muniz's photograph of Tiao, head of the Asociación de Catadores, on the trash heap at Jardim Gramacho. Tiao's pose recalls the classical painting, 'The Death of Marat' by Jacques-Louis David, portraying the French revolutionary figure who was murdered in his bath. Source: Kino (2010).
Figure 2. Tiao's portrait was recreated from garbage by the *catadores* for the 'Pictures of Trash' series. Source: Kino (2010).

The project's initial phase consisted of Muniz working with a crew of assistants to scout and develop relationships at Jardim Gramacho as the site for a major work. As a successful Brazilian-born individual, Muniz wanted to return to his country of birth to give something back to people from the lower socioeconomic classes. His goal was to demonstrate the 'alchemy of art.' The artistic product was envisioned as a set of monumental portraits of catadores made with their labor from garbage, the materials with which they typically work.

Muniz and his crew built rapport by contacting the Asociacíon de Catadores, doing research on their living and working conditions, and building warm relationships with several men and women that included interviewing them and filming their daily activities. In this initial phase, Muniz began photographing individuals on the landfill at Jardim Gramacho using found objects to recall canonical works by such masters as Botticelli, Millet, and Picasso. One photograph, for example, shows Muniz's photograph of Tiao, head of the Asociacíon de Catadores, posed in a bathtub found on the trash heap (Figure 1). Tiao's pose recalls the 1793 painting, 'The Death of Marat,' by Jacques-Louis David, portraying the French revolutionary Jean-Paul Marat who was murdered in his bath.

In the next phase, Muniz collaborated with the *catadores* to reproduce the photo portraits using garbage. This was accomplished by projecting an image from a height onto a vast warehouse floor. The individual *catadores* that were portrayed in 'Pictures of Trash' worked as a group under Muniz's direction to fill in the lines, colors and textures of their individual portraits with carefully selected recyclables. Muniz then re-photographed the huge portraits recreated with pieces of garbage and had them printed in an 8' (approx 2.5 metres) tall format. Assembling the portraits involved the pickers' skilled selection of specific materials to create the desired visual effects. In the portrait, 'Woman Ironing (Isis),' for example,

> '[Muniz] used lines of bottle caps, small steel 'o' rings, nuts and bolts to draw the woman's figure; the pleats in her skirt are a line of flip-flops; her hair is a weave of coiled rope, tires and frayed string – dreadlocks . . . From a distance, the background looks organically quilted, carefully arranged and beautiful. Up close, it's just Rio's *rejectamenta*: green and brown plastic bottles, fleshy baby doll body parts, crushed red gasoline cans, festive soda labels, toys and colored tarps.' (Lucas, 2012, p.2/4).

Similarly, Tiao's photograph was recreated on the floor of a warehouse using trash and then re-photographed (see Figure 2).

The third phase of the project was launched with the media-drenched public opening of 'Pictures of Trash' at the national museum in Rio de Janeiro, where the *catadores,* dressed for the occasion, mingled as celebrities with members of Rio's cultural elite. Next, also shown in the film, Muniz and Tiao, leader of the *catadores,* traveled to the high-end auction house in London where the prints were sold.

The artist gave his share of the proceeds, $50,000, to the *catadores* union (Kino, 2010). Muniz and the filmmakers also reportedly donated $276,000 to the cooperative 'to buy a truck and computers, found a library, provide capital funds for the cooperative and finance a small-business training program' (Kino, 2010, p. 5/5). These material benefits, however, should be viewed as spin-offs, because the transformation that Muniz was aiming to create with the 'alchemy of art' was primarily a change in perceptions of the *catadores*' humanity and worth.

This perceptual shift took place *transactionally* – that is, on two levels simultaneously, individually and collectively. On the individual level, for Tiao, the union leader, the project helped to reignite his and the other union members' fight for recognition and concessions from Rio's municipal government after a period of discouraging defeats. He also reported, with emotion and wonder, 'I never imagined I could become a work of art' (Walker, 2010). The other participants also reflected on how the film recast their self-image and affirmed their self-worth. For example, Isis, the individual portrayed in 'Woman Ironing,' faced the camera to express desire and confidence about leaving the dump to find work elsewhere, in the mainstream society.

On the collective social level, the project unified the concerns and demands of the *catadores* for social and legal recognition. It spotlighted the need to impose limits on the sprawling dump and fulfill the recyclers' union demands for municipal protections and benefits. The film played up the viewpoint of *catador* Valter dos Santos, that recyclers deserve respect for their environmental work on behalf of the planet. Similarly, the public that views the documentary film and other media are forced to question the system of consumer excess and exclusion of those who own so little: Why are the recyclers treated like garbage? Can a system that exploits natural resources, despoils the earth, and ignores the needs of workers itself be transformed?

Overlapping foundations of occupational therapy and participatory art

If there is an affinity of occupational therapy with 'Pictures of Trash,' it comes from the occupational therapy profession's overlapping conceptual foundations with participatory art. Focusing for a moment on the early years of occupational therapy in the United States, from around 1890 to 1920, social reformist theories about the use of 'occupations' – meaningful, purposeful activities – overlapped across social work, progressive education, vocational education, the Arts and Crafts movement and, of course, occupational therapy (Schwartz, 1992, 2009; Levine, 1986).

Like occupational therapy interventions, many participatory art practices are meant to trigger social change in a particular direction by means of occupations that draw the public into some form of action (N. Thompson, 2012). Participatory art is meant to alter experience, arouse awareness, prompt critical reflection and provoke action in some dimension of social life. Social occupational therapy and participatory art can be understood as fields that rely on overlapping social occupation-based practices and theories (see Figure 3 overleaf). Recognizing these overlapping foundations can support the emergence of occupational therapy practices to elicit, facilitate, and guide social participation.

Experience, situations and *occupations* are the key concepts supporting participation at the point of overlap with the arts. The American pragmatist philosopher John Dewey (1934) in his major work on aesthetics *Art as Experience* argued that the meaning of art lies not in the object, but in the lived experience that the art object

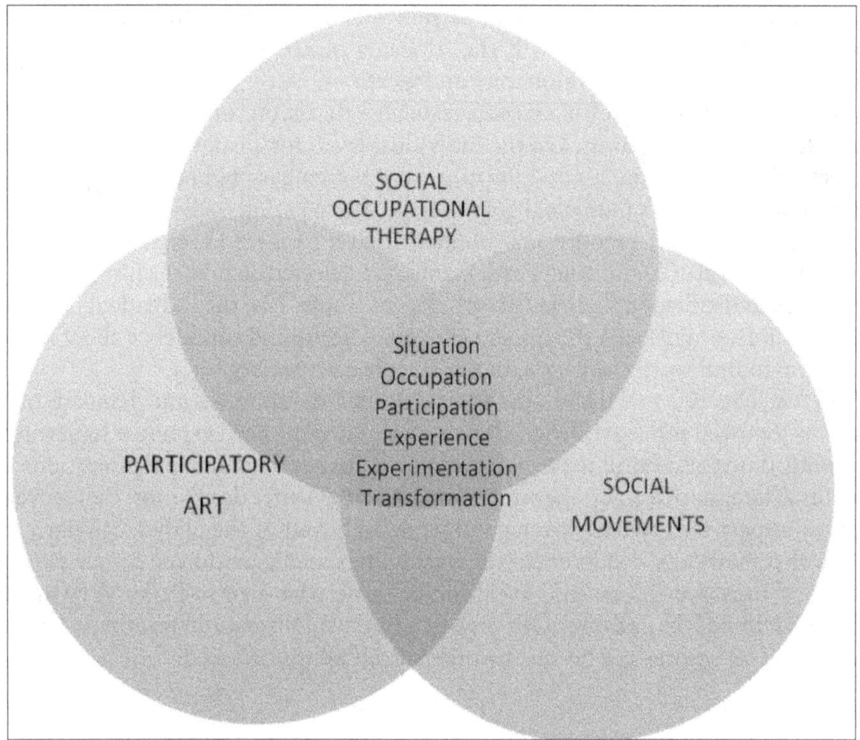

Figure 3.
Overlapping practice fields share core concepts clustered at the center of the diagram

facilitates. Dewey wrote that the primary task of aesthetics should be

> 'to restore continuity between the refined and intensified forms of experience that are works of art and the everyday events, doings, and sufferings that are universally recognized to constitute experience.' (Dewey, 1934, p. 3).

Later we will discuss how Dewey's ideas influenced mid-20th century participatory art events known as 'Happenings', but his aesthetics also illuminate an important earlier work: Marcel Duchamp's entry of a commercially made porcelain urinal into a juried exhibit in New York in 1917 (San Francisco Museum of Art, 1998). This absurd 'ready made' object that Duchamp signed and titled 'Fountain' jolted viewers' experience based on expectations of art. 'Fountain' provoked viewers to see the sculptural potential of everyday objects and experience the possibilities of mass production in a different light. From this standpoint Duchamp's gesture can be interpreted to assert that the meaning of art is not intrinsic to the object, as it was in previous centuries, but to the experience that the object evokes.

Dewey similarly put experience at the center of his theory of education. Like the Brazilian educator Paulo Freire, with whom he is often compared, Dewey (1915/1990b) focused on connecting learning to the students' life situations. He founded a laboratory school where subjects ordinarily taught by rote, such as mathematics and history, were resituated within cooperative tasks. These shared tasks or 'occupations' required problem solving while carrying them out, including all the unanticipated snags that occur when attempting to do something, whether baking a cake or building a medieval castle.

Experiences like these were intended to grow students' knowledge while expanding their capacities. Further, Dewey emphasized shared problem solving, an approach that was crucially tied to his vision of progressive politics and democratic reform in American society. The situation in the United States – with its rapid industrialization, urbanization, and expanding immigrant and ethnic populations – required a democratic form of education that created habits and dispositions in its students of cooperative social action (Pappas, 2008; Westbrook, 1991; Dewey, 1916/1997).

The concept of *situation* also overlaps in foundations of occupational therapy and participatory art. In recent decades, art has taken a 'social turn' (Charnley, 2014) that incorporates theories and concepts in European absurdist art, late Marxist philosophy, Dewey's pragmatism and various movements for civil rights and social inclusion (Finkelpearl, 2013; N. Thompson, 2012). This 'social turn' since the 1990s has been defined as a 'post-object art in which the 'medium' is social experience' (Charnley, 2014). The project, 'Pictures of Trash,' is well recognized as an exemplar of contemporary art's social turn (N. Thompson, 2012). 'Participation' (Bishop, 2006) and 'situation' (Doherty, 2009) are key concepts in art's social turn and that circle us back to Dewey. Equally important is the concept of 'anti-spectorial' art (Debord, 1967/1994).

The experimental quasi-theatrical events in the early 1960s known as 'Happenings' reflect the artist Allan Kaprow's application of Dewey's philosophy (Rodenbeck, 2011). Held in lofts and warehouses in Manhattan, 'Happenings' were situations staged by the artist with students and colleagues inviting open participation by the public (Kelley, 2004). The events involved playful provocation, unscripted live experience and spontaneous participation (Finkelpearl, 2013). Among the artist's formative influences, Kaprow's 'true intellectual father' was Dewey (Kelley, 2004, p. 8; see also Finkelpearl, 2013; Kaprow, 2003):

> 'As a young philosophy student in 1949, Kaprow kept a copy of *Art as Experience* close at hand, penciling in its margins phrases such as 'art is not separate from experience,' 'what is an authentic experience?' and 'environment is a process of interaction' – jottings that not only indicate his philosophical interest in commonplace experience, but that forecast the underlying themes of his career.' (Kelley, 2004, p. 200).

Also in the 1960s, in France, a group called The Situationalist International began creating public events called 'situations' dedicated to disrupting the hypnotic power of media and consumer culture to create public passivity (N. Thompson 2012). Founder Guy Debord (1958) defined *situations* as 'temporary fields of activity' capable of engaging and even forcing spectators to act and participate. In his book, *The Society of the Spectacle* (1967/1994), Debord argued that modern consumer societies blur the distinction between people's 'real' needs and desires and 'manufactured' needs and desires.

While the Situationalists intended their anti-spectorial methods to startle and awaken the public from its habitual passive spectatorship, a movement called Fluxus began mounting festivals and experimental performances in Europe, North America, and Asia (Schmidt-Burkhardt, 2011; Dezeuze, 2010; Sell, 2005; Higgins, 2002). These performances, known as 'Events,' brought artists, composers, musicians, designers, architects and even academics into interaction to push the boundaries of new kinds of experiences and perspectives for themselves and for audiences. Drawing on Dewey, critic Hannah Higgins (2002) explains Fluxus' modalities in terms of their 'transactional' nature.

Another anti-spectorial art form known as 'Theater of the Oppressed,' was introduced in Brazil in the 1970s by Augusto Boal (1985/2013), a director and activist influenced by Marxist humanist educator Paulo Freire's (1970/2014) pedagogy of the oppressed. In Theatre of the Oppressed, Boal (2001) began to develop an anti-spectorial approach by welcoming interventions by audience members to re-script performances addressing themes of oppression affecting their lives. This methodology, 'Forum Theatre,' evolved into a workshop format in which participants narrate situations of powerlessness that they personally experienced (Boal, 1985/2013). Situations are then enacted and reenacted by members of the workshop, introducing changes that reverse the oppressive outcome.

Occupational therapists have been showing interest in applying Theater of the Oppressed with socially vulnerable youth in Brazil (Alves et al, 2013) and with homeless people, refugees and asylum seekers in Norway (Horghagen & Jossephson 2010; Horghagen & Hocking, 2017). Horghagen and Hocking explain that 'the transformational possibilities of theatre' arise from the idea of theatre 'as a subjunctive reality, where unrealized human potential and hypothetical possibilities can be explored without the constraints of known situations and settled facts' (2017, p. 30). As in Vik Muniz's 'Pictures of Trash,' Boal's participatory, anti-spectorial methods recycle experience, by means of setting up new problem-solving situations.

The concept of *occupation* in occupational therapy and occupational science

Finally, and importantly, the concept of *occupation* is specifically articulated in occupational therapy but only implied in participatory art. Here occupational therapists have resources – a knowledge base, research and scholarship, and practice expertise with varied populations – that far exceed those of participatory art and other overlapping fields. Dewey's contribution to occupational therapy is recognized (Morrison, 2016; Schwartz, 2009; Ikiugu & Schultz, 2006; Breines 1986), but his concept of 'occupation' is not as well understood, despite the fact that wherever the profession exists, occupational therapy is defined in Deweyan terms as the use of 'meaningful' and 'purposeful' activites (AOTA, 2014; WFOT, 2010).

Dewey's philosophy holds that occupations enable people to work out solutions in problematic situations through new realizations and provisional truths. Occupational therapy theorist Mary Reilly (1962) carried forward this deeper understanding of occupation as a kind of 'work,' a dynamic process of solving problems step by step, such as how to live with a chronic illness, by trying and doing things. She retains the idea that occupation is part of a dynamic process of growth by means of experimentation leading to new experiences and self-assessments – one might even say, a process of self-realization by doing.

It is true that in his many writings, Dewey used the term 'occupation' in different ways, sometimes to mean nothing more than the typical customs and habitual actions of daily life. But his application of the concept of occupation to the psychology of education – and, by extension, its adoption in occupational therapy (Schwartz, 1992; Levine, 1986) – refers to a very particular and optimal mind-body state, one of focused attention and spontaneous engagement. The Deweyan educator tries to elicit this state by setting up learning situations in the classroom in which students collaborate in tasks to solve problems which are selected to elicit participation and growth suited to the age, interests and stage of development of particular students.

> 'The fundamental point in the psychology of an occupation is that it maintains a balance between the intellectual and the practical phases of experience. As an occupation it is active or motor; it finds expression through the physical organs – the eyes, hands, etc. But it also involves continual observation of materials, and continual planning and reflection, in order that the practical or executive side may be successfully carried on. Occupation as thus conceived must, therefore, be carefully distinguished from work which educates primarily for a trade. It differs because its end is in itself; in the growth that comes from the continual interplay of ideas and their embodiment in action, not in external utility.' (Dewey, 1915/1990a, p.131-132).

In 1989, an academic discipline, occupational science, was founded around the core concept of 'occupation' in order to counteract the profession of occupational therapy's fragmentation and lack of recognition (Clark et al, 1991; Yerxa et al, 1990; also see Clark, 2010; Kielhofner & Burke, 1977). Clark et al (1991, p.301) floated the definition of 'occupation' as 'chunks of culturally and personally meaningful activity in which humans engage that can be named in the lexicon of our culture.' But this phrasing loses the nuance in Dewey's definition of occupation as a dynamic problem-solving activity, a more subtle and unique understanding that earlier theorists sought to retain (Reilly, 1962).

Perhaps the contemporary concept that is nearest to Dewey's psychology of occupation is 'flow,' a state of consciousness while engaged in a task in which a person loses a sense of time and awareness of the outer world (Nakamura & Dubin, 2015). Descriptions of deep play in occupational therapy and in art also capture this quality of an occupation as a particular kind of experience characterized by mind-body unity, attention and engagement, spontaneous growth and creativity (Parham & Fazio, 2008; Park, 2008; Blanche, 2007; Lawlor, 2003; also see Nachmanovitch, 1990).

The next step in this chapter is to explore the sources that inform occupational therapy's recent 'social turn.' In particular, the tension needs discussion between pragmatist and new critical perspectives on occupation and social change. Both perspectives have implications for building effective social practice in relation to inclusion of marginalized and oppressed populations in a social transformation agenda.

Power and *social transformation* in occupational therapy's social turn

Occupational therapy, like contemporary art since the 1990s, has taken a 'social turn' that seeks to transform conditions that marginalize and oppress people (Sakellariou & Pollard, 2017; Whiteford & Hocking, 2012; Kronenberg et al, 2011; Kronenberg et al, 2005; Watson & Swartz, 2004). Before the emergence of this 'social paradigm' (Morrison, 2016), occupational therapy had been focused almost exclusively on treating disabilities and chronic illnesses of individuals within families and immediate environments. But the new paradigm looks for ways to apply occupational principles more radically in terms of institutions, populations, cultures, and communities in order to facilitate social change.

The social paradigm includes critique of the occupational science discipline, which ironically had been established with the emancipatory purpose to free the profession of occupational therapy from domination by medicine and positivist science (Magalhães, 2012). The discipline has been criticized on grounds of cultural imperialism, questioning its universalizing viewpoint of a privileged, autonomous 'Western' self (Kantartzis & Molineux, 2012; Hammell, 2011; Odawara, 2005; also Hocking, 2012). Others have criticized the discipline's narrowing of the study of occupations to individuals and their subjective experience. These pragmatist critics take Dewey's 'transactionalist' philosophy as their starting point, in which occupations are modes of dynamic interaction between individuals and their social situation, not simply matters of individuals' experience (Dickie et al, 2006).

Another source of occupational therapy's social turn is found in the rise of humanitarianism, philosophies of social justice and the Universal Declaration of Human Rights and its protocols after World War II (cf. Frank, 2012). Townsend and Wilcock's (2004) concept of 'occupational justice,' which assumes human dignity and the respect for human potential, falls within these perspectives. Their theory of occupational justice evokes a capabilities approach (Sen, 2000) much as the philosopher Martha Nussbaum (1995) tries to identify a set of basic universal human rights that are essential for 'human flourishing.'

In addition, Wilcock's (1998) major contribution to occupational science, a naturalistic theory of occupation and health, is very close to a Deweyan perspective: Wilcock argues that humans have an innate, evolutionary and developmental drive to engage in meaningful, purposeful occupation. Freedom to express this drive is necessary for people to experience growth, health, and wellbeing – including, as Wilcock puts it, the freedom to 'do, be, become and belong' (see Hitch et al, 2014a, b). Townsend's contribution brings to bear critical feminist sociology theories about institutional power and about the relationship between 'difference' (e.g. gender, disability) and justice (Stadnyk et al, 2010).

The occupational injustice perspective focuses on situations in which a population is denied access to a society's valued occupations because of characteristics - disability, race, ethnicity, gender, poverty, etc. – that are not essential to personhood. In this sense, occupational injustices are abuses of human rights. The typology of occupational injustice constitutes a new diagnostic language for occupational therapy focused on social exclusion (Stadnyk et al, 2010). The types of occupational injustice identified so far include 'occupational deprivation,' 'occupational marginalization,' 'occupational alienation,' 'occupational imbalance' and 'occupational apartheid' (Durocher et al, 2014). These concepts and terms help to justify socially-oriented practice as legitimate areas of concern for an otherwise medically oriented profession (Kinsella & Durocher, 2016; Hocking et al, 2015; Durocher et al, 2014).

Alongside the above sources, occupational therapists and occupational scientists are drawing on critical theories by Marx, Gramsci, Freire, Foucault, Fanon and others in the Marxist tradition to provide coherent explanations of inequality and oppression (Farias & Rudman, 2016). These theories focus on the concept of 'power' and how it operates. Critical theories set an 'emancipatory agenda' for social transformation (Farias & Rudman, 2016). Examples of critical theories include various feminist and critical race theories, disability rights discourses, and anticolonial and postcolonialist perspectives (Farias et al, 2016; Guajardo et al, 2015). They are also used reflexively in occupational therapy to critique theories and practices within the profession and discipline (Magalhães, 2012; Jackson, 2000). Critics argue, for example, that occupation science must not ignore the 'dark side' of occupation, such as gender oppression (Angell, 2014) and violence (Twinley, 2013).

The concept of 'social transformation' signals a radical frustration with the status quo in society and with conventional practice: 'Whereas *incremental* change is a variation in degree, *transformational* change is a variation in kind that involves reconceptualization and discontinuity from the initial system' (Kindler, 1979, p. 477). In general, the practices associated with critical theories can be expected to differ from those derived primarily from cultural, pragmatist, humanitarian and human rights critiques. Humanitarian interventions, for example, supply aid and assistance to relieve suffering from oppression and a return from crisis to a normal existence.

By contrast, critical interventions seek to identify and eliminate oppressive institutions and agents. They introduce alternative epistemologies into public discourse, radical education and consciousness-raising. And they call for active resistance to oppression through oppositional practices and the elimination of oppressive practices.

The next section summarizes Dewey's social thought and puts it in conversation with critical approaches. Henry Giroux (2014), a critical educator, writes:

> 'One of the most serious challenges facing teachers, artists, journalists, writers, youth, and other cultural workers is the challenge of developing a discourse of both critique and possibility' (4.3.2014).

Deweyan perspectives in a 21st century context can guide radical practice in occupational therapy with interest groups, communitiesand the public (Frank & Dos Santos, 2020; Dos Santos & Frank, Forthcoming).

Radical Deweyan practice in relation to critical theories

Some occupational scientists have argued that Dewey's pragmatism has the potential to guide social transformation (Cutchin & Dickie, 2012; also see Frank, 2016, 2012; Frank & Muriithi, 2015). This position needs updating in relation to critical theories and social transformation. The position takes up Dewey's focus on *experience* and *the problematic situation* as its starting point (cf. Cutchin, 2008). Dewey's philosophy suggests that situations emerge to disrupt the seamless functioning of habits, routines, and beliefs or 'truth.' The experimentation that follows is a mind-body process – that is occupation – that may solve the problematic situation by reconstructing conditions and consciousness to some greater or lesser degree. In focusing on habit and routine, occupational scientists have emphasized aspects of Dewey's theory that relate to functional stability (Clark et al, 2007; Garrison, 2002), at the expense of social transformation.

Dewey (1920, 1935) reconstructed the philosophy that he inherited from the Western tradition by anchoring it in everyday experience. His naturalistic standpoint was also rooted in science – particularly, Darwinian evolutionary theory and the modern cultural anthropology of his time. These frameworks demanded explanation of both social stability *and* social change, which Dewey understood to occur through public discourse and cooperative action. Dewey called this process 'social reconstruction' (Campbell, 1995). In Dewey's thought, one interpreter writes: 'The world, rather than being comprised of things or, in more traditional terms, substances, is comprised *of happenings* (recall artist Allan Kaprow) or occurrences that admit of both episodic uniqueness and general, structured order' (Field, n.d., emphasis added).

In contrast to Dewey's naturalism, critical theories – with their straightforward analysis of power inequalities – offer more immediately clear and convincing intellectual tools for diagnosing the world's problematic situations. At this moment of rising anti-democratic, racist and nationalist governments, – and of rising income inequality within nations (Lenger & Schumacher, 2015) – it is hard to dispute the perception that 'social exclusion is an increasing form of social inequity' (Malfitano et al, 2014; Frank & Dos Santos, 2020). Dewey's naturalism and faith in social democracy would seem to imply that problematic situations are already in progress of being solved cooperatively, but our experiences of the world's structural inequalities and irresolvable problems would suggest otherwise.

A radical critique from the 1960s labelled Dewey's social theory as deficient because of its 'biological' view of society, its overly optimistic faith in reason and science, and its failure to take power and inequality into account (Mills, 1964). Recent scholars of pragmatism have tried to refute these claims by reexamining Dewey's treatment of power (Wolfe, 2012; Hildreth, 2009; Rogers, 2009; Hewitt, 2002). These complicated efforts to rehabilitate Dewey's original writings may seem rather beside the point for 21st century social occupational therapies that recognize critical theories. But while Dewey's philosophical naturalism is not the handiest tool to take on social inequality, his transactional elements remain useful in a constructivist mode – that is, as guide for action (Hickman, 2009).

It is important to recognize in a general way that Dewey did not avoid questions of power, conflict and coercion, confrontation and recourse through media to public opinion. From this background the radical community organizer Saul Alinsky (1971) developed a methodology for radical social action. Dewey first began to theorize about social democracy – defined by cooperative problem solving – during the Chicago railroad workers' 'wildcat' strike against the Pullman Company in 1884 (Menand, 2001). Dewey was interested in the cooperative action by the strikers. Although the strike failed when the President sent troops to restore rail service, news of the strike – and of the brutality by private security police – changed public opinion about America's labor problems. The shift in public discourse resulted in state and federal legislation protecting workers' rights (wages, working hours, working conditions, disability insurance, etc.). Dewey continued to think and write about social reconstruction in regard to the Chinese Revolution of 1911, his years teaching in China from 1919 to 1921, the Russian Revolution of 1917, his chairing a committee to investigate Stalin's show trial of Leon Trotsky in 1937, and his own democratic socialist activism in the United States (Westbrook, 1991; also Dewey, 1968).

Alinsky turned Deweyan pragmatist sociology into a methodology for grass-roots mobilization and pressure tactics for political change (Schutz & Miller, 2015; Schutz, 2011; Schultz, 2009). 'When people are organized,' Alinsky was quoted in a 1969 interview, 'they move to the central decision-making table ... on the basis of power' (Boyte, 5.4.2015). In the book *People Power: The Community Organizing Tradition of Saul Alinsky,* Schutz & Miller (2015) describe the use of Alinsky's radical methods in the National Farm Workers boycott of wines and table grapes led by Caesar Chavez and Dolores Huerta in the 1960s. The boycott forced growers to recognize the farm workers' union and improve wages and working conditions; it is perhaps the best known of the many successful organizing efforts using Alinsky's methods (Von Hoffman, 2010). More recent 'direct action' theories (cf. Graeber, 2009) in global justice movements build on Alinsky and other radical and critical sources, as in the 1999 protest against the World Trade Organization, the 2011 Occupy Wall Street movement, and the 2014 'Yellow Umbrella' movement in Hong Kong.

Viewing Dewey's transactionalism in a constructivist manner opens up resources for practice from – and in collaboration with – participatory art and social movements. These resources are well suited to social occupational therapies because of the overlaps with the profession's expertise and knowledge base. In the Metuia project, in Brazil, for example, we see transactionalist and critical perspectives together in 'the inseparability of the collective dimension and individual needs, recognizing that individuals are agents who produce and reproduce social practices and structures' (Malfitano et al, 2014, p. 303). The Metuia project thus confronts a problematic situation: 'the need to develop specific social occupational therapy approaches for contexts where clinical, biomedical approaches are not sufficient or applicable' (p. 303).

Occupational reconstruction practice and outcomes

The occupational reconstruction framework represents a 21st century critical-constructivist development of Dewey's pragmatism for the purpose of social occupational therapy practice. The framework accepts Dewey's view of democratic social reconstruction as an egalitarian ideal. But solutions to problems in the world's authoritarian and structurally unequal regimes do not arise solely from within situations. Critical theories alert us that when people become habituated to violent and oppressive environments, their capacities for hope, desire and action to change the situation may benefit from intervention (Ramugondo, 2015). Some examples of occupational reconstruction include community development projects in post-civil war Guatemala (Frank, 2012), school-sponsored dance competitions for children suffering war trauma in Uganda and for at-risk youth in multicultural New York City (Frank, 2016) and the integration of public facilities and restoration of voting rights in the American civil rights movement (Frank & Muriithi, 2015).

Occupational reconstructions are event-structured interventions that involve shared participation. A set of seven elements introduced in this chapter's introduction begins with a critical question: What are the institutions, agents and practices that promote inequality, marginalization and oppression? This diagnostic tool enables participants to agree to an occupation or occupations that they believe could help to ameliorate their situation. It is the responsibility of social occupational therapy practitioners to guide the process with skills mostly within the existing scope of occupational therapy expertise – that is, to advise on the event structure from a knowledge base of cases; to analyze and support engagement in occupation according to participants' varied skills and abilities; to elicit and motivate participation without coercion; to coordinate action and help to manage participants' hopes and risks; to facilitate the congruence between personal and shared narratives; to recognize openings for growth, creativity and discovery; and to foster the critical reflection that is crucial to transformational experience.

Occupational reconstructions involve doing ordinary *things in* extraordinary ways. In social movements, for example, activists take ordinary actions on behalf of a cause, but use the action in ways that are no longer conventional or routine (Laverack, 2012; Martin, 2007). Singing in a choir is an ordinary occupation, but singing in jail as a protest during the American civil rights movement went beyond the usual and routine action, having a transformative impact on morale and solidarity (Frank & Muriithi, 2015). As Vik Muniz (PBS News Hour, 2011) said of *Pictures of Tras*h: 'What I really want to do is to be able to change the lives of a group of people with the same material that they deal with every day.' There is, however, no guarantee that participation in an occupational reconstruction will improve the situation. As Dewey emphasized, social reconstruction is experimental.

Some occupational reconstructions lead in a straightforward way to recognizable, tangible social change. The Black Lives Matter protest marches in the United States, for example, have led to intense public scrutiny of police shootings of unarmed African Americans and some reforms, but the situation remains volatile. While participation in itself can have empowering effects, the overall political results may remain uncertain for some time (Aldrich et al, 2016). Therefore, the idea of social transformation associated with occupational reconstructions should not be strictly limited to immediate political results or structural reforms, as important as these might be.

Rather, occupational reconstructions are hopeful attempts to ameliorate problematic situations. As with Alinsky's methods of community organizing, they may be crafted strategically to get results. But even if they should fail to improve the situation, participants are moved forward with new skills, consciousness and relationships. This experimentalism, for which social occupational therapists must prepare, allows for processes of growth through failure. The outcome of awakened desire and hopeful engagement is never solely to be understood as a technical or instrumental 'fix.' Occupational reconstructions will need forms of evaluation different from evidence-based practice in medicine based on standardized outcomes.

Occupational reconstructions may have an historical dimension in addition to the immediate effects of the intervention. The NAMES Project, conceived in 1985 when AIDS in the United States was stigmatized as 'a gay men's disease,' is an example. Federal officials refused to utter the word AIDS and recognize it as a crisis. At a memorial march in San Francisco, mourners covered the walls of San Francisco's old Federal Building with placards bearing the names of people who had died of AIDS. Cleve Jones, protégé of slain gay activist Harvey Milk, conceived of the NAMES Project as a memorial as he observed people standing for hours in wind and rain to read the names (Ruskin & Herron 1998).

The resulting project was the AIDS Quilt (https://en.wikipedia.org/wiki/NAMES_Project_AIDS_Memorial_Quilt), a public project in which mourners stitched their experiences of loss, grief and anger into a collective work of folk art. The project began in a storefront space staffed by volunteers using donated sewing machines. Friends, lovers and family members gathered there to design and create a 3 by 6 foot long panel, each a unique memorial to a loved one who had died. The AIDS Quilt was displayed on October 11, 1987 in front of the Capitol Building in Washington, D.C. at the Second National March for Lesbian and Gay Rights, an event attended by 200,000 people. Media coverage of the National March forced President Ronald Reagan to publicly acknowledge the AIDS epidemic as a public health crisis and exerted pressure on Congress to appropriate federal funds for AIDS research.

The long struggle for inclusion of marginalized groups such as the LGBTQ community includes countless occupational reconstructions, some more widely recognized than others – such as outbreak of resistance by patrons to police harassment at the Stonewall Inn, a gay bar in Greenwich Village, in 1969. Although the patrons were beaten and jailed, the event stands as the birth of gay pride and a precursor to AIDS activism. Many gays and lesbians today feel that the United States Supreme Court ruling in *Obergefell v. Hodges (2015)*, affirming the Constitutional protection of same-sex couples to marry, has been the ultimate social transformation for their experience of marginalization. This outcome could not have happened without the occupational reconstructions, like the Names Project, that turned feminist and queer critical theories into paradigm-changing collective action.

Conclusion

It is up to occupational therapy professionals to put the occupational reconstruction framework into new forms of practice (Frank & Dos Santos, 2020). The framework can be expected to support program design, theory development, and research related to the profession's concern with power and inequality. Occupational therapy's social turn has already created the environment for a more radical pragmatism to advance a critical agenda through collective occupations and collaborative action (Thibeault, 2011; Whiteford, 2005; Simó, volume 2, chapter 8).

Occupational therapists have constraints and prerogatives tied to the profession's fiduciary role in society (professional organizations, education and credentialing standards, research traditions and peer review, licensure, etc.) This chapter argues that a 21st century radical update of Dewey's pragmatist legacy stands alongside new and alternative epistemologies to move social occupational therapies forward. As Gail Whiteford (2011, p. 545) said to occupational therapists in her retrospective on social inclusion research and practice: 'The future is in your hands.'

References

Aldrich, R., White, N.A. and Conners, B.L. (2016) Translating occupational justice education into action. Reflections from an exploratory single case study. *OTJR: Occupation, Participation and Health,* 36, 4, 227-233

Alinsky, S. (1971) *Rules for Radicals: A practical primer for realistic radicals.* New York: Random House

Alves, I., Gontijo, D.T. and Alves, H.C. (2013) Theatre of the oppressed and occupational therapy: A proposed action with youth in social vulnerability. *Cadernos de Terapia Ocupacional*, 21, 2, 325-337

American Occupational Therapy Association (AOTA) (2014) Occupational therapy practice framework: Domain and process (3rd ed.) *American Journal of Occupational Therapy*, 68, 1-48, DOI: 10.5014/ajot.2014.682006

Angell, A.M. (2014) Occupation-centered analysis of social difference: Contributions to a socially responsive occupational science. *Journal of Occupational Science*, 21, 2, 104-116, doi:10.1080/14427591.2012.711230

Baranek, G. T., Frank, G. and Aldrich, R. M. (Forthcoming.) Meliorism and knowledge mobilization: Past, present, and future possibilities for occupational science. *Journal of Occupational Science*

Barros, D.D., Ghirardi, M.I.G., Lopes, R.E. and Galheigo, S.M. (2011) Brazilian experiences in social occupational therapy. in F. Kronenberg, N. Pollard, and D. Sakellariou (Eds.) *Occupational Therapy without Borders: Vol. 2. Towards an ecology of occupation-based practices.* Edinburgh: Elsevier (pp. 209–215)

Bishop, C. (Ed.) (2006) *Participation.* Cambridge, MA: The MIT Press

Blanche, E.I. (2007) The expression of creativity through occupation. *Journal of Occupational Science,* 14, 1, 21-29, doi: 10.1080/14427591.2007.9686580

Boal. A. (1985/2013) *Theatre of the Oppressed.* New York: Theatre Communications Group

Boal, A. (2001) *Hamlet and the Baker's Son: My life in theatre and politics.* New York: Routledge

Boyte, H. (2015) Community organising and the next stage of democracy. *The Huffington Post,* May 4th. [Accessed 10 September at http://www.huffingtonpost.com/harry-boyte/community-organizing-and-_1_b_7200280.html

Breines, E.B. (1986) *Origins and Adaptations: A philosophy of practice.* Lebanon, NJ: Geri-Rehab

Campbell, J. (1995) *Understanding John Dewey: Nature and cooperative intelligence.* Chicago: Open Court

Charnley, K. (2014) Criticism and Cooperation. *Art Journal,* 73, 2, 116-118, doi: 10.1080/00043249.2014.949523

Clark, F. (2010) High-definition occupational therapy: HD OT (Inaugural Presidential Address). *American Journal of Occupational Therapy*, 64, 848–854. doi: 10.5014/ajot.2010.64602

Clark, F., Parham, D., Carlson, M., Frank, G., Jackson, J., Pierce, D., et al. (1991) Occupational science: Academic innovation in the service of occupational therapy's future. *American Journal of Occupational Therapy*, 45, 4, 300-310

Clark, F.A., Sanders, K., Carlson, M.E., Blanche, E.J., and Jackson, J.M. (2007) Synthesis of habit theory. *Occupational Therapy Journal of Research: Occupation, Participation, and Health*, 27, 4, 7-23

Cutchin, M. P. (2008) John Dewey's metaphysical ground-map and its implications for geographical inquiry. *Geoforum*, 39, 1555–1569

Cutchin, M.P. and Dickie, V.A. (2012) *Rethinking Occupation: Transactional perspectives on doing*. New York: Springer

Debord, G. (1958) Preliminary problems in constructing a situation. *Internationale Situationiste*, 1. [Accessed 20 December 2016 at http://www.cddc.vt.edu/sionline/si/problems.html]

Debord, G. (1967/1994) *The Society of the Spectacle*. New York: Zone Books

Dewey, J. (1915/1990) The Psychology of Occupations. in *The School and Society* (pp. 131–154). Chicago: University of Chicago Press. Free e-book access: http://www.brocku.ca/MeadProject/Dewey/Dewey_1907/Dewey_1915c.html

Dewey, J. (1915/1990b) *The School and Society; And, the child and the curriculum*. Chicago: University of Chicago Press

Dewey, J. (1916/1997) *Democracy and education*. The Free Press. NOTE: Free e-book access: https://books.google.com/books?id=8mAWAAAAIAAJ&printsec=frontcover&dq=democracy+and+education+an+introduction+to+the+philosophy+of+education&hl=en&sa=X&ved=0ahUKEwjf_teBserQAhVHs1QKHRZ0C0MQ6AEIIzAB#v=onepage&q=democracy%20and%20education%20an%20introduction%20to%20the%20philosophy%20of%20education&f=false

Dewey, J. (1920) *Reconstruction in Philosophy*. New York: H. Holt and Company

Dewey, J. (1934). *Art as Experience*. New York: Minton, Balch

Dewey, J. (1935) *Liberalism and Social Action*. New York: Putnam

Dewey, J. (1968) *The Case of Leon Trotsky: Report of hearings on the charges made against him in the Moscow trials*. New York: Merit Publishers

Dezeuze, A. (2010) *The 'Do-It-Yourself' Artwork: Participation from Fluxus to new media*. Manchester, UK: Manchester University

Dickie, V., Cutchin, M.P. and Humphry, R. (2006). Occupation as transactional experience: A critique of individualism in occupational science. *Journal of Occupational Science*, 13, 89-93

Doherty, C. (Ed.) (2009) *Situation*. Cambridge, MA: The MIT Press

Dos Santos, V., Frank, G. and Mizue, A. (In progress). A new generation of Candangos: Occupational reconstructions and social transformation in Brasilia's periphery. *Brazilian Journal of Occupational Therapy*

Durocher, E., Gibson. B.E. and Rappolt, S. (2014) Occupational justice: A conceptual review. *Journal of Occupational Science*, 21, 4, 418-430, doi: 10.1080/14427591.2013.775692

Farias, L. and Laliberte Rudman, D. (2016) A critical interpretive synthesis of the uptake of critical perspectives in occupational science. *Journal of Occupational Science*, 23, 1, 33-18

Farias, L., Laliberte Rudman, D. and Magalhães, L. (2016) Illustrating the importance of critical epistemology to realise the promise of occupational justice. *Occupational Therapy Journal of Research: Occupation, Participation and Health*, 36, 4, 234-243

Field, R. (n.d.) *John Dewey*. Internet Encyclopedia of Philosophy. [Accessed 29 July 2016 at http://www.iep.utm.edu/dewey/]

Finkelpearl, T. (2013) *What We Made: Conversations on art and social cooperation*. London: Duke University Press

Frank, G. (2012) 21st century pragmatism and social justice: Problematic situations and occupational reconstruction in post-civil war Guatemala. in M. P. Cutchin and V. A. Dickie (Eds.) *Rethinking Occupation: Transactional perspectives on doing*. New York: Springer (pp.229-243)

Frank, G. (2016) Collective occupations and social transformations: A mad hot curriculum. in N. Pollard, and D. Sakellariou (Eds.) *Occupational Therapy without Borders, Vol II*. Edinburgh: Elsevier (pp. 596-604)

Frank, G. and Dos Santos, V. (2020) Occupational reconstructions: Resources for social transformation in challenging times. Editorial. *Brazilian Journal of Occupational Therapy*, 28, 2

Frank, G and Muriithi, B.A.K. (2015) Theorizing social transformation in occupational science: The American civil rights movement and South African struggle against apartheid as 'occupational reconstructions.' *South African Journal of Occupational Therapy*, 45, 1, 11-19

Freire, P. (1970/2014) *Pedagogy of the Oppressed* (30th anniversary ed.) New York: Continuum

Galvaan, R. (2012) Occupational choice: The significance of socio-economic and political factors. in G. Whiteford, and C. Hocking (Eds.) *Occupational Science: Society, inclusion, participation*. Oxford: Wiley-Blackwell (pp. 152–161)

Garrison, J.W. (2002) Habits as social tools in context. *Occupational Therapy Journal of Research*, 22, 11S-16S

Giroux, H. (2014) Defending higher education in the age of neoliberal savagery. *Discover Society*, 6, 4.3.2014. [Accessed 20 November 2016 at http://discoversociety.org/2014/03/04/defending-higher-education-in-the-age-of-neoliberal-savagery/]

Guajardo, A., Kronenberg, F. and Ramugondo, E. (2015) Southern occupational therapies: Emerging identities, epistemologies and practices. *South African Journal of Occupational Therapy*, 45, 1, 3-10

Guajardo, A. and Pollard, N. (2010) Occupational therapy perspectives from the southern hemisphere. *British Journal of Occupational Therapy*, 73, 6, 241

Graeber, D. (2009) *Direct Action: An ethnography*. Oakland, CA: A K Press

Hammell, K.W. (2011) Resisting theoretical imperialism in the disciplines of occupational science and occupational therapy. *British Journal of Occupational Therapy*, 74, 27–33

Hewitt, R. (2002) Democracy and power: A reply to John Dewey's leftist critics. *Education and Culture*, 18, 2, 1-13

Hickman, L.A. (2009) Pragmatism, Constructivism, and the Philosophy of Technology. in L.A. Hickman, S. Neubert, and K. Reich (Eds.) *John Dewey between Pragmatism and Constructivism*. New York: Fordham University Press (pp.143-161)

Higgins, H. (2002) *Fluxus experience*. Berkeley, LA: University of California Press

Hildreth, R.W. (2009) Reconstructing Dewey on power. *Political Theory*, 37, 6, 780-807

Hitch, D., Pépin, G. and Stagnitti, K. (2014a) In the footsteps of Wilcock, part one: The evolution of doing, being, becoming, and belonging. *Occupational Therapy in Health Care*, 28, 3, 231-246

Hitch, D., Pépin, G. and Stagnitti, K. (2014b) In the footsteps of Wilcock, part two: The interdependent nature of doing, being, becoming, and belonging. *Occupational Therapy in Health Care*, 28, 3, 247-263

Hocking, C. (2012) Occupations through the looking glass: Reflecting on occupational scientists' ontological assumptions. in G. Whiteford, and C. Hocking (Eds.) *Occupational Science: Society, inclusion, participation*. Chichester, UK: Wiley-Blackwell (pp. 54-67)

Hocking, C., Townsend, E., Gerlach, A., Huot, S., Rudman, D. L. and van Bruggen, H. (2015) "Doing" human rights in diverse occupational therapy practices. *Occupational Therapy Now*, 17, 4, 18-20

Horghagen, S. and Josephsson, S. (2010) Theatre as liberation, collaboration and relationship for asylum seekers. *Journal of Occupational Science*, 17, 3, 168-176

Horghagen, S. and Hocking, C. (2017) Shout out who we are! How might engagement in cultural activities enhance participation in everyday occupations for people in vulnerable life situations. in A.H. Eide, S. Josephson, & K. Vik (Eds.) *Participation in Health and Welfare Services: Professional concepts and lived experience*. London: Taylor & Francis (pp. 128-140)

Ikiugu, M.N. and Schultz, S. (2006) An argument for pragmatism as a foundational philosophy of occupational therapy. *Canadian Journal of Occupational Therapy*, 73, 2, 86-97

Jackson, J. (2000) Understanding the experience of non-inclusive occupational therapy clinics: Lesbians' perspectives. *American Journal of Occupational Therapy*, 54, 1, 26-35

Kantartzis, S. and Molineux, M. (2011) The influence of Western society's construction of a healthy daily life on the conceptualisation of occupation. *Journal of Occupational Science*, 18, 1, 62-80, doi: 10.1080/14427591.2011.566917

Kaprow, A. (2003) *Essays on the Blurring of Art and Life*. Berkeley, CA: University of California Press

Kelley, J. (2004) *Childsplay: The art of Allan Kaprow*. Berkeley, CA: University of California Press

Kielhofner, G. and Burke, J.P. (1977) Occupational therapy after 60 years: An account of changing identity and knowledge. *American Journal of Occupational Therapy*, 31, 10, 675

Kindler, H. S. (1979) Two planning strategies: Incremental change and transformational change. *Group & Organization Management*, 4, 4, 476-484

Kino, C. (2010) Where art meets trash and transforms life. *The New York Times*, October 21. [Accessed 28 May 2016 http://www.nytimes.com/2010/10/24/arts/design/24muniz.html?_r=0]

Kinsella, E.A. and Durocher, E. (2016) Occupational justice: Moral imagination, critical reflection, and political praxis. *Occupational Therapy Journal of Research: Occupation, Participation and Health*, 36, 4,163-166

Kronenberg, F., Simó Algado, S. and Pollard, N. (Eds.) (2005) *Occupational Therapy without Borders: Learning from the spirit of survivors*. Edinburgh: Elsevier/Churchill Livingstone

Kronenberg, F., Pollard, N. and Sakellariou, D. (Eds.) (2011) *Occupational Therapies without Borders: Towards an ecology of occupation-based practices*. Edinburgh: Elsevier/Churchill Livingstone

Laverack, G. (2012) Health activism. *Health Promotion International*, 27, 4, 429-435

Lawlor, M. C. (2003) The significance of being occupied: The social construction of childhood occupations. *American Journal of Occupational Therapy*, 57, 4, 424-434, doi: 10.5014/ajot.57.4.424

Lenger, A. and Schumacher, F. (Eds.) (2015) *Understanding the Dynamics of Global Inequality: Social exclusion, power shift, and structural changes*. Heidelberg: Springer

Levine, R.E. (1986) Historical research: Ordering the past to chart our future. *Occupational Therapy Journal of Research: Occupation, Participation and Health*, 6, 5, 259-269

Lucas, S. (2012) Talking trash: Vik Muniz: Garbage matters. Making the trek from garbage dump to gallery wall. *Creative Loafing*. [Accessed 20 November 2016 at http://clclt.com/charlotte/talking-trash-vik-muniz-garbage-matters/Content?oid=2909720]

Magalhães, L. (2012) What would Paulo Freire think of occupational science? in G. Whiteford and C. Hocking (Eds.) *Occupational Science: Society, inclusion, participation*. Chichester, UK: Wiley-Blackwell (pp. 3-7)

Malfitano, A.P.S., Lopes, R.E., Magalhães, L. and Townsend, E.A. (2014) Social occupational therapy: Conversations about a Brazilian experience/Ergothérapie sociale: Conversations au sujet de l'expérience brésilienne. *Canadian Journal of Occupational Therapy*, 81, 5, 298-307

Martin, B. (2007) Activism, social and political. in G.L. Andersen and K.G. Herr (Eds.) *Encyclopedia of Activism and Social Justice*. London: Sage

Menand, L. (2001) *The Metaphysical Club*. New York: Farrar, Straus and Giroux

Mills, C.W. (1964) *Sociology and Pragmatism: The higher learning in America*. New York: Whitman Publishers

Morrison, R. (2016) Pragmatist epistemology and Jane Addams: Fundamental concepts for the social paradigm of occupational therapy. *Occupational Therapy International*, 23, 4, 295-304

Motimele, M. R. and Ramugondo, E. (2014) Violence and healing: Exploring the power of collective occupations. *International Journal of Criminology and Sociology*, 3, 388-401, doi: 10.6000/1929-4409.2014.03.33

Nachmanovitch, S. (1990) *Free Play: Improvisation in art and life*. Tarcher, Los Angeles: Penguin

Nakamura, J. and Dubin, M. (2015) Flow in motivational psychology. in J.S. Neil and P.B. Baltes (Eds.) *International Encyclopedia of the Social and Behavioral Sciences*. New York: Elsevier (pp. 260-265)

Nussbaum, M.C. (1995) *Women, Culture, and Development: A study of human capabilities*. Oxford: Clarendon Press/Oxford University Press

Odawara, E. (2005) Cultural competency in occupational therapy: Beyond a cross-cultural view of practice. *American Journal of Occupational Therapy*, 59, 3, 325-334

Pappas, G.F. (2008) *John Dewey: Democracy as experience*. Bloomington: Indiana University Press

Parham, L.D. and Fazio, L.S. (2008) *Play in Occupational Therapy for Children*. (2nd ed.) St. Louis, Mo: Mosby Elsevier

Park, M. (2008) Making scenes: Imaginary practices of a child with autism in a sensory integration -based therapy session. *Medical Anthropology Quarterly*, 22, 234-256

PBS News Hour (2011) 'Waste Land' Explores Artist's Use of Garbage to Transform Lives in Brazil, November 17. [Accessed 20 November 2016 at http://www.pbs.org/newshour/bb/world-july-dec11-efp_11-17/]

Ramugondo, E.L. (2015) Occupational consciousness. *Journal of Occupational Science*, 22, 4, 488-501, doi: 10.1080/14427591.2015.1042516

Ramugondo, E.L. and Kronenberg, F. (2015) Explaining collective occupations from a human relations perspective: Bridging the individual-collective dichotomy. *Journal of Occupational Science*, 22, 1, 3-16, doi: 10.1080/14427591.2013.781920

Reilly, M. (1962) Occupational therapy can be one of the great ideas of 20th century medicine. *American Journal of Occupational Therapy*, 16, 1-9

Renton, L. and van Bruggen, H. (2015) Occupational therapy and European social reform: Complacent or contributing? *British Journal of Occupational Therapy*, 78, 9, 585-588, doi:10.1177/0308022614562796

Rodenbeck, J. F. (2011) *Radical Prototypes: Allan Kaprow and the invention of Happenings*. Cambridge, MA: MIT Press

Rogers, M. L. (2009) Democracy, elites and power: John Dewey reconsidered. *Contemporary Political Theory*, 8, 1, 68-89, doi: http://dx.doi.org.libproxy1.usc.edu/10.1057/cpt.2008.25

Ruskin, C. and Herron, M. (1998) *The Quilt: Stories from The NAMES Project*. New York: Pocket

Books
Sakellariou, D. and Pollard, N. (Eds.) (2017) *Occupational Therapies without Borders: Integrating justice with practice*. (2nd ed.) Edinburgh, UK: Elsevier
San Francisco Museum of Art website. [Accessed 27 May 2016 https://www.sfmoma.org/artwork/98.291]
Schmidt-Burkhardt, A. (2011) *Maciunas' Learning Machines: From art history to a chronology of Fluxus*. NewYork: Springer
Schultz, B. (2009) Obama's political philosophy: Pragmatism, politics, and the University of Chicago. *Philosophy of the Social Sciences*, 39, 2, 127-173
Schutz, A. (2011) Power and trust in the public realm: John Dewey, Saul Alinsky, and the limits of progressive democratic education. *Educational Theory*, 61, 4, 491-512
Schutz, A. and Miller, M. (2015) *People Power: The community organizing tradition of Saul Alinsky*. Nashville: Vanderbilt University Press
Schwartz, K.B. (1992) Occupational therapy and education: a shared vision. *American Journal of Occupational Therapy*, 46, 1, 12
Schwartz, K.B. (2009) Reclaiming our heritage: Connecting the founding vision to the centennial vision. *American Journal of Occupational Therapy*, 63, 6, 681-690
Sell, M. (2005) *Avant-Garde Performance and the Limits of Criticism: Approaching the Living Theatre, happenings/Fluxus, and the Black Arts movement*. Ann Arbor: University of Michigan Press
Sen, A. (2000) *Development as Freedom*. New York: Anchor Books
Smith, L.T. (2013) *Decolonizing Methodologies: Research and indigenous peoples*. London: Palgrave Macmillan
Stadnyk R., Townsend E. and Wilcock A. (2010) Occupational justice. in C.H. Christiansen and E.A. Townsend (Eds.) *Introduction to Occupation: The art and science of living*. (2nd ed.) Upper Saddle River, NJ: Pearson Education (pp. 329-358)
Thibeault, R. (2011) Rebuilding lives and societies through occupation in post-conflict areas and highly marginalised settings. in F. Kronenberg, N. Pollard, and D. Sakellariou (Eds.) *Occupational Therapies without Borders*. (2 ed.) Edinburgh: Churchill Livingston (pp. 155-162)
Thompson, J. (2012) Incredible edible: Social and environmental entrepreneurship in the era of the "big society". *Social Enterprise Journal*, 8, 3, 237-250, doi: http://dx.doi.org.libproxy2.usc.edu/10.1108/17508611211280773
Thompson, N. (2012) *Living as Form: Socially engaged art from 1991-2011*. Cambridge, MA: MIT Press
Townsend E.A. and Wilcock A.A. (2004) Occupational justice. in C.H. Christiansen and E.A.Townsend (Eds.) *Introduction to Occupation: The art and science of living*. Upper Saddle River, NJ: Prentice Hall (pp. 243-273)
Twinley, R. (2013) The dark side of occupation: A concept for consideration. *Australian Occupational Therapy Journal*, 60, 4, 301-303, doi:10.1111/1440-1630.12026
von Hoffman, N. (2010) *Radical: A portrait of Saul Alinsky*. New York: Nation Books
Walker, L. (Director). (2010) *Waste Land*. Arthouse Films. (99 min.) [Accessed 27 May 2016 at https://www.youtube.com/watch?v=QUAavzJsTBw]
Watson, R. and Swartz, L. (Eds.) (2004) *Transformation Through Occupation*. London: Whurr Publishers
Westbrook, R.B. (1991) *John Dewey and American democracy*. Ithaca, N.Y: Cornell University Press
Whiteford G. (2000) Occupational deprivation: Global challenge in the new millennium. *British Journal of Occupational Therapy*, 63, 5, 200-04

Whiteford, G. (2005) Understanding the occupational deprivation of refugees: A case study from Kosovo. *Canadian Journal of Occupational Therapy*, 72, 2, 78-88

Whiteford, G. (2011) From occupational deprivation to social inclusion: Retrospective insights. *British Journal of Occupational Therapy*, 74, 12, 545

Whiteford, G. and Hocking, C. (Eds.) (2012) *Occupational Science: Society, inclusion, participation*. Chichester, UK: Wiley-Blackwell

Wilcock, A.A. (1998) Reflections on doing, being and becoming. *Canadian Journal of Occupational Therapy*, 65, 248-256, doi:10.1177/000841749806500501

Wolfe, J. (2012) Does pragmatism have a theory of power? *European Journal of Pragmatism and American Philosophy*, 4, 1, 120-137

World Federation of Occupational Therapists (WFOT) (2010) *Statement on Occupational Therapy*. [Accessed 20 May 2016 at www.wfot.org]

Yerxa, E.J., Clark, F., Frank, G., Jackson, J., Parham, D., Pierce, D., Stein, C. and Zemke, R. (1990) An introduction to occupational science: A foundation for occupational therapy in the 21st century. in J.A. Johnson and E.J. Yerxa (Eds.) *Occupational Science: The foundation for new models of practice*. New York: The Haworth Press (pp.1-17)

Chapter 9
Advancing understandings of inclusion and participation through situated research

Robert B. Pereira and Gail E. Whiteford

Introduction

The English word *occupation* is derived from the Latin noun *occupatio* and the verb *occupare* meaning 'to occupy', 'to seize', 'to possess', 'to fill time and space', 'to take control of' and 'to employ' (Pereira, 2015a). Occupation is a multifaceted phenomenon in that it is unique to every individual or collective living and experiencing human doing in context (Njelesani et al, 2014). In occupational therapy, which is a profession focused on enabling people to participate and engage in occupations for health, wellbeing and quality of life, there are various frames of reference that guide practice, however, the focus is – or should be - on occupation as *means* and *ends* when working with individuals and collectives (Gray, 1998; Trombly, 1995).

The contemporary paradigm of occupation-focused practice aims to reclaim and advance occupation as the primary means and ends of occupational therapy intervention with individuals, families, communities, social groups and populations (Kielhofner, 2009). However, both occupational science and occupational therapy discourses are underpinned by a tacit assumption that participation in occupation is a given right for all citizens to engage in equitably (Hammell, 2008; Townsend & Wilcock, 2004). Whilst universalising occupational participation as a human right is an ideal for which we can - and should - collectively aim, when it comes to enablement, context is everything. The specific national, socio-political, cultural and economic contexts in which people engage in occupations on a daily basis impact directly and indirectly on processes that facilitate or hinder participation and whether occupation can always be achieved as an end.

Occupational engagement is dynamic and it is widely acknowledged in occupational science and occupational therapy discourse that there is a transactional relationship between the person, their environment or context, and occupation (Cutchin & Dickie, 2013; Law et al, 1996). Therefore, one can assume that when there is congruence between these three elements, optimal occupational performance will occur (Townsend & Polatajko, 2007). Nevertheless, several factors exist which can impact on the achievement of 'occupation as ends' (Gray, 1998), or occupational fulfilment (Kirsh, 2015).

Limited applied and participatory research exists that has explored the dynamic interaction between contextual drivers and the attempts of individuals and groups to achieve occupational fulfilment (Kirsh, 2015). This is especially the case amongst those who have little or no voice in mainstream discourses, i.e. people who have experienced oppression, marginalisation and deprivation of capabilities over time. In this chapter we aim to address this relative silence by presenting such a voice of a person marginalised through chronic unemployment. Rose (a pseudonym) was a participant in research conducted in Australia by the authors that focussed on the everyday realities of living with entrenched disadvantage characterised by poverty and disability (Pereira, 2013; Pereira & Whiteford, 2013; Whiteford & Pereira, 2012). Through the presentation of extracts from Rose's story, some key findings from the research are highlighted by comparing and contrasting them against key theoretical elements of social inclusion as described in interdisciplinary literature. This is done in order to highlight the complexity of achieving and promoting 'occupation as ends' in a given context (Gray, 1998). Throughout, the chapter uses moral and political philosopher Axel Honneth's (1995) theory of recognition to help situate Rose's voice and concludes with the presentation of a number of enablement strategies for occupation-focused interventions aimed at maximising social inclusion.

Occupation in context: Exploring social inclusion

Occupation comprises the things that we do in life that hold meaning, purpose and value, and accord dignity, which are never performed in a vacuum (Pereira et al, 2020). Occupation is situated: it occurs in families, workplaces, communities, and societies more broadly. And participating in occupations of choice, necessity and significance is, as we suggested earlier, a human right (Hammell, 2008; Townsend & Wilcock, 2004). However, what that means in any given context will always reflect prevailing sociocultural, socioeconomic and socio-political realities. Similar to occupation, *social inclusion* is also a concept that holds various meanings due to its multiplicity of factors that influence and enable (or constrain) its processes and outcomes (or 'means' and 'ends'). Broadly and simply, social inclusion is about having opportunities, resources and capabilities to fully participate in life, respecting one another with dignity, and being a contributing citizen in the society in which one lives (Pereira, 2017, 2015b; Whiteford & Pereira, 2012; Government of South Australia, 2009). The authors' occupational science research, as well as interdisciplinary literature into understanding social inclusion from political, social, cultural and theoretical perspectives, have highlighted key theoretical elements, or framings, of social inclusion (Pereira, 2015b; Pereira, 2013; Whiteford & Pereira, 2012). These framings are described in Appendix A.

Social inclusion, occupational justice and occupation-centred practices

The Canadian politics professor Anver Saloojee (2005) described social inclusion as a process and outcome of *democratic citizenship*, which is about 'valued participation, valued recognition and belonging' (p. 191). As social inclusion is closely linked with a rights agenda (Nelms & Tsingas, 2010; Lombe & Sherraden, 2008; Saloojee, 2005, 2001), the freedom to participate in occupations in society is as much an occupational justice concern as it is with social justice. The underlying principles of rights, inequalities and social justice that guide social and community practice (Davis, as cited in Ward, 2009) are also central to the occupational therapy profession as well as occupational justice scholarship (Whiteford et al, 2018; Whiteford et al, 2017; Whiteford & Townsend, 2011; Townsend & Whiteford, 2005). Occupational justice principles focus on 'recognising and providing for the occupational needs of individuals and communities as part [of] a fair and empowering society' (Wilcock & Townsend, 2000, p. 84). Without occupational justice, Wilcock and Townsend conceded that '...the interpersonal interactions, communities, and the world [could] experience inequalities which touch the very essence of living' (p. 84). Social inclusion and occupational therapy can be conceptualised as being philosophically aligned, as justice has been valued as a key pillar in occupational therapy's knowledge base (Whiteford et al, 2017; Whiteford & Townsend, 2011; Townsend & Whiteford, 2005). In context with the practice of occupational therapy, justice is considered as a key client-centred, occupation-based enablement foundation (Townsend et al, 2007). Elements of the 'doing of justice' (Whiteford & Townsend, 2011, p. 66) have been expressed in the Canadian Model of Client-Centred Enablement (Townsend & Polatajko, 2007) which highlights 10 enablement skills for person-centred practice through enabling occupation. Such enablement skills include advocacy, coaching, collaboration, coordination, education and engagement (Townsend et al, 2007).

Occupation as justice

Viewed through an occupational lens, being able to do, be, become and belong (Wilcock, 2006, 1998), along with having opportunities and control over occupational choices, situate occupation-based practices as direct forms and practices of justice. 'Occupation *as* justice' (Pereira, 2017, 2015b, 2013) is a nuanced approach to justice and rights within occupational justice discourse. Occupation *as* justice situates functionings (Sen, 1999), or 'occupation as ends' (Gray, 1998), at the core of justice in context with mechanisms which support, or guide the enactment of justice, rights and capabilities. Briefly, Nobel laureate for economics Amartya Sen (1999) described *capabilities* as the opportunities and freedoms to lead a life that one has reason to value. Together with leading a valued and dignified life, occupation *as* justice embraces capabilities together with the value of actually being able to do, or engage in dignified and politically recognised occupations (Pereira, 2015b; 2013). Promoters and critics of the capabilities approach alike (i.e. Barclay, 2012a; Barclay 2012b; Moss, 2012) have argued that recognising the *need* for capabilities alone cannot be considered without a concurrent focus on 'functionings', or what individuals are actually able to *do* and *be* which result from realising capabilities. This refocus within the capabilities approach itself on functionings is of significant value as it lends to theoretical and practical input from occupation-based practices. Thus, intersecting the capabilities approach with occupational justice principles is valuable for operationalising a broader vision and enactment of inclusive practices and policies (Whiteford, 2019; Pereira, 2013, Pereira et al., 2020).

Challenging assumptions: Can everyone pursue and enjoy occupation as a human right?

While it is important to acknowledge the potential of enabling occupation, some taken for granted premises about occupation need to be interrogated in order for us to address its inherent complexity. For example, the foundational premise of humans as 'occupational beings' directly refers to human engagement in, and experience of, occupations (Wilcock, 2006, 1998; Clark, 1997; Yerxa et al, 1990). This includes the need and capacity to engage in and orchestrate daily occupations in various environments and contexts over the life span (Clark, 1997; Yerxa et al, 1990). Accordingly, occupational science investigates human engagement with occupation in context with their environments; 'not as decontextualised beings' (Yerxa et al, 1990, p. 11). In this respect then, humans may be understood as human *beings* and human *doers* simultaneously - in context.

But what is the relationship between being and doing and what does this mean in everyday life for people? Everyday occupations are the mundane doings (Hasselkus, 2011; 2006) that generally go unnoticed until conditions change and they are no longer possible due to factors outside of one's control (Whiteford, 2010, 2004, 2000; Wilcock, 2006). It is within this space that we challenge another widely held premise within the profession, namely, that participating in occupation is a given right for *all* to freely pursue and enjoy. It is an ideal that they should, but it is a current global reality that injustices exist which exclude vast numbers of people – whether they be women, people with disabilities, refugees or ethnic minority groups – from participation in occupations of necessity, choice and meaning (Whiteford, 2010). Whilst some exclusions are overt and may have a legislated basis – for example as is the case in numerous countries, it is illegal for asylum seekers to enter the workforce of the country in which they are seeking asylum until their claims are processed – some are more covert. In the next section we explore this more covert form of social exclusion through the presentation of Rose's story. Before presenting aspects of her narrative for discussion, however, we foreground the theory of recognition as the theoretical lens through which Rose's struggles may be best understood.

Axel Honneth's (1995) theory of recognition: An overview

As was highlighted previously, *social inclusion as recognition* is a key framing in theories, practices and policies on social inclusion. Identity and personhood are important concepts in Honneth's (1995) theory of recognition, and play a key role in understanding how cultural, political and social recognition occur at an everyday level. Honneth's theory of recognition is related to the concept of justice, as it acknowledges the recognition, acceptance, dignity and respect of a person's or societal group's difference and diversity (Morrison, 2010; Honneth, 2001, 1995, 1992). From an ethical perspective, Honneth (2001) related recognition with 'reciprocal respect for both the unique and equal status of all others' (p. 45). In developing the theory of recognition, Honneth based his philosophical concepts of recognition on the works of moral philosopher Hegel, who portrayed recognition as a vital human need beyond mere courtesy (Deranty, 2009; Taylor, as cited in Fraser, 1995). Compared to recognition as a human rights discourse, Honneth expressed that such a discourse would be limited and not cater for associations of recognition with social esteem and loving care (Ikäheimo, 2009; Honneth, 2001). Rather, recognition in this sense was more of a moral than an exclusive human rights perspective (Honneth, 2001). Honneth (2001) also described a theory of recognition as a moral-practical philosophy to conceptualise social inclusion and exclusion:

> 'We are...dealing with the denial of rights and with social exclusion, where human beings suffer in their dignity through not being granted the moral rights and responsibilities of a full legal person within their own community. Accordingly, this type of disrespect has to have, as its corresponding relation, the reciprocal recognition through which individuals come to regard themselves as equal bearers of rights from the perspective of their fellows' (p. 49).

Social inclusion, to Honneth, is therefore recognition of equality and dignity, with self-respect as a product of an inclusive transaction between individuals or groups that takes place in moral and practical terms. According to Honneth, a 'morality of recognition' takes the form of a perfect example of the attitudes of mutual obligation that one must adopt '...to secure jointly the conditions of our personal integrity' (Honneth, as cited in Heidegren, 2002, p. 439). Furthermore, not only does Honneth's theory of recognition pronounce the essential morality of recognising another as equal (Deranty, 2009), but it also provides positive outcomes for the other from the process of being recognised as a person (Ikäheimo & Laitinen, 2010; Ikäheimo, 2009, 2007, 2002). Such outcomes include positive self-esteem, self-realisation, integrity, acceptance of egalitarian difference as well as love, appreciation for legal order and solidarity (Heidegren, 2002; Honneth, 2001).

Rose's story: Occupational challenges and the struggle for recognition

Given the paucity of research that has explored matters of recognition and misrecognition of people living with disability (Calder, 2011; Thompson & Yar, 2011), it was important to consider how occupational participation and social inclusion was experienced from people who considered themselves as marginalised. The following excerpts, directly from Rose's own narrative accounts from the authors' research, are testimony to the complexity of exploring how the phenomenon of occupation is situated within the broader sociocultural context.

About Rose

Rose is a 50-year-old Australian citizen who immigrated from Europe 25 years ago. She identifies herself as a proud mother of one daughter, a widow, a divorcee, and a dog lover. She has successfully completed tertiary education and various other training courses, lives in public housing, receives a disability support pension, and lives with several chronic health conditions including major depression, low back pain, lumbar spine degeneration, osteoarthritis and osteoporosis. She has been unemployed or underemployed for 25 years.

Wanting to do something that counts

Reflecting the notion of social recognition (Honneth, 2001), Rose's story highlights the longing to do things that are recognised by others as valuable. *Being able to participate* considers both objective and subjective aspects of doing as well as satisfaction with, and accomplishment of, participation (Anaby et al, 2011; Van't Leven & Jonsson, 2002). Being able to participate also recognises the breadth of the notion of participation from an occupational perspective, while also acknowledging that each person has unique needs for participation (Anaby et al, 2001; Van't Leven & Jonsson, 2002).

> *'So in the meantime, I go to the [Non-government organisation], say hello to people. I actually don't have any friends. I don't have any relatives. My only next of kin is my daughter. And um, and God I suppose. God is my soul mate. And it's [a] very sad life that I am living [teary] and I don't know what to do. Many times I was thinking about committing suicide. And people told me, what about your daughter? It's bad enough that the father is gone. But I, I don't know. But if I go and find a job, people come up with excuses, oh, you don't have experience or this or that. It's too long since I have been employed. I even had a forklift license. Driver's license. I could do anything like delivery, things like delivering blood or urine samples, you know, lab things. They just don't put you on. They don't trust you. You are not one of them. It's very hard to assimilate here [teary].'*

The first example of doing *for* recognition described through Rose's story above identifies some implications from lacking meaningful doing which impacted on her worker identity as a productive occupational being (Gupta, 2012). Rose also highlighted her difficulty in relating to others and fitting in, where she sought solace and connection instead with God. In this example, Rose's story exemplifies some of the effects of chronic unemployment and feeling excluded from occupational opportunities, including her negative view of finding a job despite having useful skills for employment. In context, Australia is a welfare state enabling citizens living with disability to obtain a disability support pension while also being able to seek paid employment commensurate with their abilities and functional limitations. Chronic unemployment has been found to be associated with adverse health, social and economic effects, including deleterious effects on mental health and wellbeing (Jin et al, 1995). From an occupational perspective, the lack of discretionary income from chronic unemployment can impede opportunities to engage in other meaningful occupations (Jakobsen, 2009; Whiteford, 2004, 2000) such as enabling social and productive occupations that would contribute towards meaning-making and identity reaffirmation through occupation. This is particularly pertinent in Australia and other Western countries where the impacts of poverty are compounded by consumerism and the increasing costs to participate in such occupations.

Rose's story is further complicated by feeling *othered* as well as experiencing acts of exclusion. Her constant use of 'they' describing Australian employers indicates that inclusion into mainstream Australian society through participating in the paid workforce appears to have been a significant challenge for her since migrating to Australia from her homeland 25 years ago. From her account, it appears that the constant rejection that Rose has sustained from potential employers despite her list of skills and qualifications had taken its toll on her emotional health and wellbeing. A systematic review of psychology and health science literature into the mental and physical health of unemployed individuals identified that their overall wellbeing was lower compared with employed individuals (McKee-Ryan et al, 2005). McKee-Ryan et al. also identified some qualities that were beneficial to promote mental health amongst people who were not participating in the paid workforce. These included having a valued worker role, coping resources (i.e. personal, social, financial, routine, time structure), cognitive appraisals (i.e. positive self-talk) and other coping strategies (McKee-Ryan et al, 2005).

It is evident from Rose's story above that her experiences have broadly impacted on her mental health and subjective wellbeing, as described through her expressions of feeling excluded from mainstream Australian society through being unemployed for several years. Rose's experiences of exclusion and not knowing what to meaningfully and productively *do* are echoed within the findings of occupational science research which has documented the 'destabilising effect' of being unemployed (Aldrich, 2011, p. 2). From a psychological perspective, a systematic review conducted by McKee-Ryan et al. (2005) exposed some adverse health effects related to chronic unemployment. Of note, is the effect of not having *social* types of coping resources (i.e. close family and friends), structured and productive use of time, as well as having high self-esteem and a positive outlook on life (McKee-Ryan et al, 2005). Rose's accounts, amongst many of the other participants' stories in the authors' research, appear to have experienced significant 'destabilising effects' (Aldrich, 2011) impacting on their general health, quality of life and valuing their own contributions to their communities.

Living in a community lacking compassion

For Rose and other participants in the authors' research, existential realities such as living with disability, poverty and other complex issues was further complicated by the impact of discrimination and the absence of certain social determinants of health and wellbeing. Given such adversity, the participants' stories highlighted that occupational adaptation was not sufficient or possible for more *complete* or socially recognised types of participation due to the absence of essential resources (i.e. money to purchase and cook a nutritious meal; being successful in attaining an apartment to live in). The fallout, therefore, appeared to result in incomplete occupational identities being forged. By incomplete, we infer that the essential constructs of *competence* and *mastery* for occupational adaptation (Schkade & Schultz, 1992; Schultz & Schkade, 1992) were not possible due to living day-to-day life through modes of survival. Thus, meaningful, purposeful and dignified participation in 'occupations as ends' (Gray, 1998) appeared to become more challenging, which impacted on possibilities for experiencing subjective wellbeing and realising occupational identities.

The psycho-emotional toll on Rose and other participants of not being a part of a *normal* social life was heavily affected by their impressions of living within a culture which facilitated more exclusionary effects rather than downplaying or eradicating them. As a result, participants identified elements of a *culture of exclusion*, with an apparent lack of *compassion* towards others. Thus, such experiences resulted in a deeper sense of exclusion, where participants felt relegated to a lower status along a social axis of power (Yuval-Davis, 2006). In context with these experiences, the notion of *belonging* appeared to be more redundant.

Participants provided detailed accounts which demonstrated a limited sense of belonging. The sentiment of not belonging to one's community was substantiated by participants in several ways. For example, Rose and other participants described that they experienced various forms of discrimination on a frequent basis, which resulted in feeling a diminished sense of trust and care within their community. Such feelings led participants to resort to a 'survival of the fittest' mentality. In effect, this notion of survival demystified a supposed illusion of living in a peaceful community, as well as appeared to unveil a deep cultural problem. In particular, Rose's stories of racism, exclusion and discrimination in the following accounts illuminated some complexities of what *not* belonging and living in a *culture of exclusion* meant for her:

> *'The Department of Housing put me into a complex like this, but with more density, like 15 houses in one place. And everyone watching what you're doing, what you don't do. They start to pick on you because you are not one of them. And you are not blonde and blue eyed. So they start calling me names and ah, remark about my skin and calling me 'black bitch'. I had to get out of there for me and my daughter's sake.*
> *...Every person that you see in [Western Sydney] is depressed! It's very depressing to walk in the mall in [Western Sydney]. You see all the druggies there and all the alcoholics. People spitting on the ground and coughing. It's very distressing and very depressing. The community here in [Western Sydney]. So I just try to take my stuff [food offered at Non-Government Organisation] that I need and just go.*
> *...They [white Australians] look at us [immigrants] like second-class citizens. And they are very abusive and insulting. Especially your neighbours. They tell you you have no character. And get [expletive]...They are all Australians...I feel that the Australians, they have a very cold society. And they are very rejecting. Only the ones who believe in God have compassion towards others. They are not willing to make friends. A good example is I have a neighbour that lives near me in the complex. Ten years and he has never said 'hello' to me...So I just live a very depressing life, that I have wasted 25 years of my life and I wanted to contribute something to society...The government can't help me. I have to help myself. I am not expecting anyone to help me. I am living in an unfriendly society.*
> *...Your neighbours pick on you. They don't want you around them. And it's also hard to find a job. And when you don't find a job, feel very demoralised and you say to yourself, what's wrong with me? Sometimes they said I am too smart for the job and they won't put me on. They are scared. Looks that they are scared of me. And because I am a multi-skilled woman and I speak three languages, and I can operate machines, and I can also try and translate simultaneously...I just don't find the right way to get a job and I have had enough of begging people for a job...It's a bastard of a society and they are cruel. They are very cruel. I am very demoralised. And that's how depression comes. You think you are a good-for-nothing. And why?...It's just people don't trust each other today. We need people to be more friendly, more trusting, more welcoming.*
> *...[Regarding finding a job] They don't tell you in the face they don't want you. They just don't ring you. They don't want to know about you. You are not one of them. We are the rejects. All the newcomers here with their families. They expect your children not to have an accent...And I don't think in school they teach manners. They just teach to hate each other. Racism comes from home. And I can see it. They come to the park, the Australians with their children and they don't talk to you... And it's going to get worse. Today they're only into money. Making money. Money machines. If you don't make money, you are no good. Everything is expensive. The high cost of living. The rent. The food...They are all living in charity organisations. You get sometimes fresh or second-hand food. That's how we are surviving.'*

In these stories, Rose described experiences and feelings of exclusion which affected her across several social and occupational roles; such as a being a citizen, a single mother, a woman, a public housing tenant, a person living with chronic disability and unemployment and finally as an immigrant. Rose's emotive expressions in these stories highlight her longing to contribute to society in social, cultural and occupational ways. However, feeling included was compromised by exclusionary acts by others which led her to feel undervalued. As such, the outcome for Rose's seemingly unsuccessful inclusion could instead be interpreted as living an 'othered' life in Western Sydney where denigration and misrecognition (Anna, 2018, 2012) appeared to become her norm. Misrecognition negatively impacts on the self-esteem and autonomy of a person experiencing exclusion by denying moral agency (Thompson & Yar, 2011; Laitinen, 2010). Rose's stories of exclusionary experiences which include misrecognition (Anna, 2012; Thompson & Yar, 2011; Laitinen, 2010) also revealed a sense of internalised oppression (Reeve, 2004), which she frequently described as being associated with demoralisation and depression. Rose's stories provide valuable insights into some consequences which can result from living with entrenched disadvantage such as poverty and disability with respect to the psycho-emotional toll of sociocultural exclusion.

Rose's accounts highlight the psycho-emotional impacts of living with entrenched disadvantage and not having stable and meaningful social networks and relationships. It appears that her life story in particular also holds a sense of 'failed immigration' to the 'lucky country' where having little contact with her family and having 'no friends' or 'no-one to visit' has resulted in feelings of hopelessness. She boldly stated:

'No one here for the last 25 years has invited me for a cup of coffee. No one here. It's very sad.'

It appears then, that her struggle for social recognition resonated in a simple yet taken-for-granted social act of friendship and reciprocity which is considered as important for mutual recognition and respect (Komter, 2005). Her statement about the occupation of having a cup of coffee with somebody speaks to a personal sense of deep loss affecting her everyday life. Despite Rose's social interactions with others and searching for friendship, such interactions seem to have masked a profound sadness of longing to be part of and assimilate with her broader social world.

Ways forward: Doing occupation-based practices for social inclusion

'Proper scrutiny and spirit count as much if not more than action. Successful implementation and protection of occupational rights rely obviously on the awareness and recognition of such rights, but they also depend on a vision that goes beyond the purely political into the realms of the philosophical and the ethical' (Thibeault, 2013, p. 247).

Rose's stories of her struggles for recognition and realising her capabilities to do, be, become and belong (Wilcock, 2006, 1998) point to several challenges for practice that enables occupational outcomes, or 'occupation as ends' (Gray, 1998). The taken-for-grantedness of occupational participation (Pereira & Whiteford, 2013; Hasselkus, 2011, 2006) becomes even more apparent when factors outside of one's control (i.e. tacit and explicit discrimination, racism, policy) delimit occupational possibilities (Laliberte Rudman, 2010). Therefore, cycles of disadvantage continue to perpetuate and become entrenched. However, enabling occupation holds potential to create alternative occupational realities and social recognition through adopting an ethos of moral consciousness (Wright-St Clair & Seedhouse, 2005) that can become a change agent in and of itself. Moral consciousness involves being conscious of the everyday moral dimensions of people and practice in context with the broader environment. Having politics, policies and communities that are morally conscious (Wright-St Clair & Seedhouse, 2005) can enable the occupational and wellbeing needs of citizens and occupational beings in Australian society to be recognised with dignity, equity and respect (Venkatapuram, 2011; Honneth, 1995). Recognition theory (Honneth, 2001, 1995) offers an approach to consider occupational issues of inclusion and exclusion through a morally conscious lens (Wright-St Clair & Seedhouse, 2005). As such, occupational therapists can adopt such philosophies for person- and community-centred practices (Townsend & Polatajko, 2007) that foster occupational possibilities (Laliberte Rudman, 2010) with and for people who consider themselves as marginalised and oppressed.

The political, systemic and social recognition and enactments of the key theoretical framings of social inclusion (Pereira, 2013; Whiteford & Pereira, 2012), together with working towards 'occupation as ends' (Gray, 1998), or occupational fulfilment (Kirsh, 2015), can be powerful tools for inclusive and occupation-based practices as they essentially promote principles which protect the occupational rights of individuals. Together, they can lay foundations for enabling inclusive opportunities leading to *sustainable participation*. Such principles, as suggested by Thibeault (2013, p. 250-251) include (1) examining the values, motives and attitudes of individuals; (2) adopting an occupational lens and (3) establishing fair and sustainable partnerships with communities. Each of these principles highlight a level of moral consciousness where capabilities, *occupation-as-justice* and avenues for recognition can be enacted and established in partnership with stakeholders such as community members, social institutions, policymakers, government officials and others in positions of power.

Viewing doing and being, or occupation *as* a direct form of justice, can be the starting point for ethical, moral, social and informed action influencing meaningful, purposeful and dignified participation at the everyday level (Pereira, 2013). Therefore, considering occupation and its potential, as well as adopting a morally conscious and inclusive ethic of care, *must* be on each stakeholder's agenda for sustainable participation solutions. Ultimately, therefore, the *ends* of social inclusion could become less of an ideal. In this context, the *ends* of social inclusion are those in which

> '*all* people, including traditionally marginalised and oppressed individuals, have the opportunities, resources, capabilities, choices and political recognition to achieve their human and occupational potential leading to social transformation, positive wellbeing and living a flourishing life that they have reason to value' (Pereira, 2013, p. 4).

Inclusive and occupation-based practices that hold a morally conscious ethos at their core can spearhead actions towards realising the *ends* of social inclusion. We suggest that to advance such practices, the following 'points of action' (Pereira, 2015b; 2013, p. 285-286) for sustainable and inclusive solutions should be considered:

* The pathway towards inclusion and active citizenship (doing things together) can be made real through proactively exploring with the citizens who we serve how their (1) *capabilities*, or freedoms to live a life that they have reason to value, can be enabled; (2) what *opportunities* can be made available or become possible to enable and achieve occupational fulfilment (Kirsh, 2015); (3) what *resources* can be developed, enabled or facilitated which can support occupational possibilities (Laliberte Rudman, 2010), and finally (4) how can *environments*, or the contexts which situate us as occupational beings, be made more enabling and supportive through employing our enablement skills (Capabilities, Opportunities, Resources and Environments [CORE] approach; Pereira et al, 2020; Pereira, 2017, 2015b);
* Promote sustainable participation and inclusion through community-led processes and collaborative action with key stakeholders which always involve the direct participation of citizens (Hyatt et al., 2019; Whiteford, 2019). This has the potential to recognise citizens' skills, talents and contribution potential (Whiteford & Townsend, 2011);
* Consider the diversity of disability and acknowledge that living with disability is unique to the person with disability and can be both enriching and difficult. It is also important to consider the service provider's or practitioner's own value-laden assumptions and biases towards ability and diversity to eradicate exclusionary and hegemonic practices;
* Act in ways to dispel myths about people living with entrenched forms of disadvantage, promote difference and diversity, and provide them with equitable opportunities so that they can achieve occupation-as-ends (Gray, 1998) which can be interpreted as forms of *justice in action*. There is scope within this recommendation to take a leadership and mentoring role, educating others on how to be proactive in supporting inclusion and taking a stand against discrimination and misrecognition by putting people first;
* Incorporate complementary life skills programs to capacitate individuals with the basic skills and capabilities to meet their everyday needs with dignity. Such programs could complement government activity programs and other capacity building initiatives such as learning how to cook an affordable and nutritious meal; health literacy; budgeting and money management programs; digital literacy (Hamilton et al, 2014); providing opportunities for accessible leisure and recreation; cultural diversity and awareness education; general literacy and numeracy skills, and countless other ways to create, innovate and empower;
* Recognise that there is no place for misrecognition, disablism and other forms of discrimination within society;
* Invoke a morally conscious culture of inclusion through holding and practising positive life values towards other community members which can support connectedness and a sense of belonging, and
* Recognise, respect, and promote diversity and an ethic of care within one's community, inclusive of members living in poverty with disability or other forms of adversity.

References

Aldrich, R.M. (2011) *Discouraged Worker's Daily Occupations: Exploring complex transactions in the experience of unemployment*. PhD Thesis, University of North Carolina at Chapel Hill. [Accessed 12 October 2016 at https://cdr.lib.unc.edu/indexablecontent/uuid:7a436f82-2c0a-413c-b255-274acc445ff3]

Anaby, D., Miller, W., Eng, J., Jarus, T. and Noreau, L. (2011) Participation and well-being among older adults living with chronic conditions. *Social Indicators Research*, 100, 1, 171-183

Anna, B. (2012) *Social Integration and Social Fragmentation: Axel Honneth's theory of recognition applied in everyday multiculturalism*. Paper presented at the Centre for Research on Nationalism, Ethnicity and Multiculturalism (CRONEM) Conference. Surrey, United Kingdom, 26-27 June

Anna, B. (2018) Honneth and everyday intercultural (mis)recognition: Work, marginalisation and integration, London: Palgrave Macmillan

Australian Social Inclusion Board (2010) *Social Inclusion in Australia: How Australia is faring*. Canberra: Department of the Prime Minister and Cabinet. [Accessed 12 October 2016 at http://library.bsl.org.au/jspui/bitstream/1/3170/1/Social%20inclusion%20in%20Australia%20how%20Australia%20is%20faring2012.pdf]

Bach, M. (2005) Social inclusion as solidarity: Re-thinking the child rights agenda. in T. Richmond and A. Saloojee (Eds.) *Social Inclusion: Canadian perspectives*. Toronto: Laidlaw Foundation (pp. 126-154)

Barclay, L. (2012a) Natural deficiency or social oppression? The capabilities approach to justice for people with disabilities. *Journal of Moral Philosophy*, 9, 4, 500-520

Barclay, L. (2012b) *What can Human Rights Teach us about the Capabilities Approach?* Paper presented at the Capabilities Approaches to Justice: Theory and Practice Conference, Sydney, Australia, 15 November

Buckmaster, L. and Thomas, M. (2009) *Social Inclusion and Social Citizenship: Towards a truly inclusive society*. [Accessed 10 November 2015 at http://www.aph.gov.au/About_Parliament/Parliamentary_Departments/Parliamentary_Library/pubs/rp/rp0910/10rp08]

Calder, G. (2011). Disability and misrecognition. in S. Thompson and M. Yar (Eds.) *The Politics of Misrecognition: Rethinking political and international theory*. Farnham, Surrey: Ashgate Publishing Limited (pp. 105-124)

Clark, F. (1997) Reflections on the human as an occupational being: Biological need, tempo and temporality. *Journal of Occupational Science: Australia*, 4, 3, 86-92

Cutchin, M.P. and Dickie, V.A. (Eds.) (2013) *Transactional Perspectives on Occupation*. New York: Springer

Department of Education, Employment and Workplace Relations (2009) *The Australian Public Service Social Inclusion Policy Design and Delivery Toolkit Framework*. Canberra: Social Inclusion Unit, Department of the Prime Minister and Cabinet

Department of the Prime Minister and Cabinet (2009) *A Stronger, Fairer Australia: National statement on social inclusion*. Canberra: Department of the Prime Minister and Cabinet

Deranty, J. P. (2009) *Beyond Communication: A critical study of Axel Honneth's social philosophy*. Boston, MA: Brill

Fraser, N. (1995) From redistribution to recognition? Dilemmas of justice in a 'Post-Socialist' age. *New Left Review*, I/212, 68-93

Galvaan, R. (2012) Occupational choice: The significance of socio-economic and political factors. in G. E. Whiteford and C. Hocking (Eds.) *Occupational Science: Society, inclusion, participation*. Chichester: Blackwell (pp. 152-162)

Government of South Australia (2009) *People and Community at the Heart of Systems and Bureaucracy: South Australia's social inclusion initiative*. Adelaide: Government of South Australia

Gray, J.M. (1998) Putting occupation into practice: Occupation as ends, occupation as means. *American Journal of Occupational Therapy*, 52, 354-364

Gupta, J. (2012) An issue of occupation (in)justice: A case study. *Disability Studies Quarterly*, 32, 3. [Accessed 12 October 2016 at http://dsq-sds.org/article/view/3280/3114]

Hamilton, A.L., Coldwell-Neilson, J. and Craig, A. (2014) Development of an information management knowledge transfer framework for evidence-based occupational therapy. *VINE: The Journal of Information and Knowledge Management Systems*, 44, 1, 59-93

Hammell, K.W. (2008) Reflections on...wellbeing and occupational rights. *Canadian Journal of Occupational Therapy*, 75, 61-64

Hasselkus, B.R. (2006) 2006 Eleanor Clarke Slagle Lecture. The world of everyday occupation: Real people, real lives. *American Journal of Occupational Therapy*, 60, 627-640

Hasselkus, B.R. (2011) *The meaning of everyday occupation*. (2nd ed.) Thorofare, NJ: Slack

Heidegren, C. G. (2002) Anthropology, social theory, and politics: Axel Honneth's theory of recognition. *Inquiry*, 45, 433-436

Honneth, A. (1992) Integrity and disrespect: Principles of a conception of morality based on the theory of recognition. *Political Theory*, 20, 2, 187-201

Honneth, A. (1995) *Struggle for Recognition: The moral grammar of social conflicts (trans. J. Anderson)*. Cambridge, UK: Polity Press

Honneth, A. (2001) Recognition or redistribution? Changing perspectives on the moral order of society. *Theory, Culture and Society*, 18, 43-55

Ikäheimo, H. (2002) On the genus and species of recognition. *Inquiry*, 45, 447-462

Ikäheimo, H. (2007) Recognising persons. *Journal of Consciousness Studies: Controversies in Science and the Humanities*, 14, 5-6, 224-247

Ikäheimo, H. (2009) Personhood and the social inclusion of people with disabilities: A recognition-theoretical approach. in K. Kristiansen, S. Vehmas and T. Shakespeare (Eds.) *Arguing about Disability: Philosophical perspectives*. Abingdon, UK: Routledge (pp. 77-92)

Ikäheimo, H. and Laitinen, A. (2010) Esteem for contributions to the common good: The role of personifying attitudes and instrumental value. in M. Seymour (Ed.) *The Plural States of Recognition*. Basingstoke, UK: Palgrave Macmillan (pp. 98-121)

Jakobsen, K. (2009) The right to work: Experiences of employees with rheumatism. *Journal of Occupational Science*, 16, 2, 120-127

Jin, R.L., Shah, C.P. and Svoboda, T.J. (1995) The impact of unemployment on health: A review of the evidence. *Canadian Medical Association Journal*, 153, 5, 529-540

Kielhofner, G. (2009) *Conceptual Foundations of Occupational Therapy*. (4th ed.) Philadelphia, PA: F.A. Davis Company

Kirsh, B.H. (2015) Muriel Driver lecture 2015. Transforming values into action: Advocacy as a professional imperative. *Canadian Journal of Occupational Therapy*, 82, 4, 212-223

Komter, A.E. (2005) *Social Solidarity and the Gift*. Cambridge, United Kingdom: Cambridge University Press

Laitinen, A. (2010) On the scope of 'recognition': The role of adequate regard and mutuality. in H. C. Schmidt am Busch and C.F. Zurn (Eds.) *The Philosophy of Recognition: Historical and contemporary perspectives*. Lanham, Maryland: Lexington Books (pp. 319-342)

Laliberte Rudman, D. (2010) Occupational terminology: Occupational possibilities. *Journal of Occupational Science*, 17, 1, 55-59

Law, M., Cooper, B., Strong, S., Stewart, D., Rigby, P. and Letts, L. (1996) The Person-Environment-Occupation Model: A transactive approach to occupational performance. *Canadian Journal of Occupational Therapy*, 63, 1, 9-23

Lombe, M. and Sherraden, M. (2008) Inclusion in the policy process: An agenda for participation of the marginalised. *Journal of Policy Practice*, 7, 2-3, 199-213

McKee-Ryan, F.M., Song, Z., Wanberg, C.R. and Kinicki, A.J. (2005) Psychological and physical well-being during unemployment: A meta-analytic study. *Journal of Applied Psychology*, 90, 1, 53-76

Morrison, Z. (2010) *On Dignity: Social inclusion and the politics of recognition*. Melbourne, Australia: Brotherhood of St Laurence

Moss, J. (2012) *Each to their own: Can the Capabilities Approach be legitimate and justified*? Paper presented at the Capabilities Approaches to Justice: Theory and Practice Conference, Sydney, Australia, 15 November

National People with Disabilities and Carer Council (2009) *Shut Out: The experience of people with disabilities and their families in Australia*. [Accessed 20 September 2015 at https://www.dss.gov.au/sites/default/files/documents/05_2012/nds_report.pdf]

Nelms, L. and Tsingas, C. (2010) *Literature Review on Social Inclusion and its Relationship to Minimum Wages and Workforce Participation*. Barton, Australian Capital Territory: Fair Work Victoria

Njelesani, N., Tang, A., Jonsson, H. and Polatajko, H. (2014) Articulating an occupational perspective. *Journal of Occupational Science*, 21, 2, 226-235

Pereira, R.B. (2013) *The Politics of Participation: A critical occupational science analysis of social inclusion policy and entrenched disadvantage*. PhD thesis, Macquarie University. [Accessed 10 April 2015, http:///hdl.handle.net/1959.14/282427]

Pereira, R.B. (2015a) Occupare, to seize: Expanding the potential of occupation in contemporary practice. *Australian Occupational Therapy Journal*, 62, 3, 208-209

Pereira, R.B. (2015b) *Enabling social transformation through occupation for citizens living with mental illness*. Keynote address to the Occupational Therapy Australia Mental Health Forum: Mental Health OT. Supporting participation, wellbeing and inclusion. University of Technology Sydney, Sydney, Australia, 13 November

Pereira, R. B. (2017) Towards inclusive occupational therapy: Introducing the CORE approach for inclusive and occupation-focused practice. Australian Occupational Therapy Journal, 64, 4, 429-435. doi: 10.1111/1440-1630.12394

Pereira, R. B., Whiteford, G., Hyett, N., Weekes, G., Di Tommaso, A., & Naismith, J. (2020). Capabilities, Opportunities, Resources and Environments (CORE): Using the CORE approach for inclusive, occupation-centred practice. Australian Occupational Therapy Journal. doi: 10.1111/1440-1630.12642

Pereira, R.B. and Whiteford, G.E. (2013) Understanding social inclusion as an international discourse: Implications for enabling participation. *British Journal of Occupational Therapy*, 76, 2, 112-115

Reeve, D. (2004) Psycho-emotional dimensions of disability and the social model. in C. Barnes and G. Mercer (Eds.) *Implementing the Social Model of Disability: Theory and research*. Leeds, UK: The Disability Press (pp. 83-100)

Saloojee, A. (2001) *Social inclusion, citizenship and diversity*. Paper presented at the 'A new way of thinking? Towards a vision of social inclusion' Conference, Ottawa, Canada, 9 November

Saloojee, A. (2005) Social inclusion, anti-racism and democratic citizenship. in T. Richmond and A. Saloojee (Eds.) *Social Inclusion: Canadian perspectives*. Toronto: Laidlaw Foundation (pp. 180-202)

Sayce, L. (2001) Social inclusion and mental health. *Psychiatric Bulletin*, 25, 121-123

Schkade, J.K. and Schultz, S. (1992) Occupational adaptation: Toward a holistic approach for contemporary practice, part 1. *American Journal of Occupational Therapy*, 46, 9, 829-837

Schultz, S. and Schkade, J.K. (1992) Occupational adaptation: Toward a holistic approach for contemporary practice, part 2. *American Journal of Occupational Therapy*, 46, 10, 917-925

Sen, A. (1992) *Inequality Reexamined*. Oxford: Oxford University Press

Sen, A. (1993) Capability and well-being. in A. Sen and M. Nussbaum (Eds.) *The Quality of Life*. Oxford: Oxford University Press (pp. 30-53)

Sen, A. (1999) *Development as Freedom*. Oxford: Oxford University Press

Sen, A. (2000) *Social Exclusion: Concept, application, and scrutiny*. Social Development Papers No. 1. Manila: Asian Development Bank

Sen, A. (2001) Symposium on Amartya Sen's philosophy: 4 Reply. *Economics and Philosophy*, 17, 51-66

Sen, A. (2004) Capabilities, lists, and public reason: Continuing the conversation. *Feminist Economics*, 10, 3, 77-80

Thompson, S. and Yar, M. (Eds.) (2011) *The Politics of Misrecognition: Rethinking political and international theory*. Farnham, UK: Ashgate Publishing Limited

Thibeault, R. (2013) Occupational justice's intents and impacts: From personal choices to community consequences. in M.P. Cutchin and V.A. Dickie (Eds.) *Transactional Perspectives on Occupation*. New York: Springer (pp. 245-256)

Townsend, E. and Polatajko, H. (Eds.) (2007) *Enabling Occupation II: Advancing an occupational therapy vision for health, well-being, and justice through occupation*. Ottawa, Ontario: CAOT Publications ACE

Townsend, E. and Whiteford, G. (2005) A participatory occupational justice framework: Population based processes of practice. in F. Kronenberg, S. Simó Algado, and N. Pollard (Eds.) *Occupational Therapy without Borders: Learning from the spirit of survivors*. London: Elsevier (pp. 110–127)

Townsend, E. and Wilcock, A.A. (2004) Occupational justice and client-centered practice: A dialogue in progress. *Canadian Journal of Occupational Therapy*, 71, 2, 75-87

Townsend, E.A., Beagan, B., Kumas Tan, Z., Versnel, J., Iwama, M., Landry, J. et al. (2007) Enabling: Occupational therapy's core competency. in E.A. Townsend and H.J. Polatajko (Eds.) *Enabling Occupation II: Advancing an occupational therapy vision for health, well-being, and justice through occupation*. Ottawa, Ontario: CAOT Publications ACE (pp. 87-171)

Trombly, C.A. (1995) 1995 Eleanor Clarke Slagle Lecture. Occupation: Purposefulness and meaningfulness as therapeutic mechanisms. *American Journal of Occupational Therapy*, 49, 10, 960-972

Van't Leven, N. and Jonsson, H. (2002) Doing and being in the atmosphere of the doing: Environmental influences on occupational performance in a nursing home. *Scandinavian Journal of Occupational Therapy*, 9, 4, 148-155

Vasta, E. (2010) The controllability of difference: Social cohesion and the new politics of solidarity. *Ethnicities*, 10, 4, 503-521

Vasta, E. (2011) *Migration and Solidarity: The changing fashions of inclusionary concepts.* Paper presented at the Inclusive Futures Conference, Sydney, Australia, February 17

Venkatapuram, S. (2011) *Health Justice: An argument from the capabilities approach.* Cambridge, UK: Polity Press

Ward, N. (2009) Social exclusion, social identity and social work: Analysing social exclusion from a material discursive perspective. *Social Work Education*, 28, 3, 237-252

Whiteford, G. (2000) Occupational deprivation: Global challenge in the new millennium. *British Journal of Occupational Therapy*, 63, 5, 200-204

Whiteford, G. (2004) When people cannot participate: Occupational deprivation. in C.H. Christiansen and E.A. Townsend (Eds.) *Introduction to Occupation: The art and science of living.* Upper Saddle River: Prentice Hall (pp. 221-242)

Whiteford, G. (2010) Occupation in context. in M. Curtin, M. Molineux and J. Supyk-Mellson (Eds.) *Occupational Therapy and Physical Dysfunction. Enabling occupation.* London: Churchill Livingstone (pp. 135-149)

Whiteford, G. and Townsend, E. (2011) Participatory Occupational Justice Framework (POJF 2010): Enabling occupational participation and inclusion. in F. Kronenberg, N. Pollard and D. Sakellariou (Eds.) *Occupational Therapies without Borders Vol 2: Towards an ecology of occupation-based practices.* London: Elsevier Ltd (pp. 65-84)

Whiteford, G., Jones, K., Rahal, C. & Suleman, A. (2018) The Participatory Occupational Justice Framework as a tool for change: Three contrasting case narratives. Journal of Occupational Science, 25, 4, 497-508. doi:10.1080/14427591.2018.1504607

Whiteford, G., Townsend, E., Bryanton, O., Wicks, A. and Pereira, R. (2017) The Participatory Occupational Justice Framework: Salience across contexts. In D. Sakellariou and N. Pollard (Eds.), Occupational Therapy without Borders: Integrating justice with practice. (2nd ed.) London: Elsevier (pp.163-174)

Whiteford, G. E. (2019) Sylvia Docker Memorial Lecture: Together we go further—Service co-design, knowledge co-production and radical solidarity. Australian Occupational Therapy Journal, 66, 4, 682-689. doi: 10.1111/1440-1630.12628

Whiteford, G.E., and Pereira, R.B. (2012) Occupation, inclusion and participation. in G.E. Whiteford and C. Hocking (Eds.) *Occupational Science: Society, inclusion, participation.* Chichester, UK: Blackwell Publishing (pp. 187-207)

Wilcock, A.A. (1998) *An Occupational Perspective of Health.* Thorofare: Slack

Wilcock, A.A. (2006) *An Occupational Perspective of Health.* (2nd ed.) Thorofare: Slack Incorporated

Wilcock, A. and Townsend, E. (2000) Occupational terminology interactive dialogue... occupational justice. *Journal of Occupational Science*, 7, 2, 84-86

Wright-St Clair, V. and Seedhouse, D. (2005) The moral context of practice and professional relationships. in G. Whiteford and V. Wright-St Clair (Eds.) *Occupation and Practice in Context.* Marrickville, New South Wales: Elsevier Australia (pp. 16-33)

Yerxa, E., Clark, F., Frank, G., Jackson, J., Parham, D., Pierce, D. et al. (1990) An introduction to occupational science. A foundation for occupational therapy in the 21st century. *Occupational Therapy in Health Care*, 6, 4, 1-17

Yuval-Davis, N. (2006) Belonging and the politics of belonging. *Patterns of Prejudice*, 40, 3, 197-214

Appendix A: Key theoretical framings of social inclusion (Pereira, 2015b, 2013; Whiteford & Pereira, 2012):

1. Social inclusion as *recognition*: Being treated as a valued member of the society in which one lives with mutual dignity, respect and reciprocity (Honneth, 2001); validating and recognising shared lived experiences, commonalities and aspirations (Peeira, 2013; Morrison, 2010; Deranty, 2009; Bach, 2005; Honneth, 2001; Fraser, 1995);
2. Social inclusion as *capabilities*: Having the freedoms to live a life that one has reason to value through being able to do and be (Sen, 2004; 2001; 2000; 1999; 1993; 1992);
3. Social inclusion as *opportunity*: Having opportunities to do and be leading to tangible outcomes (i.e. realising one's capabilities), (Pereira et al., 2020; Pereira, 2017; Nelms & Tsingas, 2010; Sayce, 2001; Sen, 1999);
4. Social inclusion as *resources*: Having personal, social, cultural, emotional, material, physical and/or spiritual resources that support occupational opportunities and facilitate occupational participation (Pereira, 2017, 2015b, 2013);
5. Social inclusion as *choice*: Having choices that enable occupation and participation, rather than no choice that leads to various forms of injustice (Galvaan, 2012; Whiteford, 2000);
6. Social inclusion as *participation*: Enacting and realising occupation - actual doing and being (Pereira, 2013; Pereira & Whiteford, 2013);
7. Social inclusion as *solidarity*: Sharing and celebrating social bonds, ways of cooperation, relationships, contributing to the common good, embracing difference and diversity and having the capacity to come together in ways that are mutually beneficial (Whiteford, 2019; Vasta, 2011, 2010; Bach, 2005; Saloojee, 2005, 2001; Honneth, 2001);
8. Social inclusion as *equitable access*: Removing barriers for participation, ranging from enabling physical access to places and spaces, to having accessible information that facilitates choice and control (Pereira, 2013; National People with Disabilities and Carer Council, 2009);
9. Social inclusion as *being involved in decision-making*: Being actively involved in enacting one's civic rights to respond, collaborate, participate and have one's voice heard (Australian Social Inclusion Board, 2010; Department of Education, Employment and Workplace Relations, 2009; Department of the Prime Minister and Cabinet, 2009; National People with Disabilities and Carer Council, 2009);
10. Social inclusion as *rights*: Upholding universal rights, freedoms and privileges which enable just participation in cultural, economic, political and social aspects of life (Morrison, 2010; Nelms & Tsingas, 2010; Government of South Australia, 2009; Lombe & Sherraden, 2008; Honneth, 2001); and
11. Social inclusion as *citizenship*: 'Recognising the rights, obligations and institutions that play a role in developing and supporting equality of status in the community' (Buckmaster & Thomas, 2009, p. 16); 'a commitment on the part of the state to ensure that all members of society have equal access to developing their talents and capacities' (Saloojee, 2005, p. 191)

Section 3
Shifting Perspectives

The chapters in this section explore some of the shifting perspectives taking place in occupational therapy in a variety of contexts and countries. Change is integral to the understanding of experience over time, and this effect can be perceived both historically on a broad scale in terms of the ways in which organisations, countries or communities develop, and personally in the form of loss or growth, or the acquisition of resiliency and capability. The first chapter, Opening Doors, is just that, a personal narrative told by three of the people engaged in it, through which an abused and chronically distressed woman, Ellen Ferguson, describes how she regained the capacity to open her front door to social inclusion, and become involved in community activities.

Funai's account of social enterprise, which follows, traces the development of Tayberry Enterprise Limited, UK, into a facility offering vocational rehabilitation opportunities through a canteen and education in drumming and performance skills. This developed from an idea initially put forward by students with severe and enduring mental health issues with whom she worked to create the business, and also illustrates Funai's own professional journey from working within established services to developing a social enterprise. She uses the concept of the 'fifth wave' of contemporary public health interventions to set out the challenges of putting together the structures that would themselves underpin Tayberry as a social enterprise, which now supports many local people in voluntary and employment opportunities and involves them with other businesses and organisations.

The Taieri Bloke's Shed, located in New Zealand, is a community, and a community resource, which meets the needs of retired men who have experienced a number of transitions. Sunderland and Wilson, writing with members of the Shed, describe how this example of a Men's Shed developed and, through an ethnographic research project with its members, sets out how it benefits the local community and its own members through productive craft occupations carried out in a purposeful constructive environment that also maintains a supportive social space.

Another form of health promotion is explored by Cloete, Konstabel and Duncan in their research on the consequences of the binge drinking culture amongst women workers in the wine producing area of the Western Cape, South Africa. The excessive use of alcohol produces a very high incidence of foetal alcohol spectrum disorders in children in the area, but as the chapter reveals, this is due to intergenerational conditions created through apartheid and through the practices of the wine industry, which include payment in alcohol. Cloete, Jaftha and Duncan develop a decolonising developmental approach in working with women working in the vineyards to encourage participation in transformative occupations. The women are able to critically assess their needs and to own the processes which enable them to make positive changes, such as the acquisition of work-related skills through which they can gain better working conditions and contribute to the needs of their communities.

Tongai widens the occupational perspective to an overview of how occupational therapy can promote social inclusion in Africa. He explores the limited possibilities for occupational therapists working in medical and acute settings to address the problems of unemployment, poverty, disability and stigma which are challenges facing many people, and supports the development of occupation supporting communities and groups. He explores how the growing numbers of professionals trained in Africa can bring their international experience back to the continent and encourages volunteers from the diaspora of people with African roots to develop social inclusion projects using the assets of African cultures and experience.

Finally, in another research project, Guarani and Wicks, writing from Australia, explore the opening of museum exhibits to people with visual impairments who are enabled to explore museum artefacts and art objects through touch. Participants were able to share their insights and knowledge with the author and each other, for example, and to take part in the rich experience of the appreciation of objects, works of art, and specimens which are part of the everyday sensory environment shared by less marginalised populations. Social inclusion operates on many levels and this chapter reveals the significance to health and wellbeing of personal and sensory engagement with cultural artefacts as a key experiential component of meaningful social interaction, without which people are deprived of the means of relating to cultural appreciation.

Chapter 10
Opening Doors

Ellen Ferguson, Mary Jardine, Elizabeth Firth

My name is Ellen, I am 49. I have 4 grown children that I raised alone, all of them work in the caring profession. I have Dissociative Identity Disorder (formerly known as Multiple Personality Disorder) I came from a very abusive background and ended up in care from the age of 6. My abuse was sexual, physical and emotional and by the time I was 9, I was under psychiatric care after suffering a mental breakdown. Having been in continuous therapy for over 18 years, I want to share with you how occupational therapy helped me, through the two special women whose dedication and support changed my life forever.

I approached my doctor for help as I had stopped drinking and couldn't sleep or go out. I was haunted by nightmares and flashbacks, without the numbing effect of alcohol to blot it all out.

I was exasperated with therapy.

I was planning on suicide.

Mary: Ellen had worked with the Alcohol Relapse Management team within Addiction Services and was now abstinent from alcohol use, but her anxiety remained problematic and was impacting on her functional ability, hence the referral to occupational therapy.

Having a background in Adult Mental Health, experience had taught me that many people use alcohol and or drugs either as a means of helping them cope, or to deliberately not cope, as to block out past trauma. This had underpinned my move to develop the occupational therapy role in Addictions some 9 years previously.

My colleagues were aware that the focus of occupational therapy is on the individuals' functioning (or lack of) and coping (or lack of), so if difficulties remained severe or entrenched, a referral to occupational therapy was made. As many of our referrals included working with individuals experiencing agoraphobia and the impact of resulting isolation, social inclusion is always a key issue.

At that initial visit, I was struck by many things at once. Ellen sat on a chair in her living room, shoulders hunched and her arms folded across her chest, in a very closed posture. She was dressed in jogging bottoms and a baggy sweatshirt and her personal hygiene was acceptable in so far that she was clean but she did not appear pleased with nor attentive to her appearance. Her house was clean, neat and tidy, but few family photos, none with Ellen in them, no pictures and no mirrors. She had trouble making eye contact, and her responses were very brief.

Ellen stated she did not recall the referral having being made to occupational therapy so I outlined what we do, checked that she was happy to see me again, and made another appointment. My main goal from that initial visit was building a therapeutic relationship, as no work would be done if she did not even engage with me. I knew that she was very vulnerable, had difficulty tolerating me being there, and that she had a story which had yet to be told. I wanted to hear that story, understand how I could help her to help herself move beyond her current situation if I could, but knew it would have to be at her pace. Having being trained in trauma work I suspected Ellen's background to be along these lines, but kept an open mind. 'Unconditional positive regard' is an approach we all have for the individuals we work with, but it means little if they do not feel it......

> *Ellen: Speaking as a long-term service user, I am very familiar with the mental health therapies provided. I've seen counsellors, therapists, specialists, psychiatrists and psychologists – I've seen them all. While each and every one contributed in some way towards my well-being, they were so busy trying to figure out how my mind worked, they couldn't see the more obvious problems. They helped me to understand, come to terms with, and cope with my condition. But all the talking therapy in the world could never help me to move any further forward in the real world. I needed emotional AND practical help. I needed someone to come to see me in my own space – not an office, someone to see with their own eyes what my world looked like and to help me regain a sense of self-esteem. I needed someone to help me go outside, by walking beside me and providing support.*

Mary: Several visits later, Ellen was more comfortable with me being in her space and speaking with her. I had explained that occupational therapy is about helping people to manage the everyday things in life that they may struggle with, to manage better in areas that are important to them, but that it is a joint journey to get to that point. While Ellen would tell me what she wanted to work on, I could suggest things she try in order to cope better, but that unless she tried these suggestions, we could not go anywhere. I also made it clear, that if she did try them and they did not work for her, then it was not about her, but down to me to understand why, know what to change, and to suggest something different. Activity analysis remains our core skill after all.

Ellen appeared happy with this approach, and willing to play an active part: the foundations of future endeavours had been outlined, and accepted, so our journey began....

We started off by focusing on the reasons for Ellen being referred, so had a conversation about anxiety, to help me understand how it affected her and how she coped at present. Ellen said that she 'rocked' as a means of self-soothing, something she had done for years. So how often would she do this, and for how long at a time?... The majority of each day once her daughters had gone to school, and each evening after they had gone to bed... And how did her day look above and beyond these times?... Only got washed and into clean clothes when she had to... A cleaner came in to help do housework and she only went shopping at night, accompanied by relatives... What about getting out and about to pay bills, keep appointments etc? No... cannot go to the dentist, hairdresser, anyone, and bills are paid by direct debit... So really entrenched behaviours, a severe impact on her level of function and satisfaction with how she was living at present. Her ultimate goal?... To get out and about and to do 'normal things'. A long journey ahead and every journey begins with the first step...

Ellen accepted that we should work on anxiety management as that first step, find a method that worked better for her, practice it, before moving on. We would tackle each area together, one step at a time, finding a way that worked for her... small steps that all add up.

At this point, I made it clear that this was a process, that it would be on a trial and error basis; that we may not find the right method for her at the first attempt and that it would take time as she had not arrived at this point overnight.

Ellen: I had been to see so many experts/therapists and I was exasperated with therapy. I liked that Mary was honest and down to earth.

Mary: I gave Ellen some relaxation techniques, suggesting that she try one as an alternative to her current method at least once per day, and to keep a diary of how this worked or did not work... and we would use that as a basis for the next step. I explained that I would be using a cognitive behavioural therapy approach, and what this meant: that how we think, feel and act are linked, and that we need to become aware of what we are thinking and feeling as it may throw up barriers to how we do or do not do things. As occupational therapy is related to the doing, I would need to know and understand the thinking, in order to address the barriers to the doing part. Depending on what Ellen was able to share with me would influence what I would ask her to do, and I would give her a reason why I was asking her to do it that way. This would add meaning to tasks and her engagement. However, occupational therapy is practical. This talking to understand and address the thinking is then translated into practical tasks which would be set between sessions and be reviewed. Failure to do tasks meant that I had nothing to work with, so progress would be affected. Catch 22 outlined... we needed to do our parts in order to make the journey.

Soon after that Ellen informed me she had Dissociative Identity Disorder.

Inherent in occupational therapy is the holistic approach, so an individuals' diagnosis or condition does not define the intervention, but rather provides a context for it, making the process truly person centered. However, I did more research on Dissociative Identity Disorder to ensure my approach was based on the latest evidence while keeping Ellen's experiences at the heart of everything.

I asked Ellen to tell me more about how her life has been affected, how she managed, to outline her alters, their characteristics and function, what she wanted and needed from me. Ellen stated that she had periods in life where she was very high functioning, but that she had 'switched' personalities, with the alter best suited to the situation coming out to cope.

While I continued exploring the barriers to tasks with Ellen, I asked my colleague Liz Firth (OT Technical Instructor) to continue the 'getting out and about sessions', each session with a goal, each reinforcing anxiety management techniques and improving levels of confidence.

Liz: I work for the NHS as an occupational therapist technical instructor in mental health. Mary and I met up with Ellen at her home to discuss how the three of us would work together. We quickly established a good rapport and Ellen spoke about her multiple personalities and how to recognize if any came to the fore when working with her and how each personality can be recognized by certain traits and quirks and what the likely triggers would be. It was a good sharing session for all three of us and it certainly gave me confidence in working in this new area.

When I was first asked to work with Ellen I have to admit to having some reservations on my ability to offer effective therapeutic support as I had no experience working with someone who had DID or multiple personalities and I felt I would be completely out of my depth. My overriding fear was that ultimately, I would be letting Ellen down with my inexperience.

> *Ellen: Mary was my emotional support and Liz was my practical support – I referred to them as my walking and talking therapists. Every single action I needed help with had major underlying reasons. I didn't wash because I felt dirty anyway, I couldn't go out because I was hyper-vigilant and afraid of attack, I was crippled in a world of fear and pain. I lost 4 stone in weight but still wore the same jeans, Liz persuaded me to buy a belt to hold them up. Mary persuaded me to buy new jeans, but the style was different and it traumatised me. I never managed to wear them. Quietly and patiently, Mary helped me work through it and understood that changing my style was too much – just having jeans that fitted was a major achievement! That was the 'jeansgate' drama.*

Mary: Sometimes it was two steps forward and one back, sometimes it was the other way around. At times, I had to encourage Ellen to keep going, or change things when she became stuck. At other times, I had to urge restraint as Ellen wanted to move quicker, before new ways of doing things had become part of her normal routine. There were highs and lows, which Ellen has referred to. Times when I just said 'Ok, that's not working... leave that and try this'. I think it mattered to Ellen that she could see me make mistakes too, but not get caught up in them.

> *Ellen: I think one of the biggest set-backs we had was 'mirrorgate'. In the process of building my self-esteem up, Mary asked me to look at myself in the mirror. She didn't understand that I couldn't bear to look at me/myselves while sharing all the secrets we had kept locked away. I told her I wanted to smash my face into the mirror, so ingrained was my self-loathing. That plan was binned.*

Mary: Ellen had stated that she now wanted to cope as herself, did not want to integrate her alters, but could not face living life as she had been in recent years using alcohol to block out the pain of trauma. Dealing with the trauma led to me working with Angel, the alter who was holding the trauma and pain, who was carrying out cleansing behaviours and self-harming. Letting out the story of childhood sexual, emotional, physical and mental abuse was a slow painful one for Angel and Ellen, but such an important one.

> *Ellen: Angel is the traumatised 9 yr old who had the breakdown. Angel would cut/mutilate, drank bleach and ate soap, forever trying to get clean inside. Mary gained Angel's trust and Angel started to write poems because she knew never to speak about what happened.*

> *The Attic*
> There is a special
> Place where
> They take me.
> And we only go
> There when

They need to be
Careful because
They might get
Caught
With their
Pants down
The special place is
A……..
Door on the floor
That never bangs
But they bang me on it
It never slams
But they slam me onto it
It never opens wide
Like my legs on it
It never shuts
Like my mind on it.

By Angel

Then Mary bought her paint and let her know it was another way to tell.

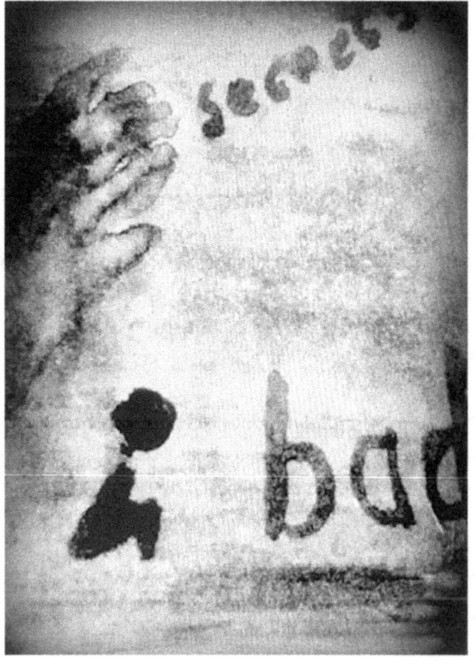

Everything Mary did to help Angel was shared with her supervisor. She stepped out of the box to take a chance and help my most dangerous personality. Angel now adores Mary, hasn't harmed me for two years. She is a more contented and happy child, having given her secrets to Mary.

Liz walked with me and built up my confidence, she helped me to be more sociable and walk with my head held high.

Mary: Angel also got homework tasks, a good behaviour chart for reducing self-injurious behaviours, changing the medium of self-expression at times, (poems, pictures, stories) finding what she liked (gardening), having positive diversionary tasks to balance all the strong negative emotions, and positive reinforcements for progress, small tangible objects associated with being accepted as the innocent one as the story unfolded.

I still worked with Ellen too though, gradually encouraging her to do more in her house until getting to the point of not needing a cleaner, working on assertiveness, to get involved in activities in the community she had expressed an interest in, and all with a bit of give and take, a laugh, and a mutual respect.

My own clinical supervision with Dr. J Stirling was vital, supporting me in reflecting on my practice and approach. He is the consultant psychiatrist in the addiction team I worked in, and oversees my trauma work with patients. He reviewed Ellen and changed her medication as required.

Liz: There were two clearly defined roles and what belonged to each therapeutic session. Mary's role centered around the PTSD context and mine was more a light-hearted approach to build confidence, social practical sessions, using positive reinforcement to halt Ellen's tendency to be self-critical. Essentially the sessions were quite simple in approach but effective in the outcome. Over two years, Ellen gradually relaxed and her self-esteem and confidence grew.

I have to say it has been a gift to work with Ellen and I feel she has benefited from this two-pronged approach. It's clear to see a much more confident, relaxed woman. I have learnt so much from her and I have nothing but admiration for the strength and courage she has shown and the positive steps forward she has taken and is still continuing to make despite her traumatic experiences early in life.

The fact that Ellen is keen to share her experiences through this book to help others with DID and to educate professionals further understand this condition is testament to the most important, erudite and kind personality that Ellen possesses – and that is herself.

Mary: It is a privilege to work as an occupational therapist. We ask individuals to let us into their most difficult moments, to trust us as we try and help them make a positive difference in their lives. I learnt so much from working with Ellen which has helped me become a better clinician. I always hope to continue learning...

Ellen: I understand that I can't be cured, but certainly have learned how to cope with life without switching all the time. My personalities won't integrate, instead they have their own internal safe havens. This suits me as they were the ones who enabled me to survive, why would I want to lose them?

Mary will forever be in my heart, I took her on a very difficult journey that was a massive learning curve, at points I felt like I was an emotional terrorist. We made it through. Without

my occupational therapists, I would still be in someone's office, talking and going round in circles. I think this service should be readily offered and available to mental health clients. I am certain that my ability to manage would have improved much sooner. In two years of occupational therapy, Mary achieved what 16 years of talking therapy couldn't. She opened the door to my mind and enabled me to open my own front door, clean and fresh, hold my head high and head out to face the world.
Ellen Ferguson

Dedication

It is with many thanks to those involved that I dedicate this chapter in loving memory to my father Thomas Shields who passed away as this was being written. Among many things, he taught me to treat others as you would like them to treat you or a loved one, a principle that serves me well in both work and life. Mary Jardine

Chapter 11
Social enterprise and occupational therapy: New ways of working and modernisation of the profession in Scotland

Gillian Funai

Introduction

What does occupation and occupational therapy as a profession mean in the 21st century? How does it fit into pushing the boundaries, promoting social inclusion and participatory approaches?

Occupational therapy development in Scotland during the 20th century is well documented by Paterson (2010). The profession began with the therapeutic use of occupation in institutions for those deemed mentally and physically unwell and disabled on both sides of the Atlantic (Paterson, 2010). Paterson suggests that occupational therapy fitted into a wider social reform with educated middle class and upper class women seeking new roles and directions in Western society. She describes the founders of the profession as social activists at the forefront of philanthropic change in early 20th century.

I have been working in National Health Service (NHS) mental health services in Scotland for many years. This chapter will discuss the challenges of providing occupation-focused interventions within a NHS and a shrinking economy, leading me to explore new ways of working. I will present chronologically my journey that has led to the development of Tayberry Social Enterprise, located in Dundee, Scotland, UK. As a social enterprise this is a non-profit making organisation, aiming to fill a gap in statutory services, related to employability (training, volunteering, unpaid or paid work) for people with significant barriers to entering the Scottish employment pipeline (Employability in Scotland, 2016).

Our work in Tayberry is closely linked to Paterson's early work on the development of occupational therapy, but also with recent discussion of public health intervention in Scotland (Lyon, 2003). It recognises the importance of occupational therapy working beyond a medical prescriptive model, towards the long-term personal development that occupation can offer.

Current discussion of public health by the Scottish Health Foundation (Lyon, 2003), describes the development of public health interventions in Western civilisations since the 1750s. It describes the ideological and socio-economical changes of the time as a series of five waves. The current fifth wave is an underpinning influence guiding my thinking and practice. This wave (which is post 1970s) focuses on doing things differently from the past medical focus. The human context is central to this wave, and while recognising the societies, organisations and science that have taken us to where we are now, uses abilities to care and be compassionate to others. This requires us to move from a consumerism model, which still governs our services and the relationship between the public and professional, towards a participative model empowering individuals and communities with a co-production approach being central. Co-production is described by the Scottish Co-production Network (2016) as a relationship between service provider and service users drawing on mutual knowledge, ability and resources to develop cost effective sustainable solutions to local issues.

Social enterprise is an alternative vocational model to the Individual Placement Support (IPS) model of employment (Priest & Bones, 2012). Whereas IPS seeks to place and train an individual in employment, a social enterprise offers the individual a number of therapeutic pre-employment and employment opportunities. Health social enterprises range from small businesses of 5 up to 500 people as described by Addicott (2011) and are placed in the communities they serve, supporting both purposeful occupation and participation (Lysaght et al, 2012). Delivering occupational therapy intervention through a social enterprise offers the individual a graded bespoke vocational pathway at all points of the vocational journey whereas IPS focuses on job search, train and place. Whilst outcomes are impressive, they do not meet the needs of those whose goal is not paid employment (Rinaldi & Perkins, 2007).

This chapter presents my journey through setting up Tayberry Enterprise Limited, its current structures and concludes with my reflections and future aspirations.

Setting up Tayberry Enterprise Limited

In 2008 I was working in statutory mental health services in a community centre providing a range of workshops and training opportunities. Despite some clients engaging and completing personal goals successfully, we did not seem to achieve long term and sustainable employment outcomes. We recognised a gap between the skills of our clients and the expectations of the local municipal authority employment partnership who were the main providers of the employment pipeline (Employability in Scotland, 2016). We were looking for alternative approaches and strategies to bridge this gap. I attended and completed a module called Introduction and How to Start Your Social Enterprise run by the Social Enterprise Academy in 2008. A business plan I wrote at the end of the module aimed to create a Lead Clinician position to develop a social enterprise that would stand alongside contemporary NHS mental health services.

In hindsight, there were two issues with this proposal. Firstly, the proposal was not fully cognisant with the shift towards a co-production approach, which includes the community or individual in decision-making, thus changing the balance of power from the professional towards the service user(s). The second issue was that policy in Scotland did not enable the establishment of social enterprises as a sustainable model of healthcare delivery. Health is one of a number of responsibilities devolved to the Scottish Government from the UK Government. As a result, there are differences in policy and delivery of those responsibilities. In England the Cabinet Office and Department of Health promoted social enterprise as a preferred model for delivering publicly funded healthcare services. This was supported by the Right to Request programme introduced in 2008, which enabled health care staff in England to put forward a social enterprise proposal to their Primary Care Trust (PCT). PCTs were required to consider these proposals and if approved, support the development of the social enterprise (Addicott, 2011). There was no similar mechanism or resource in place within Scotland to develop an employability social enterprise with support from the local health board, which affected financial viability and need to survive in the market place. Therefore, the proposal was not supported for further development.

This did not deter me from considering other ways of supporting people using NHS mental health services into employment. Since 2004 Dundee mental health services have delivered a supported-education model of education (Unger, 2007), led by myself. Called *Moving Forward*, this eight-week course is for adults with a severe and enduring mental health condition, aiming to support the transition from statutory health services to mainstream employment services. Employability outcomes for the students have been mixed. However, evaluations demonstrated students felt more confident and, if they completed the course and an exit plan, were likely to move onto volunteering and/or education. Thereafter progress into employment was in reality a significant journey, but a few did succeed. This model of supported education was recognised as a model of good practice (Scottish Government, 2010a).

During one course there was a cohort of four students who were able to function at a higher level and were more ambitious than previous cohorts. They wanted to do something different. All these students had previous employment experience working in industry and business. The aspirations of the students and creative interactions with staff delivering the course can be related to Lyon's (2003) description of the fifth wave. Lyon (2003) describes the fifth wave as creating healing reactions derived from the positive power of humans by focusing on a shared challenge. Put simply by Lyon (2003), the process of therapeutic encounters includes creativity, learning, multiple inputs from a variety of disciplines, scientific learning as well as art and respect for the other. He describes this in the context of patients in a clinical setting, rather than students in a college environment. Lyon (2003) suggests the process validates the patient in the process and moves away from considering the patient as someone with symptoms or problems. Lyon writes that the process fosters an active mind-body link between clinician and patient, yielding more satisfying and effective patent contact and decreasing burn out in the clinician. There are three main characteristics to this process- the presence, the dance and mobilising inner resources, as illustrated below.

This group of students, all of whom had a severe and enduring mental health condition, saw establishing a social enterprise as a way forward for them vocationally, as well as inspiring me through our interactions. Locally a one-day course was being held to showcase social enterprise and encourage others to become involved. Two of the students expressed an interest in attending and put in an application, which was accepted. Using Lyon's (2003) characteristics of the healing process of the presence, the dance and mobilising inner resources:

- *The Presence*
  Places were duly sought as it was free and two students plus the author attended the course. The course took the usual format of key speakers who had set up their own social enterprises and breakaway groups. Despite the fact I was attending as a fellow delegate rather than as their therapist, I was anxious as to how the students would manage in a more mainstream course. However, this anxiety was short lived (and provided food for my reflection on my position).
- *The Dance*
  The author attended the course with a business plan idea, but it was not long before the two students identified their own business idea over the course of the day.
- *Mobilising the Inner Resources*
  I asked the students how they would progress and who was going to support them with their business idea. They completed my sense of power shifting when they stated that they expected to work with me to take this forward. I was no longer their therapist, but one of five people setting out to develop a social enterprise together.

In the spirit of what is now understood as co-production, four of the students and myself developed the project proposal for an IT care and support business. A working group, led by myself, developed and identified the work plan. Tasks comprised principally market research of similar business in the area, which with some guidance the students undertook. Two of the individuals embarked on a college course in IT support, one was already an expert. Social Firms Scotland who are a third sector intermediatory, helped the group set up a legal structure, which was a company limited by guarantee with charitable status. In order to do this a model memorandum and article of association was obtained from Social Firms Scotland and amended to suit our company, called Tayberry Enterprise Limited. Prior to submitting the memorandum and article of association to Company House, who are the company regulator in the United Kingdom, and the Scottish Charity Regulator, the group identified a board of directors. This comprised myself, one of the students and two others whom the group had approached, a retired college lecturer and a serving lecturer. The remaining three students for varying personal reasons felt unable to take on these roles at that time. In continuation, Social Firms Scotland delivered training on the Scottish Charity Regulator and what our responsibilities in terms of governance were.

Tayberry Enterprise Limited (Tayberry) was launched on 23rd November 2009 with the social aim of creating pre-vocational and vocational pathways in Dundee's communities. Although the founding students did not continue their collaboration with Tayberry, they did feel listened to and the process of setting up Tayberry focused them on something real. Setting up a legal structure demanded the governance of reporting progress, minute taking and setting agendas, which were important skills they had not used in a long time. The research the group undertook demonstrated that an IT support business really needed an IT expert to take it forward. Set-up costings which the group had researched were high and there were other well-established competitors locally. Sourcing funding was unsuccessful due to high start-up costs.

In discussion with the board, on which one student remained, it was concluded that a change of direction was required. Tayberry had set up its memorandum and articles of association broadly, which stated it was a company seeking to provide vocational services for individuals with long-term conditions. Therefore, the business activity could be changed fairly easily. As an IT business was seen to be unworkable an approach was made by the occupational therapy service to move to Tayberry a successful drumming group, Drumdee, as the group's funding was ending. This group had been led by an occupational therapist and a percussionist, with considerable success in terms of the numbers of referrals and the sustained engagement of participants, who were individuals who did not normally engage in any other type of activity within the service (Cathro & Devine, 2012). In recognition of the need for ongoing employment related services for those with hard to reach long term mental health conditions, the NHS integrated service manager agreed to fund Tayberry to take on this group. This enabled the group to broaden its focus beyond a therapeutic focus to explore further its potential within a social enterprise. This group now does a number of regular public performances and workshops and members have taken on volunteer roles within the wider Tayberry organisation.

Developing Tayberry

Tayberry was and is a legal entity and there was a realisation and agreement with the board that performing arts could become the business model. At this time two other colleagues with skills in accountancy, business and drama as a performing art, expressed an interest in Tayberry's work and joined the Board. With these skills, the composition of the board was stronger. Tayberry obtained a grant from Comic Relief (a UK charity), enabling a rerun of the course the author had originally completed with the Social Enterprise Academy in the summer of 2011. The author, ten individuals who were either present or would-be directors, as well as a few other interested parties undertook this course.

Since then, Tayberry has progressed into a social enterprise run mainly by healthcare professionals. There is a growing international evidence base of healthcare professionals, particularly occupational therapists, who are using social enterprise to deliver interventions for people whom are marginalised and challenged with social participation (Lysaght & Krupa, 2011). Pollard (2011) compares the experience of occupational therapists in the UK and Europe. In the UK occupational therapists have mainly worked in the state healthcare or private healthcare, with engagement in community development roles being limited to date, whereas occupational therapists in Italy's social farms and Sweden's cooperatives has enabled them to support individuals in social enterprises which foster work integration within the communities they serve. Pollard (2011) goes on to discuss the inequalities within Latin America and how occupational therapists have embraced social enterprise principles to deliver community interventions. As Pollard (2011) acknowledged, the profession is facing challenges for survival in the more traditional environments of the UK National Health Service. Tayberry was formed at a time when day services were retracting and other educational partnerships which supported some of the occupational therapy interventions were also experiencing rationalisation of their services reducing opportunities for individuals. Additionally, the Scottish Government's *Health Quality Strategy* (2010b) favoured individual placement support (IPS) as the vocational model of choice (Priest & Bones, 2012). IPS can be described as an employability model which places individuals in employment and trains the individual once in employment. It has a significant evidence base and true IPS utilises a fidelity review scale (IPS Dartmouth Supported Employment Centre, 2016). However, local resources to develop this model were unavailable.

Regarding management and leadership, although Tayberry emerged from a dynamic service user idea and foundation, as Tayberry developed it became difficult to sustain inclusion of service users in board and management roles. This was for a number of reasons. One is the nature of the purpose of Tayberry, which is to work with those people most excluded from current vocational pathways, and who at this point in their recovery journey remain vulnerable. In addition, my own limited expertise in management of a social enterprise meant and means that I required specific expertise and experience, particularly in relation to financial expertise. Within other roles in the organisation there are multiple opportunities for service users to have input into decision making, and roles are constantly under review.

As a start-up social enterprise Tayberry is still approximately 80% dependent on grant funding to deliver much of its activity. Its turnover was in excess of £100 000 by March 2016 and at present 20% of its income is self-generated through payment to its weekly arts groups and training canteen.

Tayberry's activities

Tayberry offers a wide range of vocational opportunities, from therapeutic activities/ skill training, supportive volunteer roles, volunteer roles, trainee roles within the canteen and supported permitted work roles (where the individual can maintain their sick benefits while earning up to a maximum permitted amount and working for less than 16hrs per week). Tayberry have also taken on four trainees under the Scottish Employment Retention Incentive, which are training schemes lasting for up to one year.

Individuals accessing Tayberry's services have the options of drumming, sensory storytelling and drama as activities which develop skills, structure and routine underpinning progression to training, volunteering and employment. There are six drumming groups; four for adults with learning disabilities and two for adults with mental health conditions. Some of these individuals are now registered as volunteers and engage, with support, in public performances. There are plans to further develop these roles into facilitation roles, which will be an extension of volunteering. Three-year recurring fund from the Robertson's Trust and class fees supports financially the drumming. Additional income is earned through public performances and in the near future classes for schoolchildren will start, progressing financial stability for the drumming pathway.

Sensory Storytelling sessions are in partnership with Profound and Multiple Impairment Service (PAMIS), Dundee Repertoire Theatre and a professional storyteller. This project recently received Scottish Government funding released to take the recommendations forward for the learning disability strategic document *Keys to Life* (Scottish Government, 2013). This funding will support development of two accredited training packages - one for accredited apprentice sensory storytelling modules for individuals with a learning disability and the other for facilitators who will be trained to support the apprentices. The facilitator packs will be aimed at those aiming to return to work. These accredited training packages will be rolled out across Scotland and will be a source of further income generation.

Inform Theatre are a company of actors with learning disabilities focusing on raising awareness of disability issues and the equality agenda in partnership with Dundee Repertoire Theatre. Funding for this project comes from transitioned resources from the local Health Board.

At present 80 beneficiaries from the ages of 16 to 65 attend performing arts as a therapeutic activity. From this, 15 have registered as volunteers. Volunteer roles include public performance in drumming and assisting in the running of a tuck shop at the venue where the drumming takes place. Skills learned in the tuck shop support individuals to move onto Tayberry's training café.

Tayberry Café is a training canteen set up in partnership with Dovetail Enterprise (Dovetail) who runs a social enterprise making commercial furniture for the hotel industry, and Dundee City Council's Supported Employment Unit (SEU). Dovetail's previous factory canteen had closed. Dovetail has a high proportion of disabled men who are single, in physically demanding jobs, and whose nutritional intake did not support their daily physical requirements. The SEU as a supported employment service, were experiencing challenges in finding placements for people with long-term conditions within the local employability pipeline. Tayberry were keen to extend their existing pathways from therapeutic interventions, so individuals could move back into work. An approach was made to Tayberry to re-establish the café and due to limited resources the SEU became the partner/agent that referrals went to for placements in the café. There was an understanding that Tayberry and the SEU were essentially trying to meet the needs of the same population who were excluded due to the nature of health barriers from employment. Dovetail were keen to improve the nutrition of their workforce. This illustrates transdisciplinary working practices where three organisations who thought and worked differently, by coming together were able to achieve positive outcomes for the individuals they worked with (Wicks & Jamieson, 2014).

Tayberry considered the canteen as an opportunity to offer more training placements and paid work opportunities. External funding from NHS *Cash in Communities* enabled Tayberry to start this project and to employ two cooks over three years. Funding is being reduced over this period and thus Tayberry is exploring outside catering and expansion of this service in order to become sustainable.

Governance

Tayberry is currently managed by its five directors, who are unpaid, and come from professional backgrounds of health, finance and employability. The strategic direction, funding, administration and supervision of staff is overseen by all the directors. The board meets bi-monthly but more frequently when required i.e. working on business cases/funding applications/infrastructure etc. The directors who work in the NHS have been required to declare their interest to their employer in writing as stated in the NHS staff corporate code of governance policy. This is to ensure transparency and that there is no conflict of interest.

The board has accessed training in social enterprise and social accounting through the Social Enterprise Academy and other business training events through third sector contacts, particularly the local Social Enterprise Network. This has been a move away from health cultures and upskilling in business.

Staffing

Tayberry now employs 13 members of staff - 2 are full time, the remaining 11 are part-time. This staff groups comprises two cooks, a volunteer coordinator, a creative arts coordinator and lead percussionist. The volunteer coordinator supports individuals to develop work skills through volunteer opportunities in the company's back office functions and in performing arts. The creative arts coordinator ensures the performing groups develop skills and confidence and promotes the performing arts trading arm. The lead percussionist is responsible for dynamic, percussion-based activities, which includes African drumming, Gumboot and extended skills in performance drumming.

Of those 11 part-time members of staff, 4 are on supported permitted work opportunities which comprise admin, clerical, book keeping, and marketing roles. Additionally, under the employer's retention incentive scheme specifically for young people (aged up to 29 years old), Tayberry employed 4 young people who were trainees with additional barriers for 1 year. Tayberry's partner the SEU will offer the young people ongoing support and job coaching to enable them to move onto mainstream employment.

One of our core members of staff initially took on her role under permitted work rules, and has now completely moved off benefits (see case study 2 below). There are a total of 31 volunteers taking on a variety of tasks within the company. In total Tayberry is supporting approximately 100 individuals whatever the stage they are at in their employability journey.

In continuation, two stories are presented, written by individuals of their experiences in Tayberry.

Case Study 1 – Dorothy

'My time with Tayberry Enterprise Limited has afforded me the opportunity to journey from unemployment to fulfilling, meaningful employment. I was long term unemployed due to health conditions that had impacted on my ability to engage/ continue in my previous employment.

In 2012, I was diagnosed with bipolar affective disorder which meant my pathways to employment and my ability to engage with this type of journey was incredibly difficult and opportunities limited. However, the position of volunteer co-ordinator that presented itself with Tayberry Enterprise and the chance to move back into the work environment has allowed me to journey back into the workforce whilst in a supportive environment.

My time with Tayberry has also allowed me to personally develop and explore strategies that keep me mentally healthy in a work environment especially under stressful circumstances – this is invaluable to anyone living with a mental health condition or anxiety based disorders. I believe that my own journey informs my interactions with Tayberry's clients and volunteers and means that I have a deeper understanding of the journey to employment as well as the challenges that long-term health barriers present.
I have learnt so many new skills and developed knowledge of an industry/ sector that I had very little awareness of before. I have been afforded many training and skills development opportunities all of which have made me feel valued and challenged. The evidence of Tayberry's methodologies and investment in individuals is evident in their commitment to my journey and their support and adaptability, which has been crucial to my progression.
My time with Tayberry has been challenging, fulfilling and stressful at times but ultimately it has taught me that I am able to function, contribute and participate effectively in a working environment. It has been a pivotal point in my journey from mental ill health to mental wellbeing and value of self.'

Case Study 2 – Lynsey

'I had never had any paid employment before. I had work experience in cleaning and also a short placement in a charity shop whilst at school. I have dyspraxia which can cause fatigue and affects my ability to stand for long periods. The dyspraxia affects my confidence and I become anxious about completing tasks due to fear of failure. I claim disability related benefits. When I was on placement in the charity shop working on the till was stressful during busy periods. However, I was keen to assess my capabilities in a working environment and eager to progress towards work.
I was offered an opportunity within the Tayberry Café as a Trainee on a Work Placement. This increased my confidence, let me try new types of work within a kitchen environment and also tackle till-work in a more supportive environment. The placement began with carrying out laundry duties for the canteen, which went very well and at my request I progressed onto other duties. Tayberry staff helped me overcome my fears and anxiety to become an accomplished cashier. I moved on to serve food and carry out kitchen porter duties, safe in the knowledge that if things were too much physically, the approachable supervisors within Tayberry would be able to accommodate this.
Following excellent progress through the work placement, I was a candidate for a paid kitchen assistant position that became available within the café. After a successful application and interview, I was offered the post. I work 10 hours a week which is a limited earning allowing me to stay on my disability benefits. This allows me to make the transition into work whilst still addressing my health issues.
Tayberry Café were able to be flexible with the post in order to help fit the criteria for this Supported Permitted Work. Since commencing the job, I have taken part in extra training, World Host, Food Hygiene and Manual Handling and I also participated in a chocolate making course which I thoroughly enjoyed.'

In an environment of financial restriction, new ways of working and the integration agenda, Tayberry was set up to provide pre-employment and employment opportunities for those with significant health barriers which prevented access to existing employability provision.

Reflections

In conclusion, the journey into a social enterprise and entrepreneurialism has been a fascinating one. Tayberry was developed to fill a gap between retracting NHS day services and access to the employability pipeline (Employability in Scotland, 2016). Using a social enterprise model enabled the development of a structure that supported a wide range of pre-employment and employment activities. Although 'therapy' would not be considered by everyone an element of social enterprises, given the particular needs of the population it is serving, this was seen to be a necessity, and enabled a smooth transition into other employment roles.

Within vocational rehabilitation IPS, supported education and social enterprise are all models that have something to offer people with long-term health conditions. Social enterprise is dynamic and versatile with potential for wide-ranging practice, however, that may also threaten its stability and sound business management is required.

As an occupational therapist this has been a challenging learning experience with the development of new skills including business skills. In particular, I perceive financial skills to be a major challenge but also requirement for moving the company forward. Another important area for my development has been the transition of my therapeutic role to one of employer, and how to weave together successfully the skills of both roles.

We are in the fifth wave. The human need for purposeful occupation and spiritual development remains as strong as when the founders of the profession began their social activism one hundred years earlier. Our purpose and direction is moving beyond traditional roles and with it, our unique thinking. We need to move on and ride the fifth wave as did the activists who were our professional predecessors.

References

Addicott, R. (2011) *Social Enterprise in Health Care. Promoting organisational autonomy and staff engagement.* London: The Kings Fund

Cathro, M. and Devine, A. (2012) Music therapy and social inclusion. *Mental Health Practice*, 16, 1, 33-36

Employability in Scotland (2016) Employability pipeline. [Accessed 17 April 2016 at http://www.employabilityinscotland.com/employability-pipeline/]

IPS Dartmouth Supported Employment Centre (2016) IPS supported employment for vocational rehabilitation counsellors. Video and discussion guide. [Accessed 17 April 2016 at https://www.ipsworks.org/wp-content/uploads/2014/08/vr-video-discussion-guide.pdf]

Lyon, A. (2003) The Fifth Wave. Edinburgh: Scottish Council Foundation. [Accessed 13th

October 2016 at http://www.iffpraxis.com/u/cms/the_fifth_wave.pdf]

Lysaght, R., Jakobsen, K. and Granhaug, B. (2012) Social firms: A means for building employment skills and community integration. *Work*, 41, 455-463

Lysaght, R. and Krupa, T. (2011) *Social Business: Advancing the viability of a model for economic and occupational justice for people with disabilities, Project Final Report, Phase 1.* Vancouver: Social Enterprise Canada [Accessed 13 October 2016 at https://www.groupeconvexpr.ca/images/groupeconvexpr/publications/Projet_de_recheche_universite_Queens_Social_Business__Disablity_Study_-_Report_1.pdf]

Paterson, C. (2010) *Opportunities not Prescriptions: The development of occupational therapy in Scotland 1900-1960.* Aberdeen: Aberdeen History of Medicine Publications

Pollard, N. (2011) Working in social enterprises. *International Journal of Physiotherapy and Rehabilitation*, 1, 2, 30-37

Priest, R. and Bones, K. (2012) Occupational therapy and supported employment: Is there any added value? *Mental Health and Social Inclusion*, 16, 4, 194–200

Rinaldi, M. and Perkins, R. (2007) Comparing employment outcomes for two vocational services: Individual placement and support and non-integrated pre-vocational services in the UK. *Journal of Vocational Rehabilitation*, 27, 21-27

Scottish Co-production Network (2016) What is co-production? [Accessed 5 January 2016 at http://www.coproductionscotland.org.uk/about/what-is-co-production/]

Scottish Government (2010a) *Realising Potential. An action plan for allied health professionals in mental health.* Edinburgh: Scottish Government

Scottish Government (2010b) *The Healthcare Quality Strategy for NHS Scotland.* Edinburgh: Scottish Government

Scottish Government (2013) *Keys to Life*. Edinburgh: Scottish Government

Wicks, A. and Jamieson, M. (2014) New ways for occupational scientists to tackle 'wicked problems' impacting population health. *Journal of Occupational Science*, 21,1,81-85

Unger, K.V. (2007) *Handbook on Supported Education. Providing services for students with psychiatric disabilities.* Baltimore, MD: Brookes Publishing Company

Chapter 12
The Taieri Blokes Shed: A place of productivity and belonging

James Sunderland, Linda Wilson, and the Membership of the Taieri Blokes Shed

'Of all the clubs I've ever been in my life, and there are quite a few, this is easily the most united in its members and its aims, without doubt.' Don (Taieri Blokes Shed Member)

Introduction

The Taieri Blokes Shed, from here on referred to as The Shed, is located in Mosgiel, Otago, New Zealand, with its origins in the Men's Shed movement. It is a community where members feel valued; where they can learn and grow with the support of others; and where they can contribute to society. Shared occupations are the basis of all communities (Poplin, 1994). At The Shed the shared occupations are constructive work, where members plan, design, build and engineer together. Constructive work provides the platform for social inclusion and community contribution. Benefits are dependent on individuals finding a match between their own occupational identity and needs, and the ethos of The Shed. The Shed is non-hierarchical, self-funding, and strongly affiliated with the local community.

All members of The Shed are male. The average age of Shed members is approximately 75 years. Roughly half of the members have trades-based employment backgrounds, with others having home and community construction histories. A number are retired farmers. Over 70% live with wives and partners while others live by themselves. The members of The Shed are, in general, mobile and independent. Many manage health issues common to their age group.

The majority of the members have faced difficulties in the processes of transitioning from paid or self-employment, to retirement. In addition, a number of members have confronted transition to place, having moved to Mosgiel in their retirement. Such transitions have resulted in members being isolated from previous social networks, which accompanied work, and lacking a purpose to apply their skills and tacit knowledge to meaningful projects. The Shed, although not the solution to all of these issues, has helped members find a new balance in their retirements.

Based on an ethnographic study conducted between 2010 and 2013, this chapter provides an insiders perspective of The Shed and the benefits members perceive. Findings are presented through member's quotes, photographs, and the researchers' reflections. The aim is to give the reader a rich description of The Shed as a place of productivity and social inclusion for men who choose to engage in constructive work, in the company of others, and for the benefit of the wider community.

The authors were both academic staff at the Otago Polytechnic School of occupational therapy throughout this research.

The Men's Shed Movement

According to Misan et al (2008) community sheds were emerging in Australia in the late 1970s, with what has become known as *The Men's Shed* movement growing rapidly over the past 15 years. The movement has been adopted throughout New Zealand, Ireland, and the United Kingdom, all of which share history and strong union, light industrial, farming, and DIY (Do It Yourself) traditions. More recently the Men's Shed movement has established national associations, in these countries, which provide advice and support to individual sheds, as well as organising conferences, promoting the movement and liaising with researchers.

Men's Sheds are community based, non-profit organisations, centred on constructive trades work. Most Sheds have grass roots origins in local communities that contribute to their specific nature; some developing from already established groups while other Sheds have been driven, in the early stages, by key individuals who realised the potential benefits. Sheds often have close associations with other community services such as sports groups, health providers and religious groups (Golding, 2009; Golding et al, 2007). Sheds are predominantly, but not exclusively, populated by older males working on projects of benefit to their local community, their shed, and themselves.

There is a growing body of research on the Men's Shed Movement, predominantly based in an Australian context. Current literature, although limited, evidences Men's Sheds as meaningful community based organisations that offer health and wellbeing benefits to those who attend. Early research on the movement focused on the quantifiable health, education, and vocation benefits resulting from Shed membership (Golding, 2009, 2006; Golding et al, 2008; Golding et al, 2007). More recent research conducted by Moylan et al. (2011) established that the collaborative nature of the Men's Shed contributes to the health and wellbeing of participants as does the sense of purpose provided by the work and the structure it provides for participants. Other studies have also provided evidence of the physical, mental and emotional health benefits of the Men's Shed movement (Fildes et al, 2010; Morgan, 2010; Ormsby et al, 2010; Ballinger et al, 2009). Cordier and Wilson (2014) declared Men's Sheds have an important role to play in addressing gender health disparities for a male population experiencing higher rates of mortality and morbidity in most Western countries. This view has been recognised in the acknowledgement and funding of Men's Sheds in gender targeted health policies in Australia and Ireland. Hansji et al (2015) considered the potential of the Men's Sheds as enabling environments for Australian men living with long term disabilities.

Within the discipline of occupational science, Martin and Wicks (2008) looked at the experiences of meaningful occupation of members of one particular shed, The Berry Men's Shed. More recently Wicks (2013) has documented a transactional view of shedding, highlighting its complexity and multidimensional nature, which have associations to the findings of this research and the occupational nature of the Taieri Blokes Shed community.

The origins of The Taieri Blokes Shed

The Taieri Blokes Shed has its origins in the Australian Men's Shed movement (2014). Phil Bradshaw, a commander in the Royal New Zealand Navy, had experienced the Men's Shed movement in Australia and saw value in developing a shed, or a series of sheds, in the Dunedin region. He consulted with local organisations, and initiated public meetings, to see if there was a willingness to develop the concept. A positive reception led to a steering committee being developed and, in turn, the first two sheds (The Taieri Blokes Shed and the Kings Shed located at a local high school in Dunedin city).

The Taieri Aero Club offered the use of premises just to the north of Mosgiel in the latter half of 2007. Workshops and meeting rooms were developed which met the early requirements of constructive work as well as social activities. In 2014, due to membership growth and the demands of projects, the lease of a larger building, on the same site, was negotiated. This building is larger and allowed specific workshop areas to be constructed (woodwork, metalwork, painting) while improving the health and safety environment. By early 2015 The Shed has an active membership of over forty men who undertake a balance of community projects, shed development, and individual project work.

Research overview

When we, the researchers and co-authors of this article, first began working with The Shed in 2010 it appeared to be thriving, with positive feedback emanating from the membership and from the wider community. We sought to understand The Shed as a community focused on men's voluntary involvement in occupations of constructive work. This sought understanding was informed by Western literature and occupational therapy literature on productivity and work, where humans are deemed to be transformed by meaningful and purposeful work, investing themselves in created objects. Through work humans discover and reveal themselves to others (Kojeve, 1989). Constructive work, according to Green's (1968) definition of work, requires self-investment, skill, craft and personal judgement. Work is purposeful and meaningful and distinct from the repetition of labour, where there is little say in end results. Constructive work helps individuals and groups define who they are and how they wish to be viewed by others (Kielhofner, 2002).

In understanding the occupational structure of this community, we also sought interpretation of how participating in shared occupations of constructive work enabled social inclusion for members and perceptions of health and wellbeing. Social inclusion requires individuals to find a match between their own occupational identity and needs, and the ethos of The Shed.

Ethnographic research was undertaken between 2011 and 2013. Ethnographic methodology allows understanding of culture and meaning from the viewpoint of an insider while enabling an external analysis (Hammersley & Atkinson, 2007; Coffey, 1999; Agar, 1996). James Sunderland was a participant observer at The Shed. Participant observation incorporated involvement in, and contribution to, the life of The Shed while concurrently recording observations through writing and photographs. James' immersion in the activities of The Shed allowed for participation in the routines, roles and practices of the community while building and developing relationships. Active participation was key to him being accepted by the members and capturing their views and actions.

Additional data were later collected by undertaking theme checking qualitative interviews with members of The Shed, and through the gathering and review of cultural records and secondary sources that documented the community. All empirical materials were subjected to an analytical phase following fieldwork and qualitative interviews.

Findings

Meaningful work

> *'... to mix with people of similar ilk ... a desire for everyone to use their hands. I like being amongst people who've all got very similar interests.' Don*

Constructive work is the central occupation of The Shed and provides the purpose of this community. The Shed, like others, offers something that other, more traditional, retirement activities do not. This is not a sporting pursuit or recreation like a golf, croquet or bowls club; it is not a place to commune and engage with others who have served in the military like the Returned Service Mens' Association, and it is not based on beneficence through fundraising and business connection like the Rotary and Lions clubs. This is a place where the focus is squarely on constructive work, where members plan, design, build and engineer alongside others who share this interest, or these skills, however acquired. There is an understanding within The Shed that the main purpose of The Shed is productivity (see photo 1).

For many members, constructive work holds shared meaning and value as it directly links to their previous identities as tradesmen, farmers, or home handymen, identities that may have been compromised as a result of retirement. Constructive work provides challenge and enables them to realise their skills and knowledge. For some members, constructive work is the medium to participate in and contribute to society while finding a fit with compatible individuals.

For several members the initial attraction of The Shed was access to tools and opportunities they did not have at home due to downsizing homes and retiring from work. Yet the health and connectedness of The Shed community requires that the focus moves beyond individual gain to reciprocity in the conduct of constructive work.

With the transition from paid employment to retirement a number of members talked about finding ways of productively using their time as opposed to just passing time.

'When you work over 40 hours per week, for over 40 years of your life, it can come as a bit of a shock to the system when that finishes and you find yourself with a lot of time on your hands.' John

Attendance at The Shed helps provide structure and order to members' weeks. For some, the weekly sessions at The Shed are a highlight in their week, for others The Shed is but one component in a well-organised set of retirement activities.

For projects undertaken for groups in the local community it is not acceptable for products to be purely functional or good enough. Pride is taken in the completion of products that are fit to purpose in that they are well designed, have ease of use, durability, and aesthetic appeal. This is directly tied to the skills of the members and their ability to control production. The Shed has built a local reputation for service, helpfulness, quality and affordability. This reputation is important to the members and is actively sought and maintained. (see photo 2)

The membership has many years of experience and a wealth of (tacit) knowledge and expertise. There is robust discussion about the structure of projects, who is involved, processes, materials used, and costings.

'You have to be willing to try something or teach something.' Don

In line with qualities of generosity, team work, and dedication to a common task, there is a focus at The Shed on the sharing of knowledge. Those willing to seek help are readily taught, often as part of a project team. Often learning happens without direct instruction or explanation, through observation of the actions of others.

There is a structure to how group projects are managed. Projects, depending on size, are allocated to individuals or smaller groups. Those with the relevant skills are assigned control of projects, after group discussions during Shed meetings, and provide direction for others. Compromise is often sought when planning tasks and at times members recognise they need to forgo their opinion for the good of the collective. Continuity of those working on a task is seen as essential to a successful outcome. Associated project timeframes enforces expectations around attendance and contribution. Project leaders liaise with community groups who have commissioned work.

Longer term members know who they are comfortable working alongside. The core membership of some community projects often self-selects, based on previous successes, however there is still opportunity to bring in new members or existing members who have specific skills. New members are often initiated through inclusion in larger project groups, which helps them understand expectations around work practices while being in a structure where they can learn from others.

'What we do if we have a reasonable project is delegate a member (with the key skills) to take a lead on that and he will then ask any of the other members he feels he wants to ask to help him on that project.' Ian

The Shed community prefers to have three to four projects happening at a time to keep the membership busy and engage the range of abilities. (see photo 3)

There is active interest in recycling materials, to not waste what has potential value, and keeping project costs down. Shed members and the public regularly donate materials and equipment to The Shed. The acceptance of materials is informally monitored with future use in mind.

'We used to take everything that people donated. Now we have to be careful about what to take due to space limitations. We've got to say 'no' to some things.' Ian

There is a general knowledge amongst the members about where tools and equipment are kept which comes through involvement in projects, as well as environmental cues, and formal and informal prompts from the membership. Tool storage and maintenance are agenda items in monthly meetings and during smoko. This shared responsibility reinforces workshops routines and order.

In the early years of The Sheds development there were issues with the use of workshop spaces, tools, and the acquisition and care of materials. Workshop spaces were developed alongside the completion of projects and a steadily growing membership. This put pressure on what could be achieved safely within workspaces. The larger premises have eased such tensions as work spaces have been designed and built for specific application with attention to health and safety.

As a non-profit organisation in a country with universal accident insurance cover The Shed is not subject to workplace inspections, however there is an awareness that any serious accident has potential to put The Shed under scrutiny and could jeopardise the community.

'The reality is in this world or in the New Zealand environment if you don't have the appropriate systems in place for health and safety ... to look after your public interface you run the risk of when something goes wrong you carry the can. It's just the way it is.' Mike

Safe use of equipment in the workshop environment is based on members' work experience. There are elected health and safety officers, those with trades experience teaching those without.

At The Shed there has always been a deliberate separation of the workshop spaces from the meeting and social spaces. This physical separation is widely appreciated by The Shed as it helps set boundaries around expectations in each setting.

Support and governance work

There is a strong emphasis on equality amongst the membership. A number of The Shed members have been members of unions in their working lives, and others members of rural communities where there is an expectation of reciprocity.

'Governance of The Shed is viewed as 'responsible'. Everything is brought up and you have a chance to say something about it ... governance is the responsibility of the whole group.' Neil

The Shed has a defined governance structure. There are formal roles, including President, Secretary, Treasurer, Safety and Promotions. All Shed members are members of the committee which comes with the expectation that they contribute to decision making. The Shed's monthly meetings have a clear structure. Apologies and attendance are recorded, previous minutes reviewed, an agenda is set, presented and discussed. At times members do not see eye to eye on work or governance processes. These points of difference are openly acknowledged at The Shed, during meetings.

Although the formal governance roles call for a contribution beyond normal membership, members who take on these positions attribute meaning to them. Roles are taken on for personal satisfaction and out of a sense of responsibility to The Shed.

Social inclusion

'When you get a group of likeminded men they get along together.' Neil

A willingness to engage in constructive work, as learner, participant, or facilitator provides the platform for social inclusion. The Shed provides reason to apply skills and knowledge in the company of others for others. It is the acceptance of like-minded individuals that members value, being part of something larger than themselves. It provides an antidote to the social isolation some experienced retiring from paid employment or in moving to Mosgiel. The membership promotes this benefit to others, making acknowledgement in articles written about The Shed and in their informal conversations. It is often the case that wives and partners have read articles about The Shed and this leads to potential members initial contact.

'We've got a lot of people with a lot of experience and they're living in their little corners. I live in my shed, you live in your flat, and you do your crossword puzzle in the morning and you walk down to the shop and you walk back and you're really just decaying away health wise and mentally, and all this resource knowledge you have is not being disseminated.' Bob

'The Shed provided a chance to make new friends as we've recently moved to Mosgiel. Mosgiel properties, particularly in the new regions, all have high fences and the only time you see your neighbour is when you go in the street ... we came from the place where you had low fences and were in constant communication with our neighbours so we found it quite a struggle when we moved here.' Don

Mutual support is clearly evident in the interactions of The Shed, with members acknowledging not just differences of opinion but also differences in ability, energy, skills and health contexts.

'We've got to be generous towards each other and accept what one can and what one can't do ... I know physically there are a lot of things I can't do that others can.' Neil

'We're all there looking after each other.' Bob

Members view The Shed as a safe place to do valued work that affirms identity for those feeling marginalised by retirement, being excluded from the work force. There is a comfort in being in the presence of men who have similar interests, backgrounds and are in the same age bracket.

Members value the male-only company within The Shed, but many did not feel comfortable openly labelling The Shed a male-only community. This is due to contemporary societal views on inclusion and equal opportunity. Some members have made a point of saying The Shed is gender inclusive, yet the majority of members value working shoulder to shoulder in a setting that affirms male values and the qualities of a 'good bloke'. 'The bloke is a certain kind of Australian or New Zealand male… he is pragmatic rather than classy… he does not whinge' (Luscombe, 2000, n.p.). To be referred to as a 'good bloke' is the ultimate accolade, meaning someone who is gregarious, hospitable, generous, warm-hearted, with a good sense of humour (Walsh, 1985). There is recognition, amongst the membership, that a female presence would alter the dynamic, with a number of members feeling it might impact on their own attendance, although this has yet to be tested.

'If you had a woman in The Shed you wouldn't say a lot of what we do at smoko.' Ian

Some members thought there was nothing wrong with openly excluding female membership as there are a number of female orientated groups active in the community.

'The other thing I like about The Shed is that it's a male only place and to my way of thinking I would not like to see females introduced to it … because I don't think there's a place for them. I've got nothing against them but there are places for them.' Neil

Morning tea is commonly referred to as 'smoko' amongst the group. It is an anchor point for the daily activities of The Shed. Smoko occurs during every morning session between 10 or 10.30am. There is an expectation that all members take a break. Smoko puts the social side of The Shed to the forefront. (see photo 4)

'The social side is just as important as the working side … they all enjoy going and having a cup of tea and a cup of coffee and having a wee yarn … it's one of the few times when everyone is together.' Colin

'We put a lot of emphasis on our lounge room and having morning tea there. Just the fellowship we have in that room. People can sit beside different people at morning tea and you talk about things. That lounge or smoko room is the making of The Taieri Shed.' Don

There is a lot of good humoured banter amongst the group. The members give each other a 'hard time'. Jokes are light-hearted and often link to a member's character traits, work ethic, past history, and activities away from The Shed. The tone and manner of the humour at The Shed provides a strong indication of the member's knowledge and acceptance of each other.

'We give each other hell at times … if you dish it out you've got to be able to take it.' Neil

Smoko is a time when general Shed information is passed on to the members including up-coming out of Shed events. Wider community relationships and significant personal milestones are acknowledged at smoko and it provides a time when potential members and visitors can be introduced.

The strength of this community is evident in how members interact not only within, but also away from, The Shed. Many choose to spend time in each other's company outside of The Shed, engaged in a variety of other occupations including walking groups, fishing, and golf.

'I've met people and have relationships that I'd like to continue if The Shed closed tomorrow.' Don

Health concerns are common. Updates are provided to the general membership during smoko breaks or at monthly meetings, if someone is unwell or is coping with issues in their personal life.

The way members share information at The Shed indicates good networks of communication outside of The Shed. If someone is absent for more than a few sessions it is likely they will be rung by a Shed member.

'Anyone's only got to be sick or have a partner in the hospital or something and there are always two or three enquiring how they are, or can they help.' Colin

There is emphasis on mixing as a group with wives and partners away from The Shed. It is seen by many in the group as the key to getting to know one another.

'Involving wives in social activities to get to know each other better outside The Shed is very, very important.' Ian

Community contribution

Being of use to others in the local community is a benefit recognised by members.

'I enjoy it (membership) for the friendship, the company, and hopefully being seen as being useful.' Neil

The Shed has good relationships with community groups, businesses and services, and governing authorities in the local area. Success in a number of funding applications demonstrates the willingness to ask for assistance and external acknowledgement of the worth of The Shed to the members and the wider community.

As a non-profit organisation members are aware of not competing with local businesses but aim to be of use to other non-profit groups, and individuals, in the area. Projects are designed and built for purpose. Pride is taken to ensure projects are durable, reliable, affordable, and well finished. The membership understands that there are limits to the projects they can take on given the parameters of their own resources.

'This is a community where things get done and people know what you do. We're happy to take on community projects within our ability. It should never be an intention to do things to make money.' Neil

'It is the completion of projects that are affordable, well-constructed and visually appealing that is accepted as the best promotional tool The Shed has. Community connections come with the project work.' Neil

The Shed is conscious that it needs to be visible in its local community. It makes itself available to local media and has had regular stories published in local and regional newspapers and magazines, which helps generate new members and projects. The continued demand for project work is vital to realising the purpose of The Shed. Most members actively promote The Shed's services.

'When I'm outside The Shed, I have my name badge on… it's promoting The Shed. People out there who say 'Oh the Taieri Blokes Shed we've heard about you'. If they don't know a lot they ask a lot of questions ... we've got to keep our name and image out in the community, that way we get feedback. It also opens doors to get more projects. If people hear about us they say 'Oh you might be able to help us out', that's why they ring up.' Ian

It is common for recipients of The Shed's services to visit and give something back like materials, tools, or a morning tea as thanks. Members also make an effort to visit the organisations for which they complete projects.

Conclusion

This research focused on one Men's Shed. We described The Taieri Blokes Shed from the member's perspectives. This Shed is prospering, and is valued by its members and its local community. Benefits are recognised as flowing from meaningful occupation in constructive work.

The Shed is a place that provides occupational satisfaction, structured routine, social inclusion, self-determination, and community contribution. Benefits are dependent on individuals finding a match between their own identity and the ethos of the Taieri Blokes Shed. Membership means associating on a social level where men value each other's company, care for one another, and can tolerate difference. Although practical skills are vital to this community's work they are not a prerequisite for an individual's inclusion. Inclusion is reliant on a willingness to 'give it a go', to learn as well as teach. If an individual is not interested in learning or teaching constructive work, and is unwilling to work alongside others they will not find social inclusion at The Shed.

The findings of this study, although limited to one Men's Shed, fits with the other research on Men's Sheds. We affirm, as other research has, that constructive work is the occupational foundation on which Men's Shed communities are built.

Constructive work provides the purpose of Men's Shed in turn enabling occupations which provide social connectedness. Men's Sheds are not sheltered workshops; the product of their industry serves local communities. Men's Sheds attract men who want to be productive in the company of others, supporting one another and working towards common goals. Men's Sheds are not intended as places to hide; they are not refuges from the outside world. Men's Sheds need to be open to new projects, new members and their local community.

Looking beyond the limited scope of this research, Golding's (2015) edited book The Men's Shed Movement: The Company of Men provides a definitive overview of the development of the Men's Shed movement. He acknowledges that Men's Sheds provide social inclusion for men (commonly retired men), at the expense of others, because of the multiple benefits derived from men working in a community that does together. Individual sheds have unique origins and express unique character. Some Sheds are more inclusive than others. There have been reported, although rare, incidences of discrimination of membership based on ethnicity, sexual orientation, and religion. Conversely other Men's Sheds have actively sought inclusion of particular groups of men who are marginalised due to disability or ethnicity. What is important is finding the right match between the needs of the individual and the affordances of the particular Men's Shed community. Golding states:

> 'In practice most Men's Sheds welcome and admit men of any age or background, with a range of disabilities, though many are reluctant to take men as regular workshop participants if they require high level care without the support of a regular carer.' (2015, p. 379).

All communities, be they academic, residential or occupational, are strengthened by shared experiences, characteristics or values of the participants. The challenge is when one particular aspect becomes hegemonic. Occupational science is making a useful contribution to understanding barriers to and facilitators of participation in occupation because of the benefits of participation in occupation both to individuals and to communities. Ensuring diversity and inclusiveness whilst acknowledging or even celebrating similarity of choice in engagement is a legitimate concern worthy of more examination around the boundaries/ interactions, intersections and overlapping interests of occupational science and community development.

References

Agar, M. (1996) *Professional Stranger: An informal introduction to ethnography.* (2nd ed.) Thousand Oaks, CA: Sage Publications

Australian Men's Shed Association (2014) *What is a Men's Shed?* [Accessed 7 June 2014 at http://www.mensshed.org/what-is-a-men's-shed/.aspx]

Ballinger, M., Talbot, T. and Verrinder, K. (2009) More than a place to do woodwork: A case study of a community-based men's shed. *Journal of Men's Health,* 6, 1, 20-27

Coffey, A. (1999) *The Ethnographic Self: Fieldwork and the representation of identity.* London: Sage

Cordier, R. and Wilson, N.J. (2014) Community-based Men's Sheds: Promoting male health, wellbeing and social inclusion in an international context. *Health Promotion International,* 29, 3, 483-493

Fildes, D.L., Cass, Y., Wallner, F. and Owen, A.G. (2010). Shedding light on men: The building healthy men project. *Journal of Men's Health,* 7, 3, 233-240

Golding, B. (2006) *A Profile of Men's Sheds in Australia*: *Patterns, purposes, profiles and experiences of participants.* Paper presented at AVETRA Conference, Wollongong. [Accessed 1 June 2013 at http://avetra.org.au/ABSTRACTS2006/PA%200028.pdf]

Golding, B., Brown, M., Foley, A., Harvey, J. and Gleeson, L. (2007) *Men's Sheds in Australia: Learning through community contexts.* [Accessed 1 June 2013 at http://www.ncver.edu.au/publications/1780.html]

Golding, B., Kimberley, H., Foley, A. and Brown, M. (2008) Houses and sheds: An exploration of the genesis and growth of neighbourhood houses and men's sheds in community settings. *Australian Journal of Adult Learning,* 48, 2, 237-262

Golding, B. (2009) *The Way Sheds have Spread in Australia and Internationally.* Paper presented at the Third National Men's Shed Conference, Tasmania. [Accessed 1 June 2013 at http://www.mensshed.org/SiteFiles/mensshed2011org/HobartAMSAShedSpread.pdf]

Golding, B. (2015) Men's shed theory and practice. in B. Golding (Ed.) *The Men's Shed Movement: The company of men.* Champaign: Common Ground Publishing (pp.368-390)

Green, T.F. (1968) *Work, Leisure and the American Schools.* New York: Random House

Hammersley, M. and Atkinson, P. (2007) *Ethnography: Principles in practice.* (3rd ed.) London: Routledge

Hansji, N.L., Wilson, N.J. and Cordier, R. (2015) Men's sheds: Enabling environments for Australian men living with and without long-term disabilities. *Health and Social Care in the Community, 23*, 3, 272-281

Kielhofner, G. (2002) *A Model of Human Occupation: Theory and application.* (3rd ed.) Baltimore, MD: Williams and Wilkens

Kojeve, A. (1989) *Introduction to the Reading of Hegel: Lecturers on the phenomenology of spirit.* Ithaca, NY: Cornell University Press

Luscombe, L. (2000) Cinema: Of Mad Max and Madder Maximus. *Time.* May 5. [Accessed at http://www.time.com/time/magazine/article/0,9171,996881,00.html]

Martin, K. and Wicks, A. (2008) Meaningful occupation at the Berry Men's Shed. *Journal of Occupational Science,* 15, 3, 194-195

Misan, G., Haren, M. and Leod, V. (2008) *Men's Sheds: A strategy to improve men's health.* Parramatta, NSW: Men's Sheds Australia Ltd

Morgan, N. (2010) A room of their own: Men's sheds build communities of support and purpose. *Cross Currents: Journal of Addiction and Mental Health,* 13, 4, 12-13.

Moylan, M., Blackburn, R., Leggat, S., Robinson, P., Carey, L. and Hayes, R. (2011) *Shed Power: Collaboration for better men's health outcomes.* Paper presented at 24th Occupational Therapy Australia National Conference and Exhibition, Gold Coast. [Accessed 1 June 2013 at http://onlinelibrary.wiley.com/doi/10.1111/j.1440-1630.2011.00938.x/pdf]

Ormsby, J., Stanley, M. and Jaworski, K. (2010) Older men's participation in community-based men's sheds programmes. *Health & Social Care in the Community,* 18, 6, 607-613

Poplin, D. (1994) Theories of community. in D. Poplin (Ed.) *Communities: A survey of theories and methods of research.* (2nd ed.) New York: Macmillian (pp. 63-107)

Walsh, R. (1985) Australia observed. *Daedalus,* 114, 1, 421-438

Wicks, A. (2013) A transactional view of shedding at the Berry Men's Shed. in M.P. Cutchin and V.A. Dickie (Eds.) *Transactional Perspectives on Occupation.* Dordrecht, NL: Springer (pp.119-131)

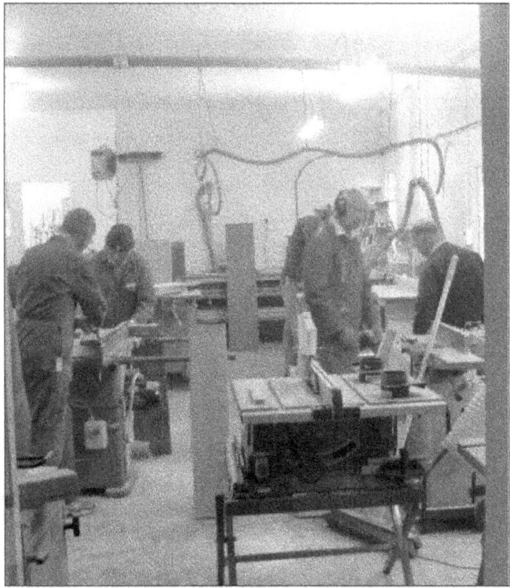

Photo 1: Main woodwork shop, March 2015

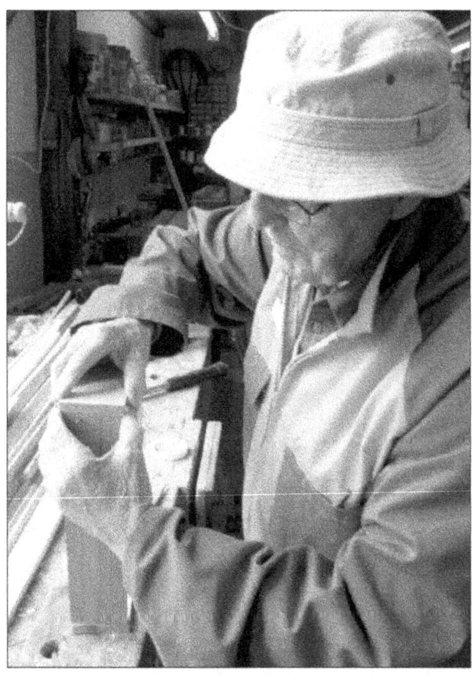

Photo 2: Construction of planter boxes for Heritage Rose Society, August 2011

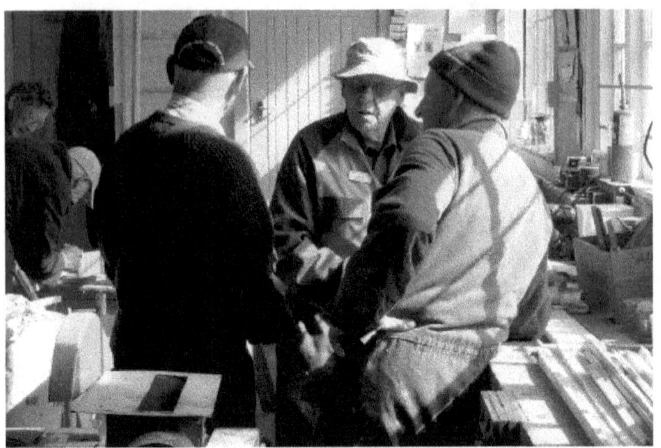

Photo 3: Project discussion, July 2011

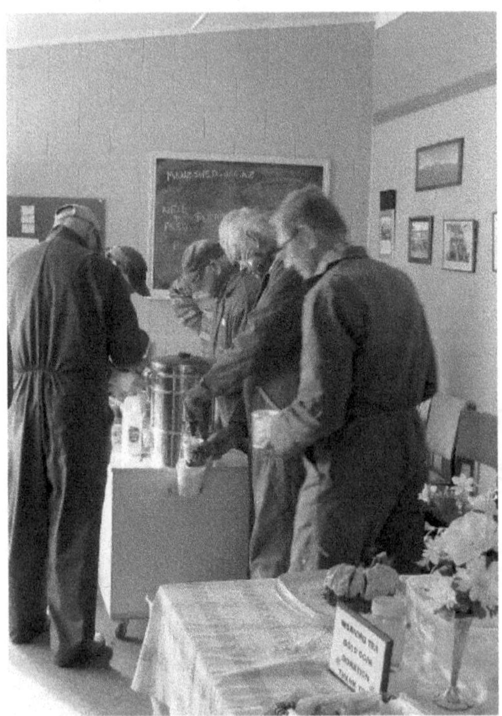

Photo 4: Smoko time, March 2015

Chapter 13
Decolonising imposed occupation: A preventative strategy for foetal alcohol spectrum disorder

Lizahn Gracia Cloete, Maria Konstabel, and Eve Madeleine Duncan

Introduction

This chapter is written by two occupational therapists and a community activist who are working in collaboration with women affected by alcohol abuse in a wine farming region of the Western Cape Province of South Africa. Cloete (2012; 2005; Cloete & Ramugondo, 2015) has been working as a clinician for five years in the region prior to embarking on occupational therapy research for the past fifteen years in communities where mothers have or are at risk of having children who present with foetal alcohol spectrum disorders (FASD). Konstabel is a community activist who grew up in a community where drug and alcohol abuse was and still is rife. She is passionate about building the capacity of women to be healthy and integrated in their communities. She commits herself to linking women with resources and structures that are located within local government and local non-governmental organisations. Duncan supervised occupational therapy students doing an honours-level study that investigated the occupational opportunities available to these women in a low socio-economic community (Mayson et al, 2014).

The authors' longitudinal, development-orientated research and practice is aimed at the prevention of FASD, a neurodevelopmental health condition that is associated with prenatal alcohol exposure (Williams & Smith, 2015). The term FASD is not intended for use as a clinical diagnosis, but rather as a description of the range of lifelong developmental disabilities that may occur due to *in utero* exposure to alcohol. Although FASD occurs in all social classes it is most prevalent in populations with poor socio-economic status, high levels of unemployment and low literacy levels, and poverty-related public health challenges such as poor sanitation, inadequate nutrition, domestic violence and maternal depression (Vythilingum et al, 2012; Setlalentoa et al, 2010; Bradshaw et al, 2007; May et al, 2005). These and other social determinants of health – such as under-developed public sector services – place pregnant women and their unborn children at occupational risk by compromising the personal, social and structural resources necessary for their human development through occupation (Wilcock, 2006).

FASD would be eliminated if all women abstained from alcohol when planning a pregnancy, as well as during pregnancy. While the right to choose sobriety resides with the individual woman, she may not be aware of the need for making such a choice in the interests of her unborn child, or she may feel unable to exercise choice, due to her life circumstances. It is difficult for pregnant women to stop drinking alcohol when they live in communities where the majority of people subscribe to excessive drinking as a culturally acceptable way of spending time (Setlalentoa et al, 2010). Excessive drinking as part of a socially normative lifestyle is known to occur in communities with a history of colonisation (Vythilingum et al, 2012; George, 2007). Drinking as an acceptable way of occupying time in these contexts has been described as an imposed occupation, because it is perpetuated through oppressive cultural practices, norms and values that are embedded in the social matrix of particular subaltern groups (marginalised people who have limited power to voice their concerns or views) (Cloete & Ramugondo, 2015; Cloete, 2012, 2005). Occupations become imposed when people's positioning in society traps them into inter-generational patterns of harmful health behaviours – including alcohol abuse. A human development approach is indicated to interrupt the perpetuation of health-compromising behaviours (Davids, 2009; Rendall-Mkosi, 2007). However, personal and social change only becomes possible by the creation of action-learning opportunities for marginalised groups. Facilitation of such action-learning spaces may enable marginalised people to empower and decolonise themselves (Salmon, 2011).

As part of a longitudinal, development-orientated research and practice project, this chapter proposes that the goal of development-orientated occupational therapy practice in the context of FASD is to work alongside women towards sobriety during pregnancy, by decolonising drinking as an imposed occupation. It describes ways in which occupational therapy can contribute to the prevention of FASD by addressing the occupational risks women face as a result of their marginalised social position. Part one of the chapter explains how the region's history of colonisation has shaped a culture of regular patterns of episodic or binge drinking as a social norm in some wine-farming communities. It describes the extent of the problem drinking that contributes to a high incidence of FASD, and explains how drinking patterns form part of a person's lifestyle. Part two of the chapter discusses drinking during pregnancy and related public health strategies, including health-promotion and development-orientated social-healing initiatives. Part three discusses the traditional and emerging contributions of occupational therapy to the prevention of FASD. It describes a participatory development process with at-risk women, aimed at decolonising drinking as an imposed occupation. The chapter concludes with the case story of the second author, who shares her personal experience of overcoming the colonising influences of alcohol abuse, and the contribution of occupational therapy towards understanding herself as an occupational being.

Excessive drinking: A colonial history

The viniculture industry is an integral part of South African history and of the economy. The roots of the South African wine industry can be traced to the explorations of the Dutch East India Company, which established a supply station in the Cape in 1652. Vineyards were planted by Dutch settlers, to produce grapes that could be used to ward off scurvy in sailors during their voyages along the spice route between Europe and the Far East. The first harvest and crushing of grapes to produce wine took place in 1659. Farm workers on wine and deciduous fruit farms were paid for their labour with tobacco, bread and large amounts of poor-quality (high ethanol content) wine. This method of remuneration was called the *dop system* – the Afrikaans word *dop* meaning a measure or drink of alcohol. The dop system laid the foundation for particular forms of alcohol use and abuse that have been passed down through successive generations of people who work and live on farms and in the surrounding communities (London, 1999). The dop system persists to this day as an institutionalised form of labour control on some farms, despite the promulgation of laws such as The Liquor Act of 1928 and the Basic Conditions of Employment Act of 1997, which sought to abolish oppressive labour practices and to improve the working and living conditions of farm labourers.

In communities such as the one from which the second author comes, drinking alcohol became an integral and structurally determined part of people's daily routine, over many generations. Farm workers organised their lives and strengthened their social networks around drinking, creating a unique cultural space that farm owners could not share (Scully, 1992). Occupying their free time by consuming alcohol together gave them a chance to joke, laugh, converse, and create meaning that was separate from – yet dependent on – their employers (De Kock, 2002; London, 1999). In the context of poor living and working conditions, alcohol use enabled a particular type of sociality to emerge – that of *drinking friendships*, in which excessive drinking became socially normative, with little or no stigma attached to drunken behaviour (Setlalentoa et al, 2010). Generations of people in the region came to view binge drinking in a social group as an acceptable form of leisure, even during pregnancy (Schneider et al, 2007; May et al, 2005; Van der Leeden et al, 2001).

Drinking patterns: The extent of the problem

A drinking pattern refers to the amount of alcohol consumed and the time period over which it is ingested. In a description of drinking patterns, Maier and West (2001) report that the total amount of alcohol consumed may be spread over a long duration (e.g. a week or a month), and individual drinks may be spaced consistently (for example, two drinks per week or one drink per day). Conversely, the same amount of alcohol may be consumed in a binge. A binge pattern means that the total alcohol consumption is compressed into a short time period (for example, an evening or a day), and the time between consumption of individual beverages is short and possibly inconsistent (e.g. a steady consumption of wine or beer interspersed with shots of hard liquor such as rum, whisky or brandy) during that binge. Thus, a woman who reports consuming seven drinks per week may consume all seven in one evening (bingeing), or consume one drink per day (not bingeing). Irrespective of an individual woman's patterns of drinking, the impact of alcohol on her unborn child and her occupational performance poses a major public health risk that adversely affects the development trajectory of both. Understanding the possible variations in drinking patterns guides the occupational therapist towards a nuanced assessment of a woman's occupational performance and occupational engagement. For example, it helps the occupational therapist ask pertinent questions about time use, drinking companions and functioning in activities of daily living prior, during and after different drinking sessions.

South Africa is in the second-highest category of countries with harmful national drinking patterns, and has the highest levels of episodic drinking for both males and females in this category (World Health Organisation, 2014). The amount of alcohol consumed per drinking person in South Africa is about 20 litres of absolute alcohol consumed per person per year (Schneider et al, 2007). An estimated 69% of the population in some Western Cape communities consume alcohol on a daily basis (World Health Organisation, 2014), including over 20% of women during pregnancy (Olivier et al, 2013). Given the extent of drinking in the region, it has one of the highest rates of FASD prevalence in the world; it is estimated that between 13.6% and 20.9% of the local population is affected (May et al, 2012).

Drinking during pregnancy: FASD, public health and social class

The diagnostic methods for identifying the signs and symptoms related to prenatal alcohol exposure differ across social groups in the South African health sector (May et al, 2012; Cloete, 2012). Children in affluent communities who have been exposed to prenatal alcohol are more likely to be diagnosed with attention deficits, behavioural difficulties and hyperactivity disorder (ADHD) than FASD. Given the dop system and the country's history of racial segregation under apartheid, children and youth from some low socio-economic communities in the Western Cape are automatically associated with prenatal alcohol exposure. Hence, the prevalence figures for the signs and symptoms related to prenatal alcohol exposure across social groups are under-represented and skewed toward historically marginalised and disadvantaged communities. In addition, there are no uniform strategies for addressing prenatal alcohol exposure across the boundaries of South African social classes. Current public health interventions fail to ensure adequate service provision for the diverse health needs of populations affected by excessive alcohol consumption (Weeramanthri & Bailie, 2015). Access to FASD prevention strategies, early diagnostic services, quality medical and antenatal care and appropriate habilitation of affected children is limited in those South African communities most at risk for maternal alcohol abuse.

While structural and developmental support for affected individuals is scarce, genetic research on prenatal alcohol exposure abounds in these communities (Weeramanthri & Bailie, 2015). The emphasis of health sector spending is on understanding and measuring the incidence of the diagnosis, rather than on addressing the social determinants that contribute to FASD. Public health programmes focus on reducing the incidence of FASD through timeous diagnosis; and in so doing, perpetuate the effects of political and economic marginalisation of vulnerable populations by limiting the amount of public funding available for social and human development. Commenting from an occupational therapy perspective on public health, Cloete (2012) suggests that reductionist biomedical interventions (such as treating the sensory and perceptual impairments of children with FASD) and individual approaches to health behaviours (such as using behaviour modification to target maternal drinking practices) may limit the outcomes of programmes aimed at FASD prevention. She argues that occupational therapists who address the health needs of children with FASD and at-risk women solely from a medical perspective may actually deepen their occupational performance problems – because the underlying social inequities and occupational risks that they face every day remain unchanged. Cloete's call for occupational therapists to counter the prevailing reductive approaches to health is addressed in the professional literature, with authors arguing for health promotion and critical social occupational therapy as an alternative (Malfitano et al, 2014; Hammell & Iwama, 2012).

Health promotion: Shifting the focus towards social healing

The World Health Organisation defines health promotion as a process for enabling people to increase control over, and improve their own health (World Health Organisation, 1986). Biomedicine exerts influence as the dominant health discourse guiding health-promotion strategies for the prevention of FASD. For example, Mundel and Chapman (2010, p.8) emphasise the importance of educating individuals to make 'healthier' lifestyle choices such as eating 'right' in order to avoid health problems or to stop drinking during pregnancy to ensure a healthy baby. For health promotion to succeed it must consider and address the contexts within which people live that make it hard for them to exercise personal control and choice. However, in the context of poverty, inequality, and historically imposed and culturally acceptable drinking practices, making the right choices and acting on them is easier said than done. An alternative health promotion discourse is therefore emerging that advocates for personal and social healing practices aimed at redressing the legacies of colonisation (Salmon, 2011).

Healing in the context of social transformation is defined as 'personal and societal recovery from the lasting effects of oppression and systemic racism experienced over generations' (Royal Commission on Aboriginal Peoples, 1996, p.107-8). The aboriginal people of Canada suffered from specific diseases and social problems, as well as 'a depression of spirit resulting from 200 or more years of damage to their cultures, languages, identities and self-respect' (Royal Commission on Aboriginal Peoples, 1996). Similar stories of colonisation and marginalisation exist among farm workers in the South African wine region (London, 1999), Australian indigenous people (Australian Institute for Health and Welfare, 2015), and colonised populations in Latin America (Althouse, 2014). The contribution of occupational therapy to the dislocation and cultural destruction of colonisation is gaining traction in the professional literature (Ramugondo, 2012, 2009, 2000).

For healing to happen, a decolonising development approach to health promotion and the prevention of health conditions is indicated (Salmon, 2011; Sherwood & Edwards, 2006). A decolonising development approach promotes the ability of individuals and their communities to identify and address personal and structural barriers (such as lack of transport and housing, poor access to health services and job opportunities, poverty, low literacy levels and poor nutrition) to their health and well-being. Drinking as occupation in motherhood should thus not be seen as an individual practice only, but also as a practice that is naturally inherent to the culture of the larger community in which mothers who abuse alcohol during pregnancy live (Cloete & Ramugondo, 2015). Programmes aimed at the prevention of drinking should therefore target – through development-orientated strategies – the impact of historical socio-political factors on people's occupations (Cloete, 2012; Frank et al, 2008).

Taking an occupational perspective: Drinking as imposed occupation

Sztompka suggests that

> 'the process of an individual becoming a social being occurs in the inherited cultural environment, the socially shared pool of ready-made templates for socialising, interpreting, framing and narrating the ongoing social praxis' (Sztompka, 1993, p.451).

The concept of drinking as an imposed occupation is based on the association that exists between historical, political and socio-economic conditions and current cultural expressions in what people do every day (Mundel & Chapman, 2010). The inherited cultural environment provides the context within which women's prenatal drinking behaviours are learnt; and in so doing, begin to mirror the social drinking patterns of the communities in which they live, work and socialise. Although culture, race and ethnicity are different concepts, they may overlap, interact or intersect with each other – for example, when historical experiences of oppression based on racial and class differences began to shape intergenerational drinking patterns among farm workers in the Western Cape.

Bucher (2010, p.2) defines culture as 'our way of life, including everything that is shared, and transmitted from one generation to the next'. Writing about excessive drinking as a culturally imposed occupation arising from intergenerational experiences of colonisation, Cloete and Ramugondo (2015) suggest that culture underlies what people decide to do, where they prefer to go, and when they would like to engage in certain activities. Drawing on the work of McGruder (1998), they point to the following six attributes of culture that influence people's occupations: it is real (and while culture is intangible, it is a powerful force that shapes the forms and meanings of changes in the social status of a group of people); it is learned and not inherited; it manifests in social interactions and takes place within a specific context, and is thus shared in human society; it is dynamic, and changes slowly over time; it drives and shapes human values; and lastly, since culture is invisible, we are often blind to how our own cultures influence what we do every day.

Repeated experiences with entering other cultural spaces, coupled with introspection, are necessary to make our own cultural assumptions visible to us. Therefore, when contributing to FASD prevention, occupational therapists should be aware of their own cultural values, as opposed to focusing only on the cultural values and practices of the clients they serve. Likewise, women who are immersed in culturally embedded drinking practices only become aware of what they are doing when they are offered opportunities to reflect on and challenge the structures that maintain their internalised oppression (Cloete, 2012; Salmon, 2011). The type of occupational therapy practice that acknowledges historical facts and incorporates knowledge of intergenerational practices into the occupational therapy process may allow practitioners to identify whether and how such practices are sustained as a legacy of colonisation; for example, a product of apartheid is internalised oppression, structural and economic violence, in the form of FASD and foreshortened life expectancy and disability-free life-years for women on wine-growing farms in South Africa (Cloete, 2012).

FASD: The contributions of occupational therapy

The contribution of occupational therapy to mitigating the disabling consequences of FASD through traditional therapeutic approaches is well-documented (Peadon et al, 2009; Franklin et al, 2008). Occupational therapists facilitate the habilitation of children and youth with FASD by helping them acquire or improve performance component skills (for example, perceptual-motor functions as prerequisites for reading and writing) and occupational performance abilities (for example, playing, learning and socialising) that may not be developing according to age-related norms. Alternative contributions of the profession – involving women, their families and communities, and which address imposed occupations – are under-reported in the occupational therapy literature. A possible reason for the limited information about FASD interventions that address occupational risk factors may be that occupational therapists have traditionally been concerned with the treatment of affected individuals, rather than with public health and social development programmes aimed at preventing the disorder from occurring in the first place.

Occupational therapists tend to use the 'lifestyle approach', which educates individuals to make 'healthier lifestyle choices' – for example, by abstaining from alcohol in order to ensure healthy pregnancies (Mundel & Chapman, 2010, p.8). Cloete and Ramugondo (2015) challenge the idea that alcohol abuse is mainly a psychological disorder, which the individual woman who drinks during pregnancy can overcome through behaviour-modification techniques. They argue that health education as the basis of FASD prevention campaigns is not enough to motivate women to modify their drinking behaviour during pregnancy, and propose that recognising alcohol abuse as an imposed occupation will locate the complexities of individual and collective alcohol consumption practices within society; thereby shifting the focus of FASD prevention strategies towards the structural inequities that perpetuate socialisation into excessive drinking.

An occupation-centred revision of understandings of alcohol abuse directs the intervention debate to three issues of concern to occupational therapists. Firstly, to women's intentions for spending time drinking (for example, drinking to get drunk, as opposed to casually enjoying a few beers with friends or family). Secondly, to the personal factors underlying women's drinking patterns (for example, low self-esteem, and limited education). Thirdly, maternal drinking as a culturally imposed practice (i.e. the intergenerational enactment of internalised social and economic oppression). Socially-orientated and occupation-based intervention strategies are indicated because women's use of alcohol as a default way of occupying themselves must be understood and addressed against the backdrop of structural and material poverty; limited economic, cultural and political opportunities; fragile social support systems; and geographic isolation (Cloete & Ramugondo, 2015; Salmon, 2011; Cloete, 2005).

Literature relating to the repertoire (range) of occupations in which women who are at risk of having children with FASD engage is scarce. Cloete (2005) found that despite their alcohol practices, mothers who are at risk of exposing their unborn babies to alcohol also have aspirations for other aspects of their lives; all of which have an occupational dimension that can be explored as part of a personal development narrative. These aspirations include finding a new home, learning an income-generating skill, starting a small garden to alleviate food insecurity, and living free of domestic violence. However, the contexts in which they live make easy access to alcohol a constant threat to the fulfilment of their aspirations. Material and social support for engagement in alternative activities enrich personal development, and enable community members to recognise how excessive drinking patterns limit their own aspirations as well as those of future generations. Occupational therapists may contribute to exploring alternative and more appropriate supportive actions and structures that enhance the health and overall well-being of marginalised populations. It is at this juncture that occupational therapy can support women, as they learn to mobilise access to development opportunities. Social and economic inclusion as a national development agenda provides the policy backdrop for action in marginalised populations. Although the entire community needs to develop a critical recognition of how their recourse to drinking is limiting their aspirations, the children with FASD may provide a key illustration and a locus for occupational therapy via mothers who drink. The route away from drinking that might be enabled through occupational therapy will tap into other intersectoral processes, such as the Departments of Labour, Rural Development and Social Development negotiating appropriate alternatives to the dop system, and employers investing in the health of their workers.

A decolonising development approach is proposed that empowers women to identify and resist structural factors that predispose them and their unborn children to life-long disadvantage and ill-health. The occupational therapy focus shifts from an individual therapeutic orientation to one that targets women's development through occupation. It seeks to support women as active contributors to social and economic transformation, by focusing on them as occupational beings and as persons who are facilitated to explore alternative identities and different engagement with their own time-use and the space available to them – outside the boundaries set by the colonising process. Occupational therapy acknowledges that the bigger issue is a system that views them as a category of person who is not a full citizen, for example, they can be paid in drink rather than in money, and without proper living, working and socialising conditions. An occupation-based focus might be part of the social and economic solution, creating opportunities for individuals and small groups of women to liberate themselves through what they do every day, i.e. their occupations.

A growing body of occupational therapy literature is emerging that theorises occupation-based development practice aimed at addressing the social determinants of health and associated occupational risk factors. For example, Whiteford and Townsend (2011) propose a participatory occupational justice framework to develop more equitable opportunities, resources, privilege and enablement for an occupationally just world. Galvaan and Peters (2013) describe an occupation-based community-development process that challenges the structural inequalities faced by minority youth in previously disadvantaged contexts. The remainder of this chapter describes a development process, aimed at decolonising imposed occupations, that is being developed by Cloete (2012) – an occupational therapy academic, clinician and researcher who has been working alongside women and children with FASD on wine farms in the Western Cape since 1997. Cloete (2012) defines decolonising development as a process whereby women who abuse alcohol and their self-identified role models who have stopped abusing alcohol become actively involved in the identification and addressing of individual, group and community barriers to their individual and collective health, well-being and development. Some occupational therapists may argue that barriers that are symptomatic of a larger economic and political system and structural violence are beyond the remit of occupational therapy. However, Wilcock's work on the occupational perspective of health paved the way for a critical approach to health when she introduced culture, economy and the policy environment as the three occupational determinants (read social determinants) of health (Wilcock, 2006). Her work broadened the scope of occupational therapy beyond biomedical symptoms to include underlying structural, economic and political causes to ill-health. Furthermore, Galvaan's work on occupational choice highlighted the importance of apartheid in South Africa as a significant historic socioeconomic force in perpetuated occupational injustice among adolescents in Lavender Hill (Galvaan, 2014). In identifying the impact of imposed occupations (Cloete & Ramugondo, 2015; Cloete, 2012) on the maternal health, well-being and participation of women who live in rural communities these studies demonstrate the role occupational therapists could play in theorising about and practicing critical occupational therapy that cuts to the heart of occupation. Ramugondo's notion of occupational consciousness (Ramugondo, 2016) draws our attention to the dynamics of hegemonic practices that impact personal and collective health and challenges occupational therapists to explore possibilities for the profession to engage in socially transformative work (Laliberte Rudman, 2015). This means that although individual, group and community action may be the start of such transformative work, occupational therapists have the obligation collaborate with clients in the planning, development and implementation of socially transformative interventions as integral part of their scope of practice. The next section explains how occupational therapists could use the decolonising development process against imposed occupations.

Decolonising imposed occupations: A participatory development process

Figure 1 depicts three phases of an iterative process of planning, reflecting, learning and acting that is being used by an occupational therapist and occupational therapy students to promote the development of women who abuse alcohol during pregnancy, in collaboration with a group of sober role models (Mayson et al, 2014; Cloete, 2012, 2005). Role models are identified by women who use alcohol during pregnancy as older women in the community who have the ability to support, educate, collaborate

Figure 1: A Decolonizing development process against imposed occupations

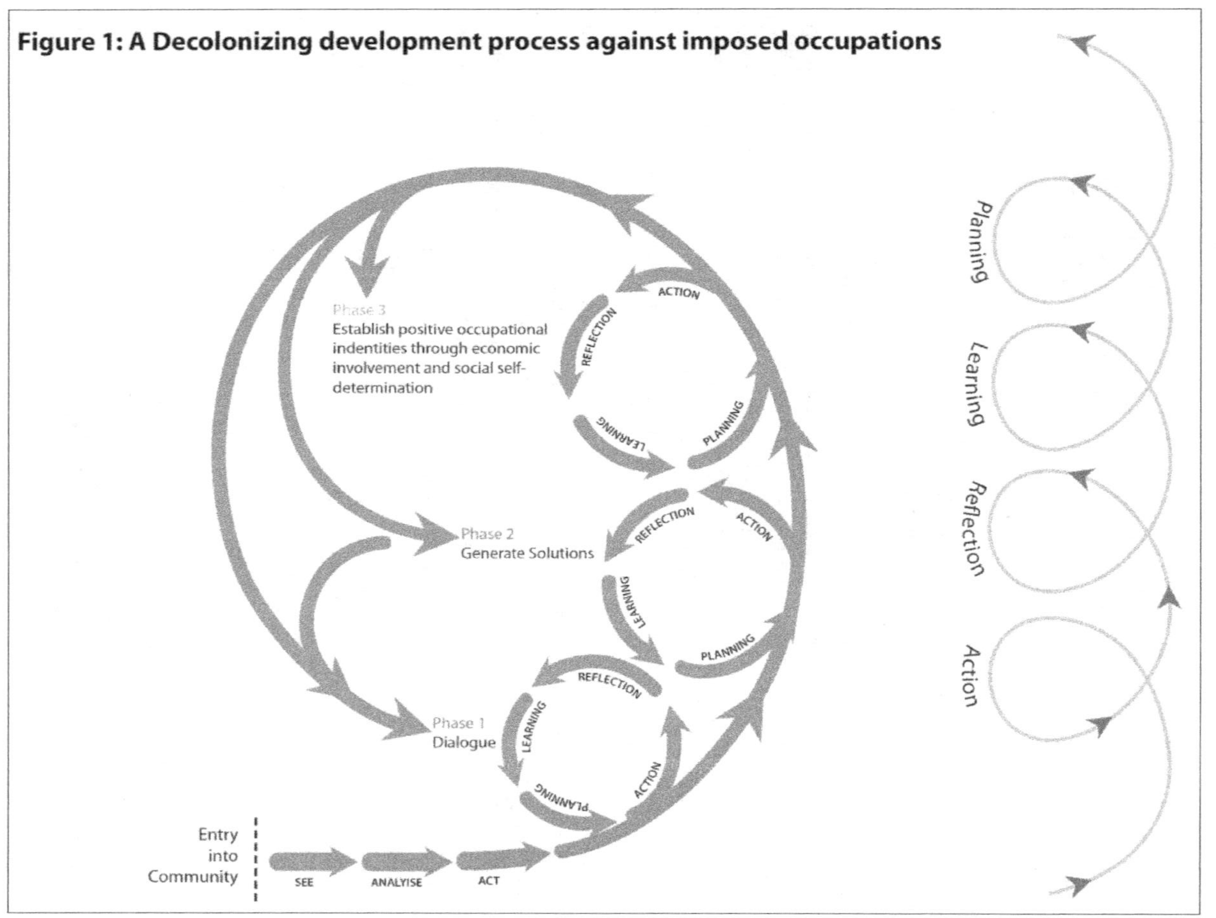

with and inspire others towards sober pregnancies. The women are identified through their affiliation to a non-governmental organisation targeting the needs of persons affected by FASD in the region. This organisation provides the occupational therapist and occupational therapy students with the infrastructure and administrative support necessary for the sustainability of the development process.

The process commenced when the occupational therapist entered the community as a researcher-clinician after requesting an appointment with the manager of the NGO. A period of time was spent *seeing* (observing, listening, learning) and *analysing* (making sense, understanding) before *acting* in collaboration with stakeholders to set three phases of participatory learning in motion. The three phases (dialogue, generating solutions, and establishing positive occupational identities) evolved iteratively and organically in response to emerging individual, group and contextual dynamics. Change has been gradual and imperceptible, with each woman progressing through the phases at her own pace. Some women have reverted to old patterns of drinking from time to time, while others have achieved significant personal goals of sobriety and alternative forms of occupational engagement with the support of their peers and mentors. In the next section we present the general steps depicted in Figure 1.

Entry into community: Starting the process

Entry into the community involves three steps: seeing, analysing and acting. The occupational therapist starts with *seeing* what the women do in their home and community environments. Observations are made as to where, how and with whom they engage in occupations – including the spaces, places and patterns of drinking, caring for self and family, and other forms of socialising. Emphasis is placed on understanding the underlying occupational determinants of FASD – such as economic opportunities, socio-political influences and dominant cultural practices – by asking women about the opportunities and barriers they experience when performing the activities of daily living. Mutual trust develops gradually, as the occupational therapist becomes familiar with and to the women.

The occupational therapist gains understanding of the women's needs and assets in the context of their daily realities, by collaboratively conducting community assessments, for example by using a community asset mapping method (Community Toolbox, 2015) as an assessment tool. She facilitates a process that enables women to assist her with step two (analysing the results from assessments), where the dynamic interactions between personal and cultural histories and prevailing personal and social circumstances are explored, discussed and recorded. During this stage, the occupational therapist does not offer a rehabilitation service by providing any treatment to women. Instead, women are seen as equal partners in exploring actions that may address the barriers identified in the previous step. Step three (acting) gradually emerges, as the occupational therapist ignites awareness of the colonising effects of drinking through posing the 'but-why' question. This flows into three phases of development: dialogue, seeking solutions, and establishing positive occupational identities. The planning-learning-action-reflection cycle (Taylor et al, 2005) is followed during each of the three phases, because it allows the women to feel in control of and accountable for their lives. The group process is complex, with interpersonal differences arising from time to time that are addressed through conflict resolution sessions facilitated by older role models. The occupational therapist remains conscious of the need for cultural sensitivity throughout all the phases, by following the strategies suggested by Galheigo (2011):

- increasing her knowledge of the women, their families, and their norms, beliefs and values, as expressed in their environment;
- initiating and developing cooperative practices, by involving the women as well as their role models in designing and implementing the change process;
- adapting interventions to be culturally appropriate and suited to the environment.

The occupational therapist reflects on professional and personally held assumptions regarding the people, the context and their occupations, through discussions with colleagues and cultural insiders. Box 1 captures an excerpt from Cloete's (2005) practice journal that illustrates how the occupational therapist strives for ethical and culturally sensitive community entry through self-reflection.

Box 1: Self-reflection

"I acknowledged my status as a visitor and a novice in the lives of participants. The value of assuming this attitude was that a rightful place was assumed by myself and the participants. It acknowledged the participants' position as primary occupants and encouraged a relationship in which participants could introduce me to people and places around the community, as well as usher me into participating in everyday community practices. I made sure that I was dressed in informal clothes that were appropriate for the context. I familiarised myself with the local dialect and avoided using professional words. Introductions, and the decision of who should be contacted first and when, were vital in determining the success of the rest of my encounter with the women. Emphasis was placed on looking for ways of helping or supporting women to have healthy pregnancies. Instead of looking for women who consume alcohol during pregnancy (a fault-finding approach), this approach fostered an optimistic atmosphere of care. Caution was exercised to avoid creating any expectations that the process could not meet."

Reflective community entry

Phase 1: dialogue

Phase 1 serves as a catalyst for critical thinking, through which women begin to question and talk about the reasons they give for excessive drinking and prenatal alcohol consumption. Dialogue (facilitated conversations) is a process during which people are able to 'name their world' (Freire, 2002). It consists of purposefully structured opportunities for women facing similar structural disadvantages to explore the underlying determinants of the everyday things that occupy their time, interest and energies, including harmful drinking patterns. Dialogue topics foreground occupations, and the choices women make or are prevented from making that place them, their children and their community at risk through what they do every day. Freire (2002, p.88-89) described true dialogue as:

> 'the encounter in which the united reflection and action of the dialoguers are addressed to the world which is to be transformed and humanised; this dialogue cannot be reduced to the act of one person depositing ideas in another, nor can it become a simple exchange of ideas to be 'consumed' by the discussants.'

By 'naming their world', the women gradually become able to transform their immediate spheres of influence. Naming makes their realities known. It reveals the world they live in and the interplay between their being in the world and the factors that determine who they represent, what positions they hold, and pertinently, how the ordinary, everyday things that occupy their time, energy and interests shape their identities, health and development. However, an occupation-focused dialogue should not leave the occupational therapist directing the process. A Freirean approach aims at liberating the women through the critical process they develop in dialogue. Box 2 below captures an excerpt from a dialogue session that illustrates a Freirean approach in dealing with emergent issues.

Box 2: Facilitating a critical dialogue

Facilitating a dialogue requires the occupational therapist firstly to be aware of the power differentials between herself as facilitator, and the participants. When entering the dialogue space, the participants are equal partners to the dialogue process. The therapist invites participants to own and co-create the space by informing them of the following norms: All participants have equal rights and responsibilities to ensure that the negotiated norms are maintained; in large groups, each participant should get an opportunity to speak once before a second turn is afforded; all contributions are voluntary; all opinions are equally important and valid, while the therapist remains impartial; participants have the ability to offer their own solutions, while the therapists ask questions to guide participants toward critical thinking in seeking solutions; the group agrees on the duration of the dialogue as well as on actions taken based on the suggestions made.

The dialogue takes the form of a conversation rather than question and answer format. The occupational therapist creates a relaxed atmosphere and asks participants how they would like to be addressed. Each participant is encouraged to name his/her own realities and not that of others. Mutual learning is a basic principle as the speaker can be both teacher and learner. The occupational therapist as facilitator stays impartial and reflects on ALL views; participants have the ability to generate their own problems should they wish. The occupational therapist does not take the responsibility to fix problems that arise in the dialogue.

By becoming conscientised (critically aware) about their personal power to resist drinking as a colonial remnant, they begin to consider alternative forms of

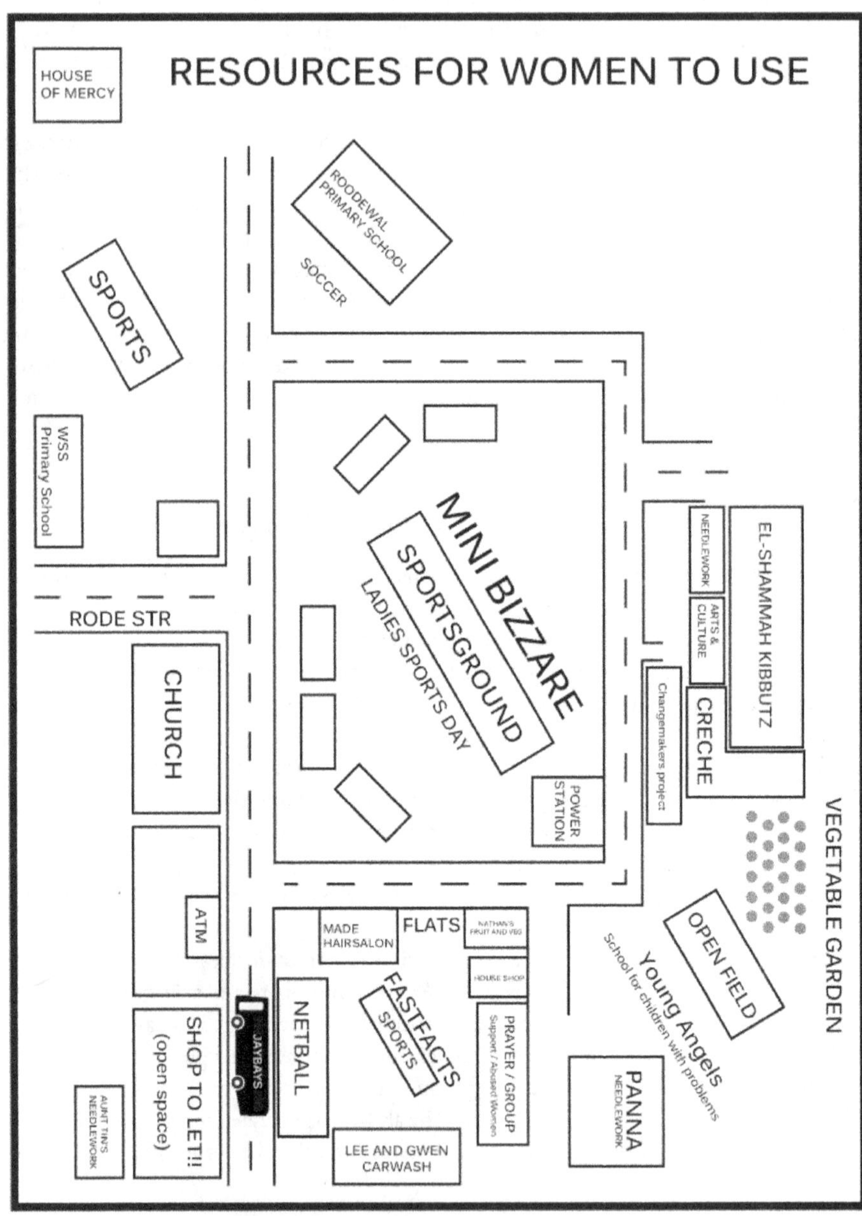

Figure 2. Community asset mapping

occupation that promote health and development, for themselves and their children. The facilitated dialogue sessions gradually transition into Phase 2 when practicable solutions begin to emerge and start to be implemented.

Phase 2: generate solutions

During Phase 2, the dialogue shifts from problem identification to solution naming. It consists of a series of workshops in which asset mapping is used to help the women generate ideas for health-promoting occupations as alternatives to drinking (Mayson et al, 2014). Asset mapping involves documenting the tangible and intangible resources of a community that can support alternative forms of occupation to replace drinking, viewing it as a place with assets to be preserved and enhanced, not deficits to be remedied. Assets may be in the form of persons, physical structures, natural resources, institutions, businesses, non-governmental organisations or informal social networks that may be accessed to promote personal and collective development (Community Tool Box, 2015). Women are affirmed as capable of identifying steps to change their personal drinking patterns, and trusted to follow through on decolonising actions when they feel ready to do so. They explore personal and collective options, opportunities and actions that may be taken, with due consideration of the constraints and barriers they face. They gradually realise that the locus of control resides within them to effect personal and social change, by tapping into available resources, skills and knowledge – for example, learning skills from each other, such as sewing, gardening, baking, reading, hairdressing and catering. Figure 2 depicts an example of a community asset map that was generated during a Phase 2 workshop.

Phase 3: Establish positive occupational identities

Some women proceed to Phase 3 by actively pursuing the solutions identified during Phase 2. They begin to engage in new occupations, such as obtaining a driver's licence, doing an accounting course, becoming an apprentice hairdresser, starting a communal garden and joining a soup kitchen to alleviate food insecurity, or finding out about municipal by-laws that support citizen rights in the fight against poor service delivery. Structural barriers are tackled by identifying training opportunities and linking women with these programmes offered at local government level. Women are also connected to non-governmental organisations that may address housing and employment needs. Some women become mentors to other women who are still drinking during pregnancy, and collaborate with and enable their mentees to access existing community resources and network with identified service providers.

Positive occupational identities start to emerge as women report back to the group about the personal, family and collective benefits of economic involvement and social self-determination. Individual and community-identified indicators, plotted and adjusted over time by the women themselves, become recognisable when an occupational perspective is adopted. Shifts in individual and collective occupational choices can be observed, measured and described. Box 3 captures Konstabel's story of establishing a positive occupational identity. It illustrates the gradual decolonising trajectory of her occupational patterns from regular intoxication to sobriety to starting her own non-profit organisation.

Box 3: a story of establishing a positive occupational identity

At first a destroyer, now a builder

More than 23 years ago, I was one of the biggest drug peddlers in my community. Due to abuse in my parents' home, I didn't ever know love. We were 21 children, and that's where everything started – there was never enough love and acceptance to go around for all of us. All of this forced me to find refuge in things that would satisfy my needs. At the age of 15 or 16 (years of age) I ended up in a relationship with a dealer who exposed me to all the dangers in life, the abuse of drugs, my first encounter with dagga (cannabis) and Mandrax. Many nights I lay awake wondering whether this was the type of life that I wanted to lead, but I didn't have a choice; everything I was searching for was served up on a plate – dagga, Mandrax, and (together with hundreds of litres of alcohol) money was always available; but it was love that was missing. There was an abundance of material things that I had never had in my life. In this relationship with my boyfriend (the dealer), I was forced to take on the role of peddler, by selling drugs and alcohol to people – yes, all the forbidden substances; and under-aged children and pregnant women were the market that I targeted. And it is at this young and tender age that you learn to experiment with these forbidden substances.

At one stage of my life, I was caught for dealing and selling of dagga, alcohol and tablets to people, and received a suspended sentence of plus/minus two years. For many years this continued, and later I married my boyfriend (the dealer), and I was abused and forced to do things that I didn't want to do; yes, I was battered and hurt repeatedly, and at times humiliated in front of his friends, I never imagined that this boyfriend whom I had once loved only wanted to use me. There was never any love, and I was only ever used to do all the dirty work.

Alcohol was one of my best sellers, and I found it easy to peddle it to youngsters and women. And pregnant mommies who at that stage of their lives also suffered in abusive relationships – I always thought that I could lessen their pain by providing them with these forbidden substances; little did I know that I was causing them harm.

I destroyed many lives, broke up many marriages, for the sake of enriching and pleasing my boyfriend. After many years of abuse in my marriage I decided to divorce this man whom I had once been in love with. I decided there and then that I was destroying other people's lives. I then focused on the community and their needs and started working with abused women, by re-building that which I had once destroyed.

In 2012 I got involved with a local non-governmental organisation that focuses on the prevention of alcohol use by pregnant women. Over time I met the occupational therapy researcher involved with the organisation, who educated us about the dangers of alcohol and the effect it has on the physical, psychological and social development of the unborn child. The support I experienced and the guidance provided by the occupational therapist will remain with me always. That is where I realised how many unborn children's lives I had destroyed, how many mommies I left in pain, and how many marriages I destroyed. There were many days I wished I could turn back the clock and put right that which I had destroyed; but yes, as the saying goes: what's done is done.

In 2014 or 2015 the occupational therapist introduced us to a group of occupational therapy students who trained us further in projects we could use to uplift our community, such as needlework, hairstyling, soup kitchens, and many more. We were taught how to deal with pregnant women who are drinking, how to approach them and how to walk by their side; and truly, we can say that what we had learned bore fruit, and God was truly with us in this work.

Many of the pregnant mommies now lead a changed life, are looking well, and continue building for the future of their children. We are thankful to be voicing our needs and contributing to build our community for our children. A seed was planted, and we are all working towards a big crop.

Conclusion

A critical occupational therapy response to the prevention of FASD is indicated; one that extends beyond a biomedical approach of health promotion and prevention that illuminates occupational determinants as causal factors of ill-health and disability. Such a response may enable occupational therapists to identify those occupations that are sustained by hegemonic (oppressive) practices, norms and values that are embedded in the social matrix of society. Dialogue using Freirean principles may facilitate subaltern groups (marginalised groups who may have lost the ability to voice their concerns or views) to generate and explore solutions in collaboration with the occupational therapy practitioner. This approach may challenge practitioners' approach to occupation-based interventions in reconstructing power relations between therapist and client, community and society. The chapter used maternal alcohol abuse to demonstrate that occupational therapy is positioned to support at-risk and vulnerable groups through the creation of participatory action spaces that interrogate taken-for-granted practices. A glance beyond individually-determined practices to the causal historical and socio-political determinants of health and participation in health-giving occupations may address the negative impact of engaging in imposed occupations.

References

Althouse, A.P. (2014) Drunkenness and interpersonal violence in colonial Michoacán. in G. Pierce and A. Toxqui (Eds.) *Alcohol in Latin America: A social and cultural history.* Tucson AZ: University of Arizona Press (pp.67-86)

Australian Institute of Health and Welfare (2015) *Fetal Alcohol Spectrum Disorders: A review of interventions for prevention and management in Indigenous communities. Resource sheet no. 36 prepared by the Closing the Gap Clearinghouse.* Canberra: Australian Government. [Accessed 18 April 2016 at http://www.healthinfonet.ecu.edu.au/key-resources/bibliography?lid=29130]

Bradshaw, D., Norman, R. and Schneider, M. (2007) A clarion call for action based on refined

DALY estimates for South Africa. Editorial. *South African Medical Journal,* 97, 438-440

Bucher, R.D. (2010) *Diversity Consciousness: Opening our minds and opportunities.* Upper Saddle River, NJ: Prentice Hall

Cloete, L. (2005) *Occupations of Women who Live and/or Work in a Rural Farming Community and who are at Risk of having Children with Foetal Alcohol Syndrome (FAS).* Cape Town: University of Cape Town

Cloete, L. (2012) *Developing Appropriate Fetal Alcohol Spectrum Disorder (FASD) Prevention Initiatives within a Rural Community in South Africa.* Cape Town: University of Cape Town

Cloete, L.G. and Ramugondo, E.L. (2015) 'I drink': Mothers' alcohol consumption as both individualised and imposed occupation. *South African Journal of Occupational Therapy,* 45, 1, 34-40

Community Toolbox (2015) Identifying community assets and resources. *Community Toolbox,* Chapter 3, Section 8. University of Kansas Workgroup for Community Health and Development. [Accessed 14th October 2016 at http://ctb.ku.edu/]

Davids, I., Theron, F. and Mapunye, K. (2009) *Participatory Development in South Africa. A development management perspective.* Pretoria: Van Schaik

De Kock, A. (2002) *Fruit of the Vine, Work of Human Hands. Farm workers and alcohol on a farm in Stellenbosch, South Africa.* M.A. thesis, Social Anthropology, University of Cape Town. [Accessed 14th October 2016 at https://open.uct.ac.za/handle/11427/10342]

Frank, G., Kitching, H.J., Joe, A., Harvey, C., Bertram, A., Bechar, R., Blanchard, J. and Taguchi- Meyer, J. (2008) Postcolonial practice in occupational therapy: The Tule River tribal history project. in N. Pollard, F. Kronenberg and D. Sakellariou (Eds.) *A Political Practice of Occupational Therapy.* Edinburgh: Elsevier (pp.223-235)

Franklin, L., Deitz, J., Jirikowic, T. and Astley, S. (2008) Children with fetal alcohol spectrum disorders. *Problem Behaviors and Sensory Processing,* 62, 3, 265-273

Freire, P. (2002) *Pedagogy of the Oppressed,* 30th Anniversary edition. (Trans. M. Bergan Ramos). New York: Continuum

Galheigo, S. (2011) What needs to be done? Occupational therapy responsibilities and challenges regarding human rights. *Australian Occupational Therapy Journal,* 58, 60-66

Galvaan, R. (2010) *A Critical Ethnography of Young Adolescents' Occupational Choices in a Community in Post-Apartheid South Africa.* Cape Town, South Africa: University of Cape Town

Galvaan, R. (2014) The contextually situated nature of occupational choice: Marginalised young adolescents' experiences in South Africa. *Journal of Occupational Science,* 21, 1-15

Galvaan, R. and Peters, L. (2013) *Occupation-Based Community Development Framework.* [Accessed 15th June 2015 at Open Education Resource http://opencontent.uct.ac.za/Health-Sciences/Occupation-based-Community-Development-Framework]

George, M.M. (2007) Bridging the research gap: Aboriginal and academic collaboration in FASD prevention. The Healthy Communities, Mothers and Children Project, Alaska. *Medicine,* 49, 2, 139-141

Hammell, K.W. and Iwama, M.K. (2012) Wellbeing and occupational rights: An imperative for critical occupational therapy. *Scandinavian Journal of Occupational Therapy,* 19, 385-394

Laliberte Rudman, D. (2015) Situating occupation in social relations of power: Occupational possibilities, ageism and the retirement 'choice'. *South African Journal of Occupational Therapy,* 45, 1, 27-33

London, L. (1999) The 'dop' system, alcohol abuse and social control amongst farm workers in South Africa: A public health challenge. *Social Science and Medicine,* 48,10, 1407-1414

Maier, S. and West, J. (2001) Patterns and alcohol-related birth defects. *National Alcohol Research, 25*, 3, 168-174

Malfitano A.P.S., Lopes R.E., Magalhaes L. and Townsend E.A. (2014) Social occupational therapy: Conversations about a Brazilian experience. *Canadian Journal of Occupational Therapy,* 81, 5, 298-307

May, P.A., Gossage, J.P., Brooke, L.E., Snell, E.L., Marais, A.S., Hendricks, L.S., Croxford, J.A. and Viljoen, D.L. (2005) Maternal risk factors for fetal alcohol syndrome in the Western Cape province of South Africa: A population-based study. *American Journal of Public Health,* 95, 7, 1190-1199

May, P.A., Blankenship, J., Marais, A., Gossage, J.P., Kalberg, W.O., Barnard, R., De Vries, M., Robinson, L.K., Adnams, C.M., Buckley, D., Manning, M., Jones, K.L., Parry, C. et al., (2012) Approaching the prevalence of the full spectrum of fetal alcohol spectrum disorders in a South African population-based study. *Alcoholism: Clinical and Experimental Research,* 37, 5, 818-830

Mayson T., Mcmillan D-L., Minnaar S., Schneider C., and Duncan M. (2014) *Women in a Low Socio-Economic Community: Exploring occupational opportunities as a preventative strategy for fetal alcohol spectrum disorder.* Cape Town: University of Cape Town

McGruder, J. (1998) Culture and other forms of human diversity in occupational therapy. in M.E. Neistadt and E. Blesedell Crepeau (Eds.) *Willard and Spackman's Occupational Therapy.* (9th ed.) Philadelphia: J.B Lippincott (pp.54-66)

Mundel, E. and Chapman, G.E. (2010) A decolonising approach to health promotion in Canada: The case of the Urban Aboriginal Community Kitchen Garden Project. *Health Promotion International,* 25, 2,166-173

Olivier, L., Urban, M., Chersich, M., Temmerman, M. and Viljoen, D. (2013) Burden of foetal alcohol syndrome in a rural west coast area of South Africa. *South African Medical Journal,* 103, 6, 402-405

Peadon, E., Rhys-Jones, B., Bower, C. and Elliott, E.J. (2009) Systematic review of interventions for children with fetal alcohol spectrum disorders. *BMC Pediatrics,* 9, 35. [Accessed 17 September at https://bmcpediatr.biomedcentral.com/track/pdf/10.1186/1471-2431-9-35?site=bmcpediatr.biomedcentral.com]

Ramugondo, E. (2000) *The Experience of Being an Occupational Therapy Student with an Underrepresented Ethnic and Cultural Background.* Doctoral dissertation, University of Cape Town. [Accessed 14th October 2016 at https://open.uct.ac.za/bitstream/item/3244/thesis_hsf_2000_ramugondo_e.pdf?sequence=1]

Ramugondo, E. (2009) *Intergenerational Shifts and Continuities in Children's Play within a Rural Venda Family in the Early 20th and 21st Centuries.* PhD. University of Cape Town. [Accessed 14th October 2016 at https://open.uct.ac.za/handle/11427/12113]

Ramugondo, E. (2012) Intergenerational play within family: The case of occupational consciousness. *Journal of Occupational Science,* 19, 326-340

Ramugondo, E.L. (2016) Occupational consciousness. *Journal of Occupational Science,* 22, 4, 488-501

Rendall-Mkosi, K.M. (2007) *Comprehensive FAS prevention programme model development in South Africa.* Conference paper delivered at the Second International Conference on Foetal Alcohol Spectrum Disorder: Research, Policy, and Practice around the World. Victoria, Canada

Royal Commission on Aboriginal Peoples (1996) Report. Volume 2, Part 2. Chapter 4, section 3. *Improving access to natural resources.* [Accessed 18 September 2017 at http://www.specific-claims-law.com/index.php?option=com_content&view=article&id=16&Itemid=18]

Salmon, A. (2011) Aboriginal mothering, FASD prevention and the contestations of neoliberal citizenship. *Critical Public Health,* 21, 2, 165-178

Scully, P. (1992) Liquor and labour in the Western Cape, 1870-1900. in J. Crush and C. Ambler (Eds.) *Liquor and Labour in Southern Africa.* Athens: Ohio University Press (pp.56-77)

Setlalentoa, B.M.P., Pisa, P.T., Thekisho, G.N., Ryke, E.H. and Loots, Du T. (2010) The social aspects of alcohol misuse/abuse in South Africa. *South African Journal of Clinical Nutrition,* 23, 3 Supplement 1, S11-S15

Sherwood, J. and Edwards, T. (2006) Decolonisation: A critical step for improving aboriginal health. *Contemporary Nurse: A Journal for the Australian Nursing Profession,* 22, 178-190

Schneider, M., Norman, R., Parry, C.D.L., Bradshaw, D. and Plüddemann, A. (2007) Estimating the burden of alcohol abuse in South Africa in 2000. *South African Medical Journal,* 97, 8, 664-673

Sztompka, P. (1993) *The Sociology of Social Change.* Oxford: Blackwell

Taylor, J., Marais, D. and Kaplan, A. (2005) *Action Learning. A developmental approach to change.* CDRA Nuggets. [Accessed 14th October 2016 at https://www.scribd.com/document/96455215/Action-Learning-a-Developmental-Approach-to-Change-August-2005-CDRA-Nugget]

Van der Leeden, M.V. (2001) Infants exposed to alcohol prenatally: Outcome at 3 and 7 months of age. *Annals of Tropical Paediatrics, 21,* 2, 127-134

Vythilingum, B., Roos, A., Faure, S.C., Geerts, L. and Stein, D.J. (2012) Risk factors for substance use in pregnant women in South Africa. *South African Medical Journal,* 102, 11, 851-854

Weeramanthri, T.S. and Bailie, R.S. (2015) Grand challenges in public health policy. *Front Public Health,* 3, 29. [Accessed 29 May 2016 at http://journal.frontiersin.org/article/10.3389/fpubh.2015.00029/full]

Whiteford, G. and Townsend, E.A. (2011) Participatory occupational justice framework (POJF 2010): Enabling occupational participation and inclusion. in F. Kronenberg, N. Pollard and D. Sakellariou (Eds.) *Occupational Therapy without Borders: Towards an ecology of education based practices* (Vol. 2). New York: Elsevier/ Churchill Livingstone (pp. 65-84)

Wilcock, A.A. (2006) *An Occupational Perspective of Health.* Thorofare, NJ: Slack

Williams, J. and Smith, V. (the Committee on Substance abuse) (2015) Fetal alcohol spectrum disorders. *Pediatrics,* 135, 5, e1395-e1406. [Accessed 17 September at http://pediatrics.aappublications.org/content/pediatrics/early/2015/10/13/peds.2015-3113.full.pdf]

World Health Organisation (1986) *The Ottawa Charter for Health Promotion.* First International Conference on Health Promotion. Ottawa. 17-21 November. [Accessed 17 September 2016 at http://www.who.int/healthpromotion/conferences/previous/ottawa/en/]

World Health Organisation (2014) *Global Status Report on Alcohol and Healt*h. Luxembourg: WHO

Chapter 14
Promoting positive collective occupations in African settings: Exploiting the latent potentials for social inclusion and well-being

Tongai Fibion Chichaya

Introduction

The author of this chapter has worked as an occupational therapist in Southern Africa specifically Zimbabwe and Namibia, both in clinical settings and at administrative level as a coordinator for a national community based rehabilitation (CBR) programme within primary health care services. The need for occupational therapy in the African communities is high; occupational disruption and exclusion as a result of socio-economic and political causes are common. The need for occupational therapy in the African communities is high; occupational dysfunctions and exclusion as a result of socio-economic and political causes are wide spread. Most occupational therapists in Africa still work in medical settings, but the majority of the people who need occupational therapy, such as the vulnerable and marginalized people, do not get these services. The circumstances mentioned result in occupational injustices whereby the affected individuals are powerless in making decisions about their own life choices, and they are restricted from participating in meaningful daily life occupations that bring them fulfilment and satisfaction (Wolf et al, 2002).

If occupational therapists continue to only focus on people referred to them with a medical diagnosis then their expertise in promoting occupational justice will not help the majority who are socially excluded (Wilcock, 1999). In Africa there is an increasing recognition of the need for occupational therapists to work to support social policies, actions, and laws that allow people to engage in occupations that have purpose and meaning in their lives (Sherry, 2010). This focus enables the occupational therapy profession to highlight the contributions it can offer to groups of persons, organizations and populations in non-clinical settings particularly those affected by marginalization and poverty (Moyers & Dale, 2007; Pollard et al, 2005; World Federation of Occupational Therapists (WFOT), 2004). Already some occupational therapists practicing in Africa have multiple roles, including designing disability related services, decision making at organizational levels and supporting and empowering vulnerable groups in societies away from the treatment rooms (Sherry, 2010).

This chapter highlights the need for social inclusion through occupation in Africa and emphasizes the necessity of refocusing the occupational therapy paradigm to meet the needs on the continent. Furthermore, the multifaceted nature of occupation is discussed including examples of positive occupations and the dark side of occupations performed collectively in the African context. Finally, the chapter presents some suggestions on how to move forward in promoting positive collective occupations as a means towards social inclusion and well-being.

The need for social inclusion through occupation in Africa

Wide spread poverty within most African communities has been documented and the impossibilities of articulating occupational therapy in Africa without addressing the extreme poverty and other challenges, such HIV/AIDS and drug resistant TB, stigma and discrimination, has been highlighted (Crouch, 2010b; Sherry, 2010; World Bank, 2007). Many people in vulnerable circumstances such as people with disabilities, people in poverty, orphans, children who drop out of schools or have never been to school, migrants, homeless individuals and people displaced by civil wars find themselves on the sidelines of societal participation and are often excluded from general community development (Townsend & Marval, 2013; Whiteford, 2004). For social inclusion to be achieved among these occupationally deprived groups approaches are required which enable them to be fully involved in making decisions about their future. Occupational therapists are strategically positioned to fill the gap as change agents (Van Bruggen, 2014).

The percentage of marginalized populations in Africa is significantly high. Africa has a population of over a billion people and has the highest percentage of people who live on less than $1.90 per day compared to other continents (World Bank, 2018). Ironically, Africa is the richest continent in terms of natural and mineral resources with about 30% of the world's minerals (Yager et al, 2012). While financial poverty in Africa decreased from 56% in 1990 to 43% in 2012, the number of people in poverty actually increased from 280 million to 330 million (Kathleen et al, 2016). Given the close association between poverty and disability, more people are likely to end up with disability if the number of people in poverty continues to increase. World Health Organization (WHO) reports indicate an estimation of more than 81 million people with disabilities in Africa, however the collection of comparable data is problematic because countries use different approaches in collecting disability data (WHO, 2011; Eide and Loeb, 2005). Among the WHO regions, Africa has the highest prevalence rate of severe disability (WHO, 2011). In 2012, orphans as a result of HIV/AIDS were estimated to be 16 million worldwide of which 14.8 million were in sub-Sahara Africa and many of them live in child headed households (UNAIDS, 2012). About 12 million people are internally displaced in Africa as a result of conflicts, violence and human rights abuses (Essoungou, 2010). The displaced populations often have no access to shelter, means of livelihoods and legal protection and often experience occupational alienation in refugee camps for example (Townsend and Polatajko, 2013; Townsend and Marval, 2013).

The current global health challenges such as non-communicable diseases (NCDs) 'silent killers', also known as lifestyle diseases, present an opportunity for a bigger impact of occupational therapy in Africa in the area of promoting healthy lifestyles.

The most common of these are cardiovascular diseases, followed by cancers, chronic respiratory diseases and diabetes. Africa has seen an increase in non-communicable diseases, being responsible for 20-30% of all deaths in many African countries. In Namibia and South Africa, they contribute to 43% of deaths for all age groups, while in Algeria they contribute 77% of deaths, surpassing communicable diseases (WHO, 2014). In parts of Africa such as Namibia, Mauritius and Seychelles non-communicable diseases contribute more than 50% of adult deaths, implying an increase in disability and ill health among the most socioeconomically productive population.

The main identified causes of NCDs are: tobacco use; physical inactivity; harmful use of alcohol; and unhealthy diet (WHO, 2014). The term lifestyle diseases imply that these diseases are a result of what people do or their occupations. In Namibia, tobacco smoking and alcohol consumption contribute 30% to the risk of NDCs among adults, which is quite high compared to other African countries (WHO, 2014). Less resourced countries are unfortunately faced with a double disease burden i.e. the increasing prevalence of non-communicable diseases and the already high prevalence of communicable diseases such as HIV/AIDS and drug resistant tuberculosis (Boutayeb, 2006).

In many African settings people with disabilities are often kept hidden in their homes, especially children. Their families fear being stigmatized and discriminated as being cursed or under some punishment from supernatural powers (Lansdown, 2002). The trends are changing as governments and the third sector continue to introduce more disability targeted programs and projects. For example, the availability of the disability grants which is a cash-based safety net in countries like Namibia and South Africa has encouraged persons with disabilities to register with statutory services so that they can access the benefits.

Refocusing on the occupation paradigm in African settings

The history of how occupational therapy came to Africa presents challenges that require occupational therapists practicing in Africa to shift from a predominately medical model to the occupation paradigm, both individually and collectively. History shows that between 1940 and 1950, the occupational therapy profession together with other health professions, was entering the biomechanical phase with a focus on how the body functions. As a result attention to occupation was to a greater extent diverted towards the mechanist paradigm (Kielhofner, 2009; Joubert, 2010). Unfortunately, it was during this period that occupational therapy came to South Africa, initially through the then colonial masters. It later began spreading to other African countries, such as Zimbabwe, Namibia, Zambia, Malawi and Lesotho in southern Africa; Kenya, Uganda, Tanzania and more recently Rwanda in eastern Africa; Nigeria, Burkina Faso, and Burundi in Western Africa (Crouch, 2010c). Currently the Occupational Therapy Africa Regional Group (OTARG), which is a WFOT regional group, has a membership of 17 countries (OTARG, 2014). While other African countries are not OTARG members they have occupational therapy presence, for example Tunisia, Egypt, Algeria and Morocco in North Africa. As a result of the mechanist paradigm, most of occupational therapists in Africa work in referral hospitals which are mostly situated in urban areas and are often absent in rural areas where the needs are even higher when considering for example that the percentage of people with disabilities is higher in rural areas compared to urban areas.

However, the ethos of occupational therapy focuses on the innate desire of all humanity to want to do and to be and by so doing, to become more of oneself. The need at population level should be to ensure that individuals find belonging to their communities where they are viewed as equal members making decisions on issues that affect them and participating in occupations of their choice and need (Wilcock, 2006). However, in developing countries there are few practicing occupational therapists, often less than one per 10,000 population (WHO, 2011). For example, Nigeria reported 20 occupational therapists for a population of more than 174 million (WFOT, 2014; World Bank, 2014). In countries like Lesotho and Zambia, where only five occupational therapists were reported to be working in each country respectively, there can be a more significant impact in working for social inclusion for many vulnerable groups through engaging and collaborating with stakeholders in the community (WFOT, 2014; Watson & Swartz, 2004).

The reality of working for social inclusion among occupational therapists in many African settings is challenging for a number of reasons. Firstly, there is a lack of employment opportunities in such roles meaning that there is need work for creation of these roles. Secondly, working for social inclusion is often not situated in places of comfort e.g. slums, poverty-stricken communities, high crime areas, under developed rural areas and sometimes working with stigmatized populations. Despite these challenges, applying knowledge of occupation in social inclusion work has been found to be rewarding and satisfying for occupational therapists who are willing to remain true to the foundations of the profession and work to empower marginalized groups (Sherry, 2010; Stickley, 2015).

Evidence shows that the vicious cycle of poverty, disability and discrimination can be broken by taking strategic steps in education, health, social and developmental sectors (WHO, 2011). In education for example, the application of the occupation-based community development framework (ObCD), has shown success in promoting social inclusion and education among vulnerable adolescents through collaboration in a low socio-economic setting with deep rooted apartheid ideologies in South Africa (Galvaan & Peters, 2013; Galvaan, 2010). Through getting education and better performance, the adolescents will have more opportunities to make decisions about their future, get work and consequently a way out of poverty leading to better quality of life. While it is equally important for occupational therapists to help those who need help in medical settings, it is important to think differently and find creative ways of addressing the huge need of the excluded populations without neglecting the current service users. Some possible considerations are addressed towards the end of this chapter.

In order for greater impact to be created towards social inclusion through occupation, occupational therapists have key roles to play at societal level. They can use their skills in problem solving, group dynamics, advocacy and being change agents. These skills can be used to promote societal well-being through participation in culturally relevant and meaningful occupations, as evidenced by the way some occupational therapists working in South African townships with extreme poverty have innovated (Watson & Swartz, 2004). However, there is still not enough evidence on the impact of occupation in social inclusion in African settings, despite the fact that by the use of occupation, occupational therapists are making a positive impact on the continent (Crouch, 2010a). Possible reasons for the limited evidence on the importance of promoting social inclusion through occupation in African settings could be lack of research expertise, and limited time and resources among occupational therapists (Upton et al, 2014).

Occupation needs to be propagated in terms of human existence rather than in terms of the mechanistic paradigm or a functional - dysfunctional continuum. This chapter takes the stance that occupation is the essence of human existence and every person deserves an equal opportunity for optimum occupational participation despite disability, developmental stage, or socio-cultural, economic or political background. Occupational therapists need to reflect on the way they apply occupation individually and how it can be articulated to address prevailing pressing social, health and community development needs in order to promote health, well-being and social inclusion. Wilcock (1999) further highlights that occupational therapists may end up with feelings of powerlessness because they have not viewed themselves as a profession with expertise on the occupational nature of human beings. Some writers postulate that the survival of the occupational therapy profession is under threat if it remains focused on institutional practice and not moving more towards the community, where many people experience occupational injustice and exclusion from participating in meaningful occupations (Thew et al, 2011).

There is a challenge when articulating occupation and related constructs because occupational therapists use common words but with different meanings from those used in African contexts. If the general population is asked about what is occupation they will most probably refer to employment or having a job, yet occupation is everything people do, including self-care and leisure activities, from an occupational therapist's perspective. The concept of self-care and associated tasks can vary widely in the African context. For example, bathing to the ovaHimba women in Northern Namibia, entails covering themselves with a blanket and having a smoke bath from burning certain plants, because in their culture women do not bath with water at all, in fact it is considered a disgrace for a woman's body to be washed with water (Coussement, 2015). In other communities taking a bath entails a lot of cognitive and physical performance components required for walking a long distance to fetch water in a bucket from a river or some form of water point. These perspectives are a huge contrast with the notion of bathing as self-care in the developed countries where the term originated and refers to someone getting into the bathroom and using running water from a shower or bath tub to execute the occupation of bathing.

In many African languages the terms such as occupation, activities, and tasks are just the same word (Ramukumba, 2014). Their meaning can even further extend to other terms such as behavior. It therefore calls for linkages of terminology used across societal strata to ensure a common understanding when communicating among agents of social reform and the local communities, preferably using more descriptions and explanations than just terms (Kronenberg et al, 2005; Bowen, 2001). Occupational therapy education in Africa needs to increase emphasis on empowering the students and professionals on the use of terminologies that are understood by the local communities and are culturally relevant without diluting the focus on occupation as underpinned by occupational therapy and occupational science (Lorenzo et al, 2006).

The different faces of occupation and social inclusion

Historically, occupation has been conventionally embraced as the good things people do, with the outcomes of enhancing good health and well-being. However, this perception has been confronted with evidence that not all occupations are positive or can lead to good health, and that occupation is multidimensional including the occupations that are considered to be damaging, having negative effects on health, deviant or antisocial occupations also described as the dark side to occupation (Twinley, 2012). A broader understanding of the multifaceted nature of occupations is important for occupational therapists when taking steps to promote positive social inclusion. Occupations can be performed either individually or collectively in groups.

Some examples of antisocial occupations include crimes such as stealing, street fighting and substance misuse. In high-density suburbs and informal settlements of most African countries, for example, shebeens and other unlicensed liquor outlets selling potentially harmful homemade brews are located within the residential areas and children are exposed to alcohol use and cigarette smoking. When patrons are drunk they may use foul language and engage in more antisocial occupations. As a result children are socialized to follow suit as they grow and the vicious cycle of antisocial occupation continues.

One sheeben patron said:

'I can't get a job, I failed school, its better I come here to drink so that I forget my problems... for the whole day I will at least find someone to buy for me 1 or 2 (beers)...'

Of major concern in many African countries is the breakdown of the moral fiber popularly known as "Ubuntu" or "Unhu" in parts of Southern Africa. The same philosophy is shared in Africa despite different terms used depending on the local language. Ubuntu basically means humanity to others. In essence the philosophy is about social inclusion in the sense that no one should be excluded and everything done by individuals should ultimately be for the good of all in the society (Bangura, 2005; Higgs, 2003). This implies the collective nature of African life that governs participation in positive occupations. In this chapter positive collective occupations are those occupations that people engage in as groups to promote the common good of the society (Fogelberg and Frauwirth, 2010; Ramugondo, 2015).

Another form of an emerging antisocial collective occupation is xenophobic protesting. Anti-immigrant protests that have been reported in South Africa seem to be an unresolved issue. Some migrants were killed in the protests while about 2000 migrants from Malawi, Zimbabwe, Mozambique and Burundi were displaced in the 2015 attacks (South African History Online, 2015). Thousands of foreign nationals residing in the high density suburbs around Durban and Johannesburg fled to refugee camps, their businesses and livelihoods were destroyed which is a disruption of prosocial occupations by antisocial occupations. Xenophobia is a complex issue related to poverty and territorial demands on scarce economic resources. It therefore appears to be a battle of occupations and it necessitates further research by occupational therapists and occupational scientists.

In contrast to anti-social collective occupations, there is evidence of some positive collective occupations that benefit the whole community among poor communities. For example in a rural community in Limpopo, South Africa community members were mobilized to engage in a project for constructing a secondary road for themselves with support from International Labour Organization (ILO) and Council for Scientific and Industrial Research (CSIR) in South Africa (ILO, 2013). There is no evidence of occupational therapist's involvement in this particular project. However, involvement of occupational therapy in such projects can ensure inclusion of community members who might be discriminated for example based on impairments, whereby appropriate tasks will be assigned to accommodate a diverse population. Similarly in Zimbabwe, food for work programmes were introduced whereby in times of famine villagers who needed drought relief food were required to come up with projects. The projects could be constructing and maintaining feeder roads or water control projects like dam and weir construction or rehabilitation. In turn the government would provide drought relief food aid. This approach was taken to prevent a dependency mentality and to promote ownership of community development (Webb, 1995). Collective occupations of this nature can further be promoted or inspired by occupational therapists in similar settings while ensuring that groups such as people with disabilities are also included.

Establishing community groups for parents of children with disabilities can be useful in promoting the social inclusion of the children with disabilities and their families in community development and participation in cultural activities. However, experience shows that such groups need to have a component of meeting basic needs or livelihoods because if people are in poverty they are more driven to participate in activities that can lead to escaping poverty (Chichaya, 2012a; WHO, 2010). This can be illustrated by an example in which mothers could not bring their children with cerebral palsy to a community rehabilitation center as they prioritized seeking for piecework. The moment the centre decided to start offering support with capital for starting small businesses to mothers, attendance improved and the community outcomes were satisfactory (Bowler, 2010). Similarly, the author of this chapter has used community based approaches with parents of children with disabilities an impoverished rural community in Namibia to promote play and social interaction among the children while empowering the parents with practical skills and knowledge on stimulating development of their children.

It is no longer a shame in this small society for a child with disabilities to be brought out of the house or to be seen by other people. In addition, the same group of parents is involved in income generating gardening activities utilizing a communal water point and taking turns to look after their children with disabilities (Chichaya, 2012b). This brings the important factor of meeting the basic need of food without abandoning therapeutic groups for their children in search for food elsewhere. My involvement with this group and similar groups of CBR committees in Namibia reveals some evidence that both parents and children can move towards social inclusion through occupation-based interventions. According to participants in this group, these interventions have also brought dignity to the family members of people with disabilities in this community; they can participate freely in religious and cultural activities within their community. Most importantly the children with disabilities get exposed to the external environment where they can interact with other people, animals and objects they rarely saw when they were kept indoors. As expressed by one of the mothers: 'My child can now associate the sounds of singing birds with the birds themselves, their colors and how they eat and fly'.

Another example of positive occupations is for young people who are engage who run an informal business at an open market in a high-density suburb of Windhoek in Namibia. In an environment of very low employment rates, engagement in positive occupations has resulted in meaningful livelihoods for individuals especially people with disabilities and those with very low education levels who will otherwise face difficulties in obtaining formal employment. The youths from the urban area go to the rural areas to get traditional foods and agricultural products prepared using traditional methods and bring them for sale to the urban dwellers. Most of these food stuffs are natural grains which are healthy compared to processed foods often found in supermarkets. Consumption of these traditional food stuffs can bring positive health outcomes considering that they are natural and healthier sources of nutrition. Unfortunately, many people in Africa are abandoning these foods in favour of processed foods (Udeze, 2009). Most of the processed foods are readily available, do not take time to prepare, are well advertised and look more attractive but their consumption perpetuates the prevalence of non-communicable diseases because of the high levels of fats, sugar, salt, trans-fats and saturated fats (United Nations, 2014).

In this case a group of youths from the urban area go to the rural areas to gather traditional foods and agricultural products prepared using traditional methods and bring them for sale to the urban dwellers. Most of these food stuffs are natural grains which are healthy compared to processed foods often found in supermarkets. Consumption of these traditional food stuffs can bring positive health outcomes considering that they are natural. Unfortunately. many people in Africa are abandoning these foods in favour of processed foods that were introduced during Western colonization (Udeze, 2009). Most of the processed foods are readily available, do not take time to prepare, are well advertised and look more attractive but their consumption perpetuates the prevalence of non-communicable diseases because of the high levels of fats, sugar, salt, trans-fats and saturated fats (United Nations, 2014).

One youthful vendor said:

> *'It is better for me to sell traditional food than stay at home without earning a living...otherwise I will end up stealing so that I can have money for myself...'*

Another example is the use of occupation in a women's support group, in which female occupational therapy students from disadvantaged families in Uganda have been enrolled. In this support group, the students apply their acquired skills about occupation while interacting with other vulnerable women in income generating projects and simultaneously generating income to pay for their education (Awolo, 2015).

Positive occupations relevant to local context and cultural practices are an antidote to prevailing health and social challenges in less resourced settings. Health promoting occupations encompassing what types of food and drink people consume and maintenance of healthy bodies, minds and souls can be used in developing low-cost high-impact interventions. Pressing societal needs that are a result of anti-social occupations should be replaced with positive or pro-social occupations, where the same group of people derive meaning and positive outcomes in occupationally just societies.

How to move forward

Occupational therapists require a strong voice to address global health needs but do not have a strong enough power base to make an impact. This can be developed through successful networks and collaboration with community members, policy makers and other stakeholders. These networks will then be the platforms through which the effectiveness of occupational therapy can be demonstrated and communicated (Brintnell, 2014). In Africa, the involvement of policy makers, government and traditional leaders to properly address occupation as a vehicle for social inclusion is required. Initial steps could be the establishment of policies that support social inclusion and necessary budgetary allocations underpinned by international frameworks such as the Universal Declarations for Human Rights (1948), the UN Convention of the Rights of Persons with Disabilities (2006) and the Sustainable Development Goals (2015). Occupational therapists have an important role in pushing the occupation agenda as a means to social inclusion as well as addressing the social determinants of health (Van Bruggen, 2014).

Proper planning at governmental level is required in many developing countries instead of a focus on lack of resources. For example in Namibia, between 2011 and 2013 a total amount of N$4 billion (approximately US$83 million) was returned to the treasury unutilized by different government ministries (Immanuel, 2015). This money was meant for different community development initiatives, which were not implemented while many people are suffering in poverty. The ministries that returned the most money to the treasury were the Ministry of Agriculture, Ministry of Health and Social Services, Ministry of Education, Ministry of Youth and Ministry of Gender Equality. The main reasons cited for the under expenditure were shortage of staff and poor planning by officials (GRN, 2014). Surprisingly, these are key ministries in addressing the needs of many who are socially excluded.

Some successful examples of influence on government departments for them to ensure inclusive education among children with different needs including children with disabilities have been observed in countries such as Rwanda, Uganda, Namibia, and Ghana through professionals including occupational therapists working for social inclusion (VSO International, 2006). The dimension of addressing advocacy issues with community leaders, politicians, and the local business community calls for increased political awareness among occupational therapists and further skills in social enterprises, poverty reduction and community development.

Often occupational therapists in Africa perceive themselves as apolitical and are hesitant to address the social determinants of health, even though they are frequently faced with the reality of occupational injustice (Chichaya, 2015). From the perspective of politics as a struggle for scarce resources utilizing available power, occupational therapists in Africa need to be political. This is being political, not in the sense of government bureaucrats (big 'P' politics), even though it will be welcome, but in the sense of promoting equality in resource allocation for vulnerable groups of society this is also referred to as small 'p' politics in the political practice of occupational therapy (Pollard, Sakellariou and Kronenberg, 2008).

Social enterprises are an interesting and rewarding opportunity for occupational therapists to utilize occupation to promote well-being and address socioeconomic inequalities (Stickley, 2015). The aim of social enterprise is to empower vulnerable members of the society who are marginalized by providing creative solutions to problems of social exclusion (Organization for Economic Co-operation and Development (OECD), 2013). Therefore, the expertise of occupational therapists in occupation and addressing occupational injustices can be well applied through social enterprises to serve marginalized groups such as people with disabilities, children living on the streets, displaced populations and impoverished communities.

There is some evidence of involvement of occupational therapists in African social enterprises. For example, in Lesotho, Morocco, South Africa, and Uganda occupational therapists have been involved in social enterprises such as piggery, sewing and tuck shop projects for people with disabilities and their families mainly through non-governmental organizations (African Leadership Network, 2015; Stickley, 2015; O'Leary, 2008). Acting as change agents and advocates, occupational therapists in Africa could help marginalized communities in lobbying for planning and funding of social enterprises by governments. In Namibia, the funds that have been returned to the treasury as mentioned previously could, for example, have been used to seed fund social enterprises.

The ObCD framework has provision for use with diverse populations, and occupational therapists can explore and possibly expand the application of this framework in social enterprises. The four phases of the iterative processes of the ObCD framework i.e. Initiating Intervention, Designing, Implementation and Monitoring, Reflection and Evaluation are applicable in designing and running social enterprises (Galvaan & Peters, 2013). Furthermore, the suggested critical questions for each phase are useful in encouraging decision making and guiding the application of this framework among marginalized groups in which the occupational therapists play the roles of facilitators and equal partners.

Other steps that can be taken by occupational therapists in Africa include volunteering. This can be an initial step to provide evidence to governments and communities on the impact of the use of occupation in addressing inequalities and social injustices to promote health and well-being, for example in local municipalities, spending time with the vulnerable and marginalized groups of society. By spending time with such groups, occupational therapists are well positioned to understand the context and needs of the marginalized groups and collaborate with them towards performance of occupations that can promote social inclusion through prosocial occupations. These activities have been done in South Africa, Zimbabwe, Namibia and Kenya but at a low scale and mostly publicized during the celebrations of the World Occupational Therapy Day, and there is a need for scaling these up.

Many African occupational therapists who are working overseas have been trained in countries such as South Africa, Zimbabwe, and Kenya amongst others.

They are a good resource to form coalitions of diaspora volunteers so as to bring their international exposure and skills for social inclusion back to Africa. Such local capacity building approaches are also being explored by the African Union through the African Diaspora Volunteer Corps Project (African Union, 2015). Ultimately, the roles of occupational therapists should be paid roles whereby governments establish structures through which occupational therapy can be provided at population level.

To a greater extent there is need for occupational therapists in Africa to create synergies with community stakeholders in order to harness resources that are already in existence. For example, community playgrounds in some townships of Windhoek, Namibia only need to be modified to allow access for children with disabilities to safely participate in age appropriate play and to socially interact with their peers on equal basis. This will promote playfulness among children with physical and or cognitive disabilities who are often excluded from such outdoor play, as have been seen in some parts of informal settlements in Cape Town, South Africa (Bross et al, 2008).

Recycled materials, and natural materials can be used to create toys and other objects of play sometimes at no cost. Uys and Samels (2010) propose a wide range of toys that can be made from waste cloth materials, wood, everyday objects such as empty tins, old utensils and appropriate paper technology to address problems such as poor coordination; poor hand function and sensory problems as well as stimulating development among children without disabilities in the same community. However, an understanding of the politics of engaging the responsible local authorities to either improve the designated play grounds or establish them in communities where they are absent is required.

Folk tales are an inherent part of most African cultures as a vehicle for teaching young generations about life (Ryan, 2012). African occupational therapists themselves can modify old folk tales in their culture or work with poets and artistes to embed messages about social inclusion and ensuring the creation of just societies through poetry and folk tales. The ObCD framework can also be applied in this context because it involves challenging the routine ways of thinking and doing things so that disadvantaged people make decisions in removing occupational injustices that they face, promoting their own health and well-being (Galvaan & Peters, 2013). Educational dramas on healthy living by, for example, unemployed local youths help raise awareness on addressing the social determinants of health and well-being issues in the communities. In rural Ghana folk media has been successfully utilized in HIV/AIDS prevention (Panford et al, 2001). Furthermore, radio dramas in Tanzania have been found to be effective in effecting behavior change among illiterate population groups particularly if the dramas incorporate cultural values and beliefs of the local communities (Van Slyke, 2008).

Conclusion

There are vast opportunities for occupational therapists to use their understanding of occupation to promote social inclusion in Africa. While it is challenging to find paid employment in these areas, volunteerism can raise awareness of the contributions of positive occupations towards health and well-being for all in communities. Furthermore, expansion of the scope of focus from individual treatments to populations is a necessary mindset shift for occupational therapists in Africa where sometimes the therapeutic gains of therapy are lost because people return to the same unjust society where the problems were initially created. To a greater extent occupational therapy is perceived as a clinical profession and this is an injustice to a profession with such a broad scope. Hence the need for occupational therapists in Africa to utilize their latent skills in promoting social inclusion through positive occupations.

The ObCD framework presents an opportunity to turn aspirations of social inclusion into practical results as evidenced by the encouraging results in South Africa. The training of occupational therapists needs to empower students and practitioners with ways of translating occupational therapy language when communicating with people outside the profession in their local contexts. The use of social enterprises by occupational therapists to address occupational deprivation as a result of poverty, presents another latent opportunity in Africa. There is a critical need for occupational therapists in Africa to document the use of occupation as a vehicle for social inclusion in their local contexts and diverse cultures to create a credible evidence base.

References

African Leadership Network (2015) *African Awards for Entrepreneurship 2015 Recognizes Outstanding Social Entrepreneurs.* [Accessed 30 December 2015 at http://africanleadershipnetwork.com/2015/10/23/aae2015-recognizes-outstanding-social-entrepreneurs/]

African Union (2015) *Mission Report on African Diaspora Volunteer Corps Project Technical Workshop*, Ottawa, Canada, 11-13 May 2015. Ethiopia: AU. [Accessed 17 September at https://au.int/web/sites/default/files/newsevents/workingdocuments/27380-wd-mission_report_on_african_diaspora_volunteer_corps_project_technical_workshop_3.pdf]

Awolo, J. (2015) *Participation in Income Generating Activities to Support Occupational Therapy (OT) Education, Professional Development and Creativity.* Presentation on the 9th Occupational Therapy Africa Regional Group Congress, 10 September 2015, Kampala, Uganda

Bangura, A.K. (2005) Ubuntugogy. An African educational paradigm that transcends pedagogy, andragogy, ergonagy, hentagogy. *Journal of Third World Studies*, 22, 2, 13- 53

Boutayeb, A. (2006) The double burden of communicable and noncommunicable diseases in developing countries. *Transactions of the Royal Society of Tropical Medicine and Hygiene,* 100, 3, 191-199

Bowler, K. (2010) Working together to change lives through a multidisciplinary approach to occupational therapy. in V. Alers and R. Crouch (Eds.) *Occupational Therapy: An African perspective.* Johannesburg: Sara Shorten (pp.80-81)

Bowen, S. (2001) *Language Barriers in Access to Health Care.* Ottawa, ON: Health Canada Publications

Brian H., Cook, S., Taylor D., Freeman L., Mundy T., and Killaspy H. (2015) Occupational therapists as change agents in multidisciplinary teams. *British Journal of Occupational Therapy,* 78 , 9, 547-555

Brintnell, S. (2014) *Seizing the Future: Occupational therapy's readiness for the Global Health Stage.*

Inaugural WFOT Lecture delivered at the 16th World Federation of Occupational Therapists Congress, Yokohama, Japan 18-21 June

Bross, H., Ramugondo, E., Taylor, C., & Sinclair, C. (2008) Children need others: Triggers for playfulness in pre-schoolers with multiple disabilities living within an informal settlement. *South African Journal of Occupational Therapy*, 38, 2, 3-7.

Chichaya, T.F. (2012a) *Factors Associated with Approval and Rejection of Disability Pensions in Khomas Region, Namibia*. Master of Public Health Thesis, University of Namibia

Chichaya, T.F. (2012b) *Report on the Community Based Rehabilitation Training for Hoachanas,Mariental District Namibia*. Unpublished report Ministry of Health and Social Services, Namibia

Chichaya, T.F. (2015) *Occupational Therapy and Politics in African Settings: Who gets what when and how?* Congress presentation on the 9th Occupational Therapy Africa Regional Group Congress, Kampala, Uganda, 9 September

Coppala, D.P. (2015) *Introduction to International Disaster Management*. Oxford: Elsevier

Coussement, R. (2015) Five interesting facts about the Himba. *African Geographic Magazine*. [Accessed 22 November 2015 at http://africageographic.com/blog/5-interesting-factsabout-the-himba/]

Crouch, R. (2010a) The relationship between culture and occupation in Africa. In V. Alers and R. Crouch (Eds.) *Occupational Therapy: An African perspective*. Johannesburg: Sara Shorten (pp.50-59)

Crouch, R. (2010b) The impact of poverty on the service delivery of occupational therapy in Africa. in V. Alers and R. Crouch (Eds.) *Occupational Therapy: An African perspective*. Johannesburg: Sara Shorten (pp.98-110)

Crouch. R. (2010c) What makes occupational therapy in Africa different? *British Journal of Occupational Therapy*, 73, 10, 445

Eide, A.H. and Loeb, M.E. (2005) *Data and Statistics on Disability in Developing Countries. Disability knowledge and research*. [Accessed 12 June 2015 at http://r4d.dfid.gov.uk/pdf/outputs/disability/thematic_stats.pdf]

Essoungou, A. (2010) *Africa's Displaced People: Out of the shadows*. [Accessed 10 January 2016 at http://www.un.org/africarenewal/magazine/april-2010/africa%E2%80%99s-displacedpeople-out-shadows]

Fogelberg D., Frauwirth S. (2010) A complexity science approach to occupation: Moving beyond the individual. *Journal of Occupational Science*. 3, 131–139.

Galvaan, R. (2010) *A Critical Ethnography of Young Adolescents' Occupational Choices in A Community in Post-Apartheid South Africa*. Health and Rehabilitation Sciences: Division of Occupational Therapy, University of Cape Town [Accessed 17 September at https://open.uct.ac.za/handle/11427/10504]

Galvaan, R. and Peters, L. (2013) *Occupation-Based Community Development Framework*. [Accessed 10 October 2015 at https://vula.uct.ac.za/access/content/group/9c29ba04-b1ee-49b9-8c85-9a468b556ce2/OBCDF/index.html]

Government of the Republic of Namibia (GRN) (2014) *Office of the Auditor General: Financial reports*. [Accessed 31 December 2015 at http://www.oag.gov.na/CG_FINREPORT_MAIN.html]

Higgs, P. (2003) African philosophy and transformation of educational discourse in South Africa. *Journal of Education*, 30, 67-94

Immanuel, S. (2015) Permanent secretaries urged to plan properly. *The Namibian*, 29

April 2015 (p.1). [Accessed 17 September https://www.namibian.com.na/index.php?id=136390&page=archive-read]

International Labour Organisation (ILO) (2013) *Construction of Low Volume Sealed Roads: Good practice guide to labour-based methods.* Pretoria: ILO

Joubert, R.W.E. (2010) Exploring the history of occupational therapy's development in South Africa to reveal the flaws in our knowledge base. *South African Journal of Occupational Therapy,* 40,3, 21-26

Kathleen, B., Christiaensen, L., Dabalen, A. and Gaddis, I. (2016) *Poverty in a Rising Africa. Africa poverty report overview.* Washington: World Bank

Kielhofner, G. (2009) *Conceptual Foundations of Occupational Therapy Practice.* Philadelphia: F.A Davis Company

Kronenberg, F., Simo Algado, S. and Pollard, N. (Eds.) (2005) *Occupational Therapy without Borders: Learning from the spirit of survivors.* Oxford: Elsevier/Churchill Livingstone

Lansdown, G. (2002) *Disabled Children in South Africa: Progress in implementing the Convention on the Rights of the Child. Disability awareness in action.* [Accessed 3 January 2015 at http://www.daa.org.uk/uploads/pdf/SA%20Childrens%20report%20.pdf]

Lorenzo, T., Duncan, M., Buchanan, H. and Alsop, A. (2006) *Practice and Service Learning in Occupational Therapy. Enhancing potential in context.* Chichester: Whurr

Moyers, P.A. and Dale, L.M. (Eds.) (2007) *The Guide to Occupational Therapy Practice.* Bethesda, MD: AOTA Press

Occupational Therapy Africa Regional Group (2014) *December 2014 Newsletter* [Accessed 15 October 2015 at http://www.otarg.org.za/Files/Newsletters/Newsletter%20Dec2014.pdf]

Organisation for Economic Co-operation and Development (OECD) (2013) *Policy Brief on Social Entrepreneurship: Entrepreneurial activities in Europe.* Luxembourg: European Commission/OECD [Accessed 17 September at https://www.oecd.org/cfe/leed/Social%20entrepreneurship%20policy%20brief%20EN_FINAL.pdf]

O'Leary, E. (2008) *Twinning the Kingdoms Field Report.* [Accessed 10 January 2016 at http://www.eileenoleary.com/docs/Project_Update_3-08.pdf]

Panford, S., Nyaney, M.O., Amoah, S.O. and Aidoo, N.G. (2001) Using folk media in HIV/aids prevention in rural Ghana. *American Journal of Public Health,* 91,10, 1559–1562

Pollard, N., Alsop, A. and Kronenberg, F. (2005) Reconceptualising occupational therapy. *British Journal of Occupational Therapy,* 68, 11, 524-526

Pollard N., Sakellariou D., Kronenberg F. (Eds.) (2008) *A Political Practice of Occupational Therapy.* Edinburgh, Elsevier Science

Ramugondo, E., L. (2015) Occupational consciousness. *Journal of Occupational Science.* 22, 4, 488–501.

Ramukumba, A. (2014) *Vona du Toit Memorial Lecture: 2014.* Video. [Accessed 18 June 2015 at https://www.youtube.com/watch?v=JYMBdt_nHv0&feature=youtu.be]

Ryan, C. (2012) *Black History Preserved in African Folk Tales.* [Accessed 30 December 2015 at http://www.howtolearn.com/2012/02/black-history-preserved-in-african-folk-tales/]

Sherry, K. (2010) Voices of occupational therapists in Africa. in V. Alers and R. Crouch (Eds.) *Occupational Therapy: An African perspective.* Johannesburg: Sara Shorten (pp.26-47)

South African History Online (2015) *Xenophobic Violence in Democratic South Africa.* [Accessed 28 December 2015 at http://www.sahistory.org.za/article/xenophobic-violence-democraticsouth-africa]

Stickley, A. (2015) *An Exploration of Occupational Therapy Practice in Social Enterprises in the UK.*

Doctoral thesis. The University of Northampton [Accessed 17 September at http://nectar.northampton.ac.uk/7482/]

Thew, M., Edwards, M., Baptiste, S. and Molineux, M. (2011). *Role Emerging Occupational Therapy: Maximising occupation-focused practice.* Chichester: Wiley-Blackwell

Townsend, E. and Marval, R. (2013) Can professionals actually enable occupational justice? *Canadian Journal of Occupational Therapy,* 21,2, 215-228

Twinley, R. (2012) The dark side of occupation: A concept for consideration. *Australian Occupational Therapy Journal,* 60, 4, 301-303

Udeze, B. (2009) *Why Africa? A continent in a dilemma of unanswered questions.* USA: Xlibris Corporation

UNAIDS (2012) *Global Report: UNAIDS report on the global AIDS epidemic 2012.* WHO [Accessed 3 January 2015 at http://files.unaids.org/en/media/unaids/contentassets/documents/epidemiology/2012/gr2012/20121120_UNAIDS_Global_Report_2012_with_annexes_en.pdf]

United Nations (1948) *Universal Declaration of Human Rights.* [Accessed 28 December 2015 at http://www.un.org/en/universal-declaration-human-rights/]

United Nations (2006) *The Convention on the Rights of Persons with Disabilities.* [Accessed 28 December 2015 at http://www.un.org/disabilities/convention/conventionfull.shtml]

United Nations (2014) *Unhealthy Foods, Non-Communicable Diseases and the Right to Health.* Report of the Special Rapporteur on the right of everyone to the enjoyment of the highest attainable standard of physical and mental health, Twenty sixth session. UN General Assembly. [Accessed 17 September at http://www.who.int/nutrition/events/2014_Report_SP_RtH_report_unhealthyfoodsandNCDs.pdf?ua=1]

United Nations (2015) The Sustainable Development Goals. [Accessed 28 December 2015 at http://www.un.org/sustainabledevelopment/sustainable-development-goals/]

Upton, D., Stephens, D., Williams, B. and Scurlock- Evans, L. (2014) Occupational therapists' attitudes, knowledge, and implementation of evidence-based practice: A systematic review of published research. *British Journal of Occupational Therapy,* 77, 1, 24-38

Uys, K. and Samuels, A. (2010) Early childhood intervention in South Africa: Minimising the impact of disabilities. in V. Alers and R. Crouch (Eds.) *Occupational Therapy: An African perspective.* Johannesburg: Sara Shorten (pp.206-231)

Van Slyke, C. (2008) *Information Communication Technologies: Concepts, methodologies, tools and applications.* New York: IGI Global

Van Bruggen, H. (2014) Turning challenges into opportunities: How occupational therapy is contributing to social, health and educational reform. *World Federation of Occupational Therapists Bulletin,* 70, 1, 41-46

VSO International (2006) *A Hand Book on Disability Mainstreaming.* London: VSO UK

Watson, R. and Swartz, L. (2004) *Transformation through Occupation.* London: Whurr

Webb, P. (1995) Employment programs for food security in rural and urban Africa: Experiences in Niger and Zimbabwe. in J. Von Braun (Ed.) *Employment for Poverty Reduction and Food Security.* Washington DC: International Food Policy Research Institute (pp.174-200)

Whiteford, G. (2004) When people can't participate: Occupational deprivation. in C. Christansen and E. Townsend (Eds.) *Introduction to Occupation: The art and science of living.* Upper Saddle River NJ: Prentice Hall (pp. 221-242)

Wilcock, A.A. (1999) Reflections on doing, being and becoming. *Australian Occupational Therapy Journal,* 46, 1-11

Wilcock, A.A. (2006) *An Occupational Perspective on Health.* (2nd ed.) New Jersey: Slack

Wolf, L., Ripat, J., Davis, E., Becker, P. and MacSwiggan, J. (2002) Applying an occupational justice framework. *Occupational Therapy Now,* 12,1, 15-18

World Bank (2007) *Voices of the Poor.* New York: World Bank

World Bank (2014) Nigeria Population, Total. [Accessed 5 January 2016 at http://data.worldbank.org/country/nigeria]

World Bank (2018) *Poverty and Shared Prosperity.* New York: World Bank

World Federation of Occupational Therapists (WFOT) (2004) *Position Paper on Community-Based Rehabilitation.* Forrestfield, Western Australia: WFOT

World Federation of Occupational Therapists (2014) *WFOT Human Resources Project 2014.* Forrestfield, Western Australia: WFOT

World Health Organization (2010a) *Global Status Report on Noncommunicable Diseases.* Geneva: World Health Organization

World Health Organization (2010b) *Community Based Rehabilitation Guidelines: Introductory booklet.* Geneva: World Health Organization

World Health Organization (2011) *World Report on Disability.* Geneva: Author

World Health Organization (2014) *Noncommunicable Disease Country Profiles.* [Accessed 4 January 2016 at http://www.afro.who.int/en/clusters-a-programmes/dpc/non-communicablediseases-managementndm/overview.html]

Chapter 15
Including people with vision impairments in museums

Beaux Guarini and Alison Wicks

cherry tree
even the blind woman
picks blossoms
(Clement, 2006)

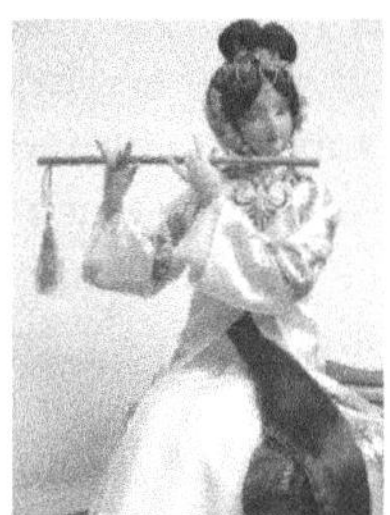
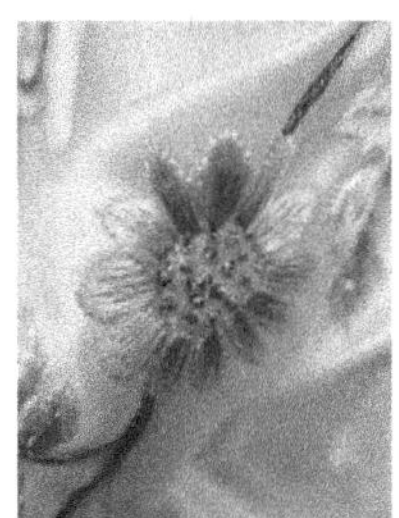
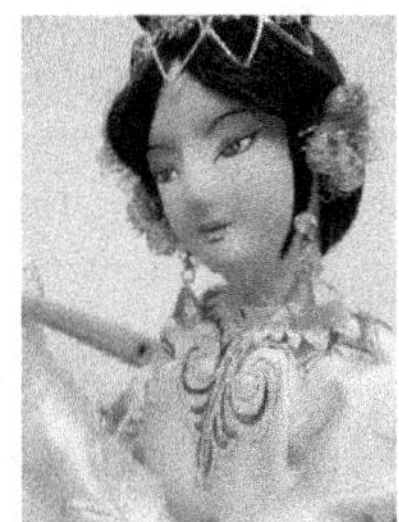
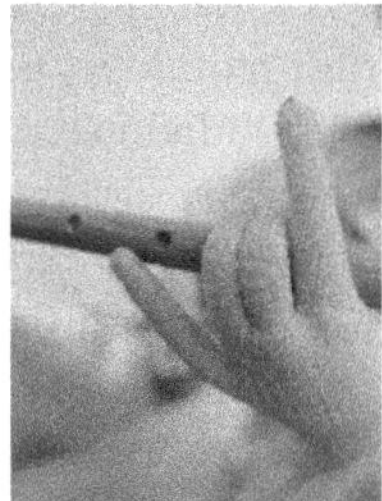

Prologue: The doll's vignette

A Japanese doll, a cultural artefact, is one object in a university's collection of varied and vibrant things. She looks resplendent, dressed in cascading silks of cream and plum. A bamboo flute with crimson tassel is held in her hand. Home is a metal shelf alongside the jagged edges of partially conserved porcelain tea cups.

Like most objects in museums, the bulk of her time is spent in a store room - veiled from public view. Sheltered from intense exhibition lights, fluctuating temperatures and fluxes in relative humidity, the doll remains safe from the spoiling oils of inquisitive human hands.

One sunny day, she is transported to another place...

...Melodic tones of folk song can be heard. The sweet aroma of cherry blossom waft by. An invited audience waits to engage with her, and perhaps with each other?

Soon, a hand moves cautiously toward the doll: reaching out to stroke a soft, delicate robe; a chrysanthemum-studded tiara; and a finely wrought flute. The immediacy of touch reveals something previously unknown or triggers a thing once known but forgotten or, perhaps, an aspiration never shared publicly.

Comfortably seated around a table, adults with vision impairments are entranced by object, melody, scent and conversation. At times, they are wilful receivers of authorised knowledge. More often, they share their own thoughts and opinions. The doll induces reflection and, frequently, laughter.

Introduction

The chapter describes ongoing doctoral research that validates how promoting social inclusion in a museum setting positively affects the health and well-being of adults with blindness or low vision. Conditions affecting sight, whether by birth or through lived experience, are considered in this study as *vision impairments*. Underpinning the case study are the beliefs that all people have a right to participate in a museum and that humans are sensory beings, living in a world of aromas, flavours, sounds, textures and sights. Consequently, we have intentionally set out to evoke the sensory world we all live in by scattering a series of vignettes throughout this chapter. Based on transcripts and field notes from the study, these extracts offer one interpretation of the participants' and objects' experiences.

The chapter is informed by a qualitative-driven pilot study undertaken by the first author. Although excluding the expanded study's ethnographic component of accompanying participants with vision impairments throughout museum exhibitions, the preliminary investigation included group workshops and semi-structured interviews with individual participants. Using objects from the University of Canberra's cultural heritage program in a group setting, the first author was keen to explore the potential benefits that may arise from two-way exchanges between museums and audiences with vision impairments. This interpersonal model is therefore founded largely on the principles of reciprocity. Also respecting the *nothing about us without us* maxim that some espouse (Charlton, 2000; Werner, 1997), the first author makes no claims to be a *disability expert*. Rather, he supports museums which advocate cultural access for all. Cultural accessibility is defined by Joseph Wapner (2013) as:

> '...programs and services [which] are designed to optimize the visitors' opportunities for equal access to the informational content and services offered by organizations to the public.'

The Australian transdisciplinary study involves or is informed by key theorists in the fields of disability and museum studies, museum practitioners, academics and community organisations - their managers and occupational therapists - as well as adults with vision impairments. For the pilot study, the Royal Society for the Blind -Canberra Blind Society- facilitated access to five adult research participants. Serving Australia's capital city, the mission of this not-for-profit organisation is to:

> '...maximise the personal resources and ability of people...whose lives are affected by blindness or low vision, by responding to their needs through care, communication and support' (RSB-CBS, n.d.).

In view of the Society's alignment with the study's focus on social inclusion, it continues to be an ideal partner. Brought together in a single two-hour sensory workshop, held onsite at the Society, participants touched and looked at objects from the University's collection. Opportunities to smell and taste foodstuff as well as listen to music and oral histories connected to the objects were also provided. Group discussions as well as individual interviews were completed soon after the workshop.

Background

An 'inclusive museum' (Sandell, 2002) embodies the features of an inclusive society: tolerance, respect for diversity, social justice, equity and equality (Australian Human Rights Commission, 2013; United Nations, 2000). Representing over 20,000 cultural institutions across 136 countries, the International Council of Museums (ICOM) challenges its members to 'act in the service of society and of its development' (ICOM, 2013, p. 15). Rather than a tick-a-box corporate exercise masquerading as responsible social citizenship, this leading body's commitment to communities can be traced to around the time of the Santiago Declaration (Chile) facilitated by ICOM in 1972 (Giménez-Cassina, 2013). The signatories, all from Latin America, impelled local museums throughout their respective countries (and later globally) to work within their communities to resolve issues of social inequality (Assunção, 2013). Reframing the museum as a socio-political institution in the service of society - one that plays an active role in informing and shaping societal discussions - the champions of the *integral museum* sought to redefine the very purpose of contemporary museums.

The touchstones of an inclusive society offer a stark challenge to museums to attract people frequently excluded from many of the social and cultural aspects of community life, such as people with vision impairments. Across the world, 39 million people are blind and 246 million people experience low vision (World Health Organization, 2014a). In Australia, blindness affects approximately 120,400 people and low vision impacts around 598,600 (Australian Bureau of Statistics, 2009). These figures indicate that 3.4% of the national population has a vision-related impairment. The conventional aesthetics of contemporary exhibition design and object interpretation in museums hamper the participation of people with vision impairments. Many artefacts remain enclosed within glass cabinets safely beyond harm's reach (or we could say arms' reach); low levels of lighting mitigate deterioration of objects but also hinder viewing; and information labels are rarely in large print or Braille or offered as audio guides. By and large, museums continue to privilege people with near-perfect sight (Candlin, 2004).

The wider doctoral study questions the *Do Not Touch* doctrine upheld in many museums today. A close examination of historical museum practices reveals that the contemporary *hands-off* ethos was pre-dated, at least in Britain, by an acceptance of visitors touching, stroking, feeling, rubbing and handling artefacts, specimens, and exotic curios (Candlin, 2010; Cassim, 2007; Classen, 2007; Pye, 2007). In other words, the earliest public museums of the late 1600s through to early 1800s were places for transformative encounters - people touched objects, and in turn, objects touched people. We argue that the contemporary and normative practice of imbuing museum objects with near-sacred status can obstruct people connecting with the collective cultural heritage of humanity. In response, we support a doctrine that invites closer encounters with objects in museum collections, which enable all people to assert their right to social and cultural participation.

However, we rebuff notions that touch alone can reveal to people with vision impairments the varied and vibrant stories of museum objects. Instead, we endorse a range of sensory encounters between audiences and objects, alongside dialogic exchanges between museum practitioners and their audiences. In this form, (new and old) understandings can be acquired, shared, challenged and co-constructed. High-cost technologies such as touch-sensitive digital displays, immersive soundscapes or elaborate light shows are not necessary to ensure such basic cultural rights are met. We claim that the majority of museums already have the capacity to create opportunities for people with vision impairments to engage with collections. Through innovative yet low-cost approaches, where the *intellectual* museum object is also recognised as a *social* museum object (Simon, 2010), museums can provide opportunities for cultural access for all.

Based on participation, rapport and trust, *person-centred* approaches to the social work of museums have been shown to create opportunities for personal reflection and social connection (Simon, 2010; Arigho, 2008; Phillips, 2008). Such participatory approaches use museum objects, including art works, artefacts, specimens, manuscripts and archives, to promote learning as well as provide inspiration and aesthetic enrichment. These are the goals museums usually have for their visitors (Burcaw, 1997). Through these encounters, individuals are empowered to connect with themselves as well as with family, friends, museum practitioners and other members of the community. Some museums, which recognize the potential benefits of linking past memory to present well-being (Arigho, 2008), welcome groups of senior citizens to handle objects for triggering reminiscences. Some universities provide objects to hospitals for therapeutic benefit for patients, such as women with cancer (Lanceley et al, 2012). We suggest that providing opportunities for people to access museum objects through multisensory encounters affords one meaningful way to prise open frequently inaccessible collections.

Mindful of their role as public custodians for future generations, museum staff can be apprehensive about visitors handling objects for fear of damaging collections. This anxiety is exemplified by a director of an Italian art gallery who stated, 'In a globalised world like ours, the fundamental rules for visiting a museum have been forgotten, that is, "Do not touch the works"' (Hall, 2013, n.p.). David Rice (Candlin, 2004, p. 76), chairperson of the United Kingdom's Art Through Touch, holds a contrary opinion:

> 'Being totally blind the only way I can appreciate the national heritage is by touch. You keep saying it's being saved for future generations, well I'm sorry but this is my generation and I need to appreciate my national heritage.'

Given that the *Do Not Touch* doctrine is not as foundational to museum practice as is thought by some experts in the field, we believe the argument against this doctrine is more compelling. The tangible benefits arising from equitable forms of access, safely enacted within a controlled environment overseen by trained museum personnel, outweigh hypothetical concerns for damaging the cultural inheritance of future generations. Without doubt, the right to cultural access is an issue of ethical practice. Museums are obliged to provide people with impairments the same rights to cultural participation as enjoyed by others (United Nations, 2006).

So, while handling objects like the Japanese doll mentioned in the prologue invites social and cultural participation, the museum experience can be augmented with additional sensory encounters. According to Paul Pagliano (2012, p. 6), if people are denied multisensory encounters, then they are 'starved of their own humanity… [as such stimulation]… supplies the very building blocks of who we are and who we become'. Consequently, our sensory encounters affect our identity, which informs us and others who we are and where we belong in the world (Silverman, 2010). Our sense of identity also provides us with a sense of place within our communities. In turn, a positive self-identity contributes to health and well-being. The World Health Organization (2014b) defines health as a 'state of complete physical, mental and social well-being and not merely the absence of disease or infirmity'. Rebecca Jones (2014, pers.comm., 18 December), occupational therapist at the Canberra Blind Society, states that:

> '...in the Maori language there's...[a]...term called *hauora*, which means, essentially, *health and well-being*. [It is] looked at as a house [with] four walls: social, physical, emotional, and mental. If one of the walls falls down, the next one will fall.'

Accordingly, community-based action to address inequalities experienced by people with impairments respects their right to social and cultural participation (Cultural Ministers Council, 2009). We contend that a community and sensory based museum praxis, as the study described in this chapter illustrates, can contribute to the stability of the *hauora* house by supporting the well-being dimensions of health for people with vision impairments.

About the study

The participants

The voices of the five participants in the study are heard throughout the chapter: four women, Helina, Ursula, Mara, and Abbie, and one man, James. At the time of the study they were aged between twenty-five and seventy-five years old. Mara lost all vision over a period of time (adventitious blindness), Ursula was blind since birth (congenital blindness) and James was blinded in an accident. In contrast, Helina lost most functional sight progressively (adventitious low vision) and Abbie experienced substantial loss of vision through injury. All participants were *legally blind* however. Legal blindness is a clinical diagnosis for when a person cannot see at six metres that which a person with normal vision can see at 60 metres and or where a person's field of vision is less than ten degrees in diameter in the better eye (Vision Australia, 2007).

The process

The pilot workshop was held at the office of the Canberra Blind Society. Selected objects from the University of Canberra's cultural heritage collection were transported to the Society's office. Participants sat around a table while the workshop mediator, also the first author, introduced each object to the group. The aim of the mediator was to facilitate free-flowing discussions about each object and, in turn, explore the capacity of objects to spark the sharing of reminiscences and aspirations. Critical to the success of the study was a relaxed, open and supportive environment.

A comfortable setting was achieved, in part, by the mediator distancing himself as the primary holder of *authorised knowledge*. More so, participants were invited to reject notions of themselves as passive absorbers of information. Rather than wear the museum educator or curator hat from the outset, the mediator presented information about each object to participants only on request. The participants, who were encouraged to control the direction of dialogue, generated and sustained thought-provoking and often humorous conversations.

Findings

Humour

Mara's vignette

'In anticipation of handling the Japanese doll, Mara smiles. Pressing her hands slowly forward, she gently grasps the doll's chestnut stained wooden pedestal. With care but conviction, she traces its smoothness before moving on to a ruby tasseled-shoe. While brushing the back of her hand over a petite embroidered motif of a cherry blossom, Mara pauses to gather her thoughts. Her fingers encounter another tassel: this time tiny silver bells hanging from a cream kimono. She gently strokes the garment, moving slowly from ankles to knees to waist. Feeling the doll's thighs, Mara pauses again, but this time smiles and states 'She is a very shy girl…because of the legs'. After she quickly explains that the thighs of the doll are pressed firmly together, in tasteful probity, a peal of laughter fills the room.'

Humour, including risqué quips made in jest, can positively contribute to health and well-being (Cann & Kuiper, 2014). Lucille Nahemow (cited in Harries, 1995, p. 984) describes humour as 'a key element in the human repertoire, so much so that many consider it as a defining human attribute'. Mara's jovial icebreaker helped create a non-judgmental environment centred on trust, rapport and warmth that respected the individuality and personal choices of participants (Arigho, 2008). Throughout the workshop, it was evident that laughter was a powerful means of fostering group cohesion amongst people from differing age groups and genders as well as social and cultural backgrounds.

Reinforcing the ideals of the public museum (ICOM, 2013, p. 15) as a place for 'study, education and *enjoyment*' (authors' emphasis), the response of participants suggested that museums and their collections can be used to support personal edification as well as pleasure. Pleasure is theorised by some cognitive psychologists as an emotional state related to sadness, fear, anger and happiness (Eysenck & Keane, 2010). Museums which, through their collections, empower visitors to create, share and connect with each other (Simon, 2010) facilitate human expression. Laughter is one such universal expression of personhood. The use of humour by participants opened doors to further conversation and, in turn, awakened reminiscences.

Reminiscences

Accepting the premise that knowledge is socially constructed and results in divergent and multiple realities (Bryman, 2012), our understanding of the world is moulded through the interchangeable meanings that we attach to objects and things (Creswell, 2013). A sensory exploration of objects, a vital component of the study, assisted participants to create and share their own meanings as well as embrace new understandings. Augmenting the handling experience, participants were able to handle an Australian Aboriginal *dilly bag* (typically woven from plant fibre) and were introduced to the scent of ground lemon myrtle (an Australian native tree with aromatic and flavoursome leaves). The aroma reminded James of his childhood:

> *'We used to have a passion fruit tree at our old child care centre at mum and dad's. [They] didn't last too long on the vine. We used to put it with vanilla ice cream. It was beautiful.'*

Consistent with the Proust phenomenon, the triggering of memories by specific odours (Eysenck & Keane, 2010), James' wistful recollection induced questions about a youth filled with mischief. In contrast, tasting a rosella (a native bush fruit) reminded Abbie of once living in Fiji, 'I wanted to taste to see if [it was] the same thing. They make jam out of it.' Abbie took centre stage for nearly five minutes, and enjoyed fielding queries on the finer details of Fijian jam making. She demonstrated her skill as a *knowledge expert* rather that being a passive receiver of imparted information.

The participants' comments exemplify the benefits of museum practitioners encouraging two-way exchanges with their audiences. Instead of adopting a top-down communication approach, participants and the workshop facilitator co-created the museum experience. We suggest however that such an organic praxis does not diminish the mystery of the collected object, the cultural authority of the museum as a respected public institution or the knowledge and expertise of museum practitioners. Laura Phillips (2008) suggested in her pilot study of reminiscence work with senior citizens, that museums can use their cultural capital for promoting the development of knowledge, for enhancing creative thought and for building personal confidence. In the same vein, permitting participants to share anecdotes from their own lives enriched the experience of the workshop for all.

Understandings

Each participant wanted to know about the objects being explored: what they were; who made them; when they were made; how they were made; where they were made; and why they were made. They were eager to find out who originally collected the artefacts and why, what made them significant as objects for research and how they were cared for by the university. Such intellectual conversations are not dissimilar to those had by Australian museum curators when assessing objects for possible acquisition (Russell & Winkworth, 2009). Australian curators generally evaluate the significance of objects by contextualising their historical, aesthetic, social, spiritual and scientific research values. Further deliberations may be given to their interpretive capacity, rarity or representativeness, physical condition or completeness in addition to provenance. The final analysis results in a written summary of their meaning, value and importance. Participants therefore instigated many of the same talking points as curators, only less formally. Instead of a stream of information directed at participants, conversations ebbed and flowed in a somewhat naturalistic fashion.

All conversations ultimately led back to the object under exploration, despite participants having license to control the direction of workshop discussions. Consequently, our study suggests that opportunity for intellectual engagement with objects, shared with others, contributes to personal well-being. As stated by James, 'it is good to share [my thoughts] and hear about other people's [ideas]'. The inference is that social and intellectual connection reinforces a positive sense of identity and affirms a sense of place within the community. Nina Levent and Alvara Pascual-Leone (2014, p. xiii) support multilayered museum experiences where the:

> '...end result might be learning, wonder, reflection and relaxation, sensory stimulation, conversation with friends, new social ties, creating of lasting memories, or recollection of past events.'

Intellectual encounters are identified as an integral component of the journey. For that reason, we support a praxis that respects the traditional role of museums as producers of knowledge and acknowledges the contemporary rights of people to challenge or add to those understandings through conversation.

Access

Ursula's vignette

'While the last object was being handled and when conversations from curious minds shrunk to a murmur, a clear voice with conviction rings out. 'I don't go to exhibitions of paintings anymore' says Ursula, 'because I feel too frustrated'. Looking inquisitively around the table, I attempt to gauge the response of participants. 'People can explain [the paintings] until they are blue in the face but...it's not a beautiful experience at all'. Acknowledging the hum of agreement, Ursula continues, 'I remember taking another blind person to the gallery, and after we'd been around half way listening to the audio description of each painting, he said, 'Oh, for God's sake, let's go and have a beer'.'

Defining the concept of *access* was complex and multi-faceted, as exemplified by the group discussion held immediately after the workshop. Echoing the remarks of the Australian Government Cultural Ministers Council (2009), participants also highlighted the frustration of the environmental barriers associated with premises as well as attitudinal and social barriers. Ursula's reflections exemplified all participants' concerns that access to high quality museum services meant more than wheelchair ramps and Braille signage on toilet doors.

When we unpack Ursula's comments, which are consistent with the experiences of other participants, it is apparent she clearly enjoys the social benefits of participating in a friendship group (which includes people with and without vision impairments).

Like other Australians, she is motivated to participate in the cultural life of the nation. Between 20% and 24% of Australians with impairments visited at least one art gallery or museum during 2006 (Australian Bureau of Statistics, 2011) in comparison to around 23% of their sighted peers aged fifteen years old or over (Australian Bureau of Statistics, 2008). Framing the exhibition space as a social and intellectual experience, Ursula expressed her deep frustration when museum hosts or guides (the American *docent*) talk *at* visitors rather than encourage an exchange of ideas. Even with the introduction of technical aids intended to augment visitor experiences, such as handheld and headphone audio guides, Ursula's comments suggest that museums have yet to consistently develop a descriptive visual language which captures the imagination of people with vision impairments.

In contrast, acknowledging that some museum hosts are excellent at conducting *touch tours* for the vision impaired – facilitating access to objects normally forbidden to visitors - Helina was at times disappointed. During some tours, she found herself segregated from her sighted friends. Eager to participate in recreational activities with her peer group, Helina stated, 'It's disappointing that I can't walk around with my friends and they can't experience the same as what I was experiencing'. Like other community members, social interaction is a significant element of the museum experience (Vartiainen & Enkenberg, 2014). Vying with other forms of recreation, some centred on technology and interaction, museums are competing to attract newer audiences while retaining their traditional audiences. Museum practitioners are well aware that their institutions are now part of the leisure industry.

Leisure is synonymous with 'enjoyment, relaxation, rejuvenation or recreation... that enhance people's lives in some way' (Australian Bureau of Statistics, 2006, n.d.). Participants suggest that museums, as sites for recreation and leisure, are more appealing when they provide accessible services. Just as for sighted people, museums can be places where participants connect with peers. They can walk and talk, ponder and laugh and sit down to share a meal. Helina declared that 'one thing blind people have been fighting for years is to be integrated into the normal world.' For Ursula, her presence in the museum makes her visible to the wider community. Partaking in museum events can therefore positively contribute to health and well-being and, perhaps, shatter stereotypes of people with impairments.

Reflections

There were some limitations to the study. For example, while five participants may be viewed as a small sample size, the decision to focus on the perspectives and experiences of a limited number of people is consistent with an in-depth qualitative case study approach (Creswell, 2013). The participants affirmed that the small workshop group resulted in a group dynamism and richness of individual experience that may have been difficult to achieve within a larger group. Going forward, participants felt that workshop groups of five to eight people would be ideal. While the first author's doctoral research is limited to people with vision impairments, participants were open to potential museum programs involving all community members.

An important lesson for the first author, as someone without a vision-related impairment or who did not know anybody with legal blindness prior to the study, was that people with vision impairments wish to be seen as ordinary people. They are everyday people doing everyday things, desirous to participate in the social and cultural aspects of community life. Equally, he came to appreciate that people with vision impairments are not a homogenous group. No two conditions affecting sight offer the same lived experience. For example, people with adventitious blindness may have capacity to recall the visual properties of objects whereas people with congenital blindness do not. Therefore, sensory preferences differ significantly amongst people with contrasting vision impairments. This diversity, in itself, does not negate the identified benefits of promoting inclusive museum practices however.

Conclusion

The case study described how a selection of objects conventionally found in a museum collection positively enhanced the sensory, personal and social experiences of a group of people with diverse impairments of sight. The inclusive *person-centred* approach adopted by the first author as workshop mediator reinforced the message to participants that museums belong to every person in the community, not just sighted people. At the same time, the potential for museums to contribute to the health and well-being of people with vision impairments became apparent during the study. Exploring the mutual benefits of two-way exchanges between museums and conventionally overlooked audiences, we identified social and cultural opportunities latent in the objects collected by museums.

During the study, participants derived particular satisfaction from encountering museum objects through novel means. They enjoyed opportunities to touch, hear, smell, taste and see. Participants also derived pleasure from sharing knowledge through conversations they generated. Compared to high cost technology-driven museum programs, the cost of this study using existing objects from a collection was modest. Comments from participants also reinforced the observation that museum objects can be useful for supporting their health and well-being.

Significantly, the study suggests that museum programs embracing a range of sensory encounters with collections afford opportunities to engage with other community members in a welcoming and supported social setting. While participants in this study shared their memories and listened to stories, often with humorous results, they also at times became *museum experts*. They educated others in the group, including the workshop mediator, about the cultural significance of particular objects. Summing up the benefits of the study, the voice of Mara concludes the chapter:

> *'[Today], we used our sense of smell. We used our sense of thinking, sense of feeling [and] sense of touch. We have only lost our sense for sight but the rest of our senses – they become our eyes now. When this program is running, I'll be there in the museum every week. As long as it's free!'*

References

Arigho, B. (2008) Getting a handle on the past: The use of objects in reminiscence work. in H. Chatterjee (Ed.) *Touch in Museums: Policy and practice in object handling.* Oxford; New York: Berg (pp. 205-212)

Assunção, P. (2013) Introduction: To understand New Museology in the 21st Century. in P. Assunção and J. Primo (Eds.) *Sociomuseology 3: To Understand New Museology in the XXI Century.* Lisbon; Universidade Lusófona de Humanidades e Tecnologias (pp. 5-10)

Australian Bureau of Statistics (2001) *Measuring Wellbeing: Frameworks for Australian social statistics, 2001, cat. no. 4160.0.* Australian Bureau of Statistics. [Accessed 26 February 2015 at http://www.abs.gov.au/ausstats/abs@.nsf/Latestproducts/B8784B639DB52193CA2571B9001E1458]

Australian Bureau of Statistics (2008) *Arts and Culture in Australia: A statistical overview, 2008* (2nd ed.) cat. no. 4172.0. Australian Bureau of Statistics. [Accessed 26 February 2015 at http://www.abs.gov.au/ausstats/abs@.nsf/Products/8B93DE630D02E68BCA2574E90012E7E6?opendocument]

Australian Bureau of Statistics (2009) *National Health Survey: Summary of results 2007- 2008,reissue, cat. no. 4364.0.* Australian Bureau of Statistics. [Accessed 13 February 2015 at http://www.abs.gov.au/ausstats/abs@.nsf/mf/4364.0]

Australian Bureau of Statistics (2011) *Social Participation of People with a Disability 2011, cat. no.4439.0.* Australian Bureau of Statistics. [Accessed 13 February 2015 at http://www.abs.gov.au/AUSSTATS/abs@.nsf/productsbyCatalogue/C6C921A387266B2DCA2578B600134812?OpenDocument]

Australian Government Cultural Minsters Council (2009) *National Arts and Disability Strategy.* Barton, ACT: Cultural Ministers Council

Australian Human Rights Commission (2013) *Social Inclusion and Human Rights in Australia.* Australian Human Rights Commission. [Accessed 10 February 2015 at https://www.humanrights.gov.au/news/speeches/social-inclusion-and-human-rights-australia]

Bryman, A. (2012) *Social Research Methods.* Oxford: Oxford University Press

Burcaw, G. (1997) *Introduction to Museum Work.* Walnut Creek, CA: AltaMira Press

Candlin, F. (2004) Don't touch! Hands off! Art, blindness and the conservation of expertise. *Body & Society*, 10, 1, 71-90

Candlin, F. (2010) *Art, Museums and Touch.* Manchester: Manchester University Press

Cann, A. and Kuiper, N. (2014) Research on the role of humor in well-being and health. *Europe's Journal of Psychology*, 10, 3, 412-428

Cassim, J. (2007) The touch experience in museums in the United Kingdom and Japan. in E. Pye (Ed.) *The Power of Touch: Handling objects in museum and heritage contexts.* Walnut Creek,CA: Left Coast Press (pp. 163-182)

Charlton, J. (2000) *Nothing about Us without Us: Disability oppression and empowerment.* Berkeley, CA: University of California Press

Classen, C. (2007) Museum manners: The sensory life of the early museum. *Journal of Social History*, 40, 4, 895-914

Clement, R. (2006) *Best International Poem, 2006 Winning Haiku*, Vancouver Cherry Blossom Festival, Vancouver. [Accessed 28 Janurary 2015 at http://www.vcbf.ca/haiku-invitational/winning-haiku/2006-winning-haiku]

Creswell, J. (2013) *Qualitative Inquiry and Research Design: Choosing among five approaches.* Los

Angeles: Sage Publications

Cultural Ministers Council (2009) *National Arts and Disability Strategy.* Cultural Ministers. [Accessed 8 January 2015 at http://mcm.arts.gov.au/sites/default/files/arts-disability-0110. pdf]

Eysenck, M. and Keane, M. (2010) *Cognitive Psychology: A student's handbook.* Hove; New York: Psychology Press

Giménez-Cassina, E. (2013) 'Who am I?' An identity crisis. Identity in the new museologies and the role of the museum professional. in P. Assunção and J. Primo (Eds.) *Sociomuseology 3: To Understand New Museology in the XXI Century.* Lisbon: Universidade Lusófona de Humanidades e Tecnologias (pp. 23-37)

Hall, J. (2013) Don't touch the exhibits! American tourist accidentally snaps finger off priceless 600-year old statue in Florence. *The Independent,* 6 August. [Accessed 15 January 2015 at http://www.independent.co.uk/news/world/europe/dont-touch-the-exhibits-americantourist-accidentally-snaps-finger-off-priceless-600yearold-statue-in-florence-8747878.html]

Harries, G. (1995) Use of humour in patient care. *British Journal of Nursing,* 4, 17, 984-986

International Council of Museums (2013) *ICOM Code of Ethics for Museums.* International Council of Museums [Accessed 2 February 2015 at http://icom.museum/fileadmin/user_upload/pdf/Codes/code_ethics2013_eng.pdf]

Lanceley, A., Noble, G., Johnson, M., Balogun, N., Chatterjee, H. and Menon, U. (2012) Investigating the therapeutic potential of a heritage-object focused intervention: A qualitative study. *Journal of Health Psychology,* 17, 6, 809-820

Levent, N. and Pascual-Leone, A. (2014) Introduction. in N. Levent and A. Pascual-Leone (Eds.) *The Multisensor Museum: Cross-disciplinary perspectives on touch, sound, smell, memory, and space.* Lanham, MD: Rowman and Littlefield (pp. xiii-xxvi)

Pagliano, P. (2012) *The Multisensory Handbook: A guide for children and adults with sensory learning disabilities.* London: Routledge

Phillips, L. (2008) Reminiscence: Recent work at the British Museum. in H. Chatterjee (Ed.) *Touch in Museums: Policy and practice in object handling.* Oxford: Berg (pp. 199-204)

Pye, E. (2007) *The Power of Touch: Handling objects in museum and heritage contexts,* Walnut Creek, CA: Left Coast Press

Royal Society for the Blind - Canberra Blind Society (n.d.) *Home - Canberra Blind Society,* Canberra Blind Society. [Accessed 14 January 2015 at http://www.canberrablindsociety.org.au]

Russell, R. and Winkworth, K. (2009) *Significance 2.0: A guide to assessing the significance of collections.* Adelaide: Collections Council of Australia

Sandell, R. (2002) Museums and the combating of social inequality: Roles, responsibilities, resistance. in R. Sandell (Ed.) *Museums, Society, Inequality.* London; New York: Routledge (pp. 3-23)

Silverman, L. (2010) *The Social Work of Museums.* New York: Routledge

Simon, N. (2010) *The Participatory Museum.* Santz Cruz, CA: Museum 2.0

United Nations (2000) *World Summit for Social Development.* United Nations. [Accessed 1 February 2015 at http://www.un.org/documents/ga/conf166/aconf166-9.htm]

United Nations (2006) *Convention on the Rights of Persons with Disabilities.* United Nations. [Accessed at 29 January 2015 at http://www.un.org/disabilities/convention/conventionfull. shtml]

Vartiainen, H. and Enkenberg, J. (2014) Participant-led photography as a mediating tool in object-oriented learning in a museum. *Visitor Studies,* 17, 1, 66-88

Vision Australia (2007) *Deafblindness: Information for families, carers and health professionals.* No place of publication: Vision Australia

Wapner, J. (2013) Mission and Low Vision: A visually impaired museologist's perspective on inclusivity. *Disability Studies Quarterly,* 33, 3, n.p. [Accessed 18 January 2015 at http://dsq-sds.org/article/view/3756/3290]

Werner, D. (1997), *Nothing about Us without Us: Developing innovative technologies for, by, and with disabled persons.* Palo Alto, CA: Healthwrights

World Health Organization (2014a) *Visual Impairment and Blindness, Fact Sheet no. 282, updated August 2014.* World Health Organization. [Accessed 2 February 2015 at http://www.who.int/mediacentre/factsheets/fs282/en/]

World Health Organization (2014b) *Mental Health: Strengthening our response, Fact Sheet no. 220, updated April 2014.* World Health Organization. [Accessed 2 February 2015 at http://www.who.int/mediacentre/factsheets/fs220/en/]

Index

Note: Page locators in *italic* refer to figures or photographs.

adult learning community 80–81, 84
Africa 201–216
  developing social inclusion through occupation 209–211
  marginalised populations 202
  need for social inclusion through occupation 202–209
  non-communicable diseases (NCDs) 202–203
  understanding terminologies 205–206
  see also Algeria; Namibia; South Africa
AIDS 121, 202, 211
  Quilt 121
Algeria 7, 203
Alinsky, S. 118, 119
Alzheimer Scotland 41
Ancient Greece 3
antisocial occupations 81–82, 206–207
Arendt, H. 75, 82, 83, 85, 86, 87
Aristotle 26–27, 85
Arnstein, S. 15, 85
art, participatory
  conceptual foundations overlapping with occupational therapy 111–114
  'Pictures of Trash' 108–111, *109*, 113, 120
asset mapping *194*, 195
Australia
  Men's Shed movement 168–169
  Rose's story 133–137
  see also museums, including people with visual impairments in

Barros, D.D. 37, 87, 107
bathing, different understandings of 205
belonging, sense of 45, 79–80, 82, 135–137
Black Lives Matter 120
Boal, A. 114
Bourdieu, P. 28
Brazil
  Metuia project 119
  'Pictures of Trash' 108–111, *109*, 113, 120
  social occupational therapy 37, 87, 107
  'Theater of the Oppressed' 114
Bruggen, H. van 41, 66, 107, 202, 209

Burgman, I. 40

Capabilities Approach 17–18, 29, 30, 91, 131, 182
capitalist labour 63–65
catadores (trash pickers) 108–111, *109*, 113, 120
Chicago railroad workers' strike 118–119
citizenship 75–90
  context and 87
  dis- 78
  in French tradition 8–9
  idea of 76–79
  inequalities 77–78
  models 76–77
  occupation transforming 79–86, 86–87
  as an occupational practice 79
  participation in political life 85–86
  rights 8, 75, 76, 82
  social inclusion/exclusion and 78, 79, 130, 145
  spaces in which to practice 84–85
  tests for migrants 8
civic society, occupation and rebuilding of 83
Collective Health 61, 62, 69, 71n3
collective occupation 27
  in African settings 206–209
  case studies of transformational change and 79–81, 84, 85
  recognition, equal dignity and 81–83
  a way of doing in world with others 83–84
Colombia, farmers in 79–80, 82, 84
colonisation 5–7
  decolonising imposed occupations 189–197
  and excessive drinking 182–184
  social healing to redress legacies of 185–186
community development, occupation-based *see* Occupation-based Community Development (ObCD) framework
compassion, a lack of 135–137
conscientization 42–43, 48
Cordoba, A.G. 66, 69
critical epidemiology 62
critical reflexivity 42
critical storytelling 101–102
critical theory 117, 119
  in contrast to Dewey's social theory 117–119
  to frame domestic work 93–95
crusades 5
cultural
  accessibility 218, 220

difference and social inclusion/exclusion 5–8, 9, 10–11, 13
influences on people's occupations 186–187
culture of exclusion 135–137

David, J.-L. *109*, 110
Debord, G. 113
dehumanization 82–83
Delors, J. 9
Dementia Friendly Communities 41
democratic citizenship 130
Dewey, J. 28, 45
concept of occupation 114–115
meaning of art 111–112, 113
social thought in relation to critical theories 117–119
theory of education 112–113
dialogue 192–195
Dickens, C. 48
Diggles, T. 32, 44–45, 57–60
dis-citizenship 78
disabilities
attitudes in Africa to 203
community groups for parents of children with 207–208
enabling social participation of children with 40
Mitchell's Plain Workgroup for persons with physical 95–97
prevalence in Africa 202
Rose's story of struggle for recognition living with 133–137
social inclusion and 12–13
Tayberry's activities for people with learning 161–162
see also museums, including people with visual impairments in
disability movement 28, 37
dissociative identity disorder, occupational therapy for a person with 149–155
domestic work, critical race theory to frame 93–95
dop system 183
Dovetail Enterprise 162
drug users, working with 66–67, 69–70
Duchamp, M. 112
Dundee City Council Supported Employment Unit (SEU) 162
Dundee Repertoire Theatre 162
Durkheim, E. 8

Eastern Europe 38–39
ELSiTO European Learning Partnership 44, 45, 46, 48, 49
emancipatory occupation 66–67, 67–69
examples 69–70
ENOTHE (European Network for Occupational Therapy in Higher Education) 38
environment

human flourishing and 30–31
planetary citizenship and 76–77
ergo 25
European Union 7–8, 9, 12
everyday occupations 48, 132
experience, concept of 111–113, 118

farmers in Colombia 79–80, 82, 84
feminist theory 28, 116
Ferguson, E. 149–155
'fifth wave' of public health interventions 156–157, 158
Fluxus 114
foetal alcohol spectrum disorder (FASD) 181–182
colonial history of excessive drinking 182–184
drinking as imposed occupation 186–189
drinking during pregnancy 184–186
health promotion strategies to prevent 185–186
occupational health programme to prevent 189–197
dialogue 192–195
entry into community 191–192
establishing positive occupational identities 195–197
generating solutions *194*, 195
striving for ethical and culturally sensitive behaviour 192
prevalence 184
public health programmes 184–185
folk tales 211
food
project for selling of traditional, healthy 208
for work programmes 207
Fordism 64
'Fountain' 112
France
North African migrants 7
republican ideology 7, 8–9
The Situationalist International 113
Frank, G. 107, 108, 116, 117, 118, 120, 121, 186
Fraser, N. 17, 43, 83, 84, 132, 145
Freire, P. 42, 48, 75, 82–83, 86, 87, 114, 192

Galheigo, S. 66, 79, 87, 98, 107, 192
Galvaan, R. 43, 91, 93, 95, 97, 98, 99, 107, 145, 189, 204, 210, 211
Georgia 38–39
Giroux, H. 117
Golding, B. 168, 177
Gray, J.M. 129, 130, 131, 135, 137, 138, 139

Hamilton, M. 81
'Happenings' 113
hauora house 221
health
  -disease process, social determination of 62
  emancipatory practice and 66–67
  musculoskeletal injuries 68
  non-communicable diseases (NCDs) 202–203
  occupation and ix–x, 29–32, 47
  occupations detrimental to 27
  sensory encounters supporting well-being and 220–221
  social inclusion/exclusion and 11–12
  see also mental health
health services, capitalist need for 65–66
Herzlich, C. 31
HIV/AIDS 202, 211
Hocking, C. 24, 27, 28, 87, 114, 116, 117
Honneth, A. 16, 17, 43, 84, 130, 132–133
Hoskins, B. 76, 77
Human Development Approach *see* Capabilities Approach
human flourishing 29–31, 116
human rights
  citizenship and 8, 75, 76, 82
  occupation and 28, 116, 129, 131–132
  of people with disabilities 12
Human Scale Development 29–30

Ikamva Labantu (IL) 101
imposed occupation 182
  decolonising 189–197
  drinking as 186–189
Individual Placement Support (IPS) model 157, 161
Inform Theatre 162
International Council of Museums (ICOM) 219, 222
Ircland 5, 7

Japan 6–7
Jewish communities 4, 5
Jones, R. 220
justice
  occupation as 131, 138
  occupational 38, 39–40, 41–42, 68, 116–117, 130–131, 188–189

Kantartzis, S. 26, 27, 40, 44, 45, 116
Kaprow, A. 113
Kelley, J. 113

Kelly, B. 13
Kirsh, B.H. 129, 138, 139
Kronenberg, F. 27, 28, 38, 66, 67, 68, 82, 95, 107, 108, 116, 205, 210

Labonte, R. 14, 18
Labour 61
  as a central ontological category of social being 63
  as conceptual basis for occupation-based social practices 67–69
  as distinct from capitalist labor 63–65
  as an element in social determination of health-disease process 62
labour, occupation as an element of social division of 65–67
Lenoir, R. 8
Levent, N. 224
LGBTQ community 121
literacy 48–49
  Pecket project for adult 80–81, 84
Lucas, S. 110
Lukács, G. 63, 71n1
Lyon, A. 156, 158

madhouses 4
manifesto for occupation ix–xi
Marat, J.-P. *109*, 110
Max-Neef, M. 29–30
Men's Shed movement 168–169, 176–177
  Taieri Blokes Shed 167–180
mental health 12
  centres for drug users 66–67, 69–70
  history of confinement for problems with 4
  NHS services 156, 157–158
  occupational therapy case study 149–155
  photography supporting wellbeing and 57–60
  services in the community 40–41, 45
  social enterprise service *see* Tayberry Social Enterprise
  unemployment and impact on 134–135
Mental Health, Social Inclusion and the Arts programme 40
Metuia project 119
migrants 7–8, 40
  domestic workers 93–95
  experiencing a culture of exclusion 136
  xenophobic protests against 206–207
Milner, P. 13
misrecognition 17, 137
Mitchell's Plain Workgroup 95–97
moral consciousness 138
Moral Treatment movement 27

Morrison, R. 40, 114, 116
Moving Forward 158
Muniz, V. 108–111, *109*, 113, 120
Muriithi, B.A.K. 43, 108, 117, 120
musculoskeletal injuries 68
museums, including people with visual impairments in 217–229
  access 218, 224–225
  background 219–221
  Do Not Touch doctrine 219, 220
  high-cost technologies 220
  humour 222
  methodology 221–222
  participants 221
  person-centred approaches 220
  reminiscences 223
  sensory workshop 217, 218, 219–220, 222–225
  touch tours 225
  understandings 223–224
Muslim communities 4, 5, 7

NAMES Project 121
Namibia
  children with disabilities 207–208
  community development funding 209
  community playgrounds 211
  non-communicable diseases 203
  OvaHimba women 205
  project for selling of traditional, healthy food 208
National Social Inclusion Programme (NSIP) 40
Native Americans 5–6
needs, production of 68–69
negative occupations 81–82, 206–207
neighbourhood 11, 46
neoliberalism 12, 65
New Zealand *see* Taieri Blokes Shed
non-communicable diseases (NCDs) 202–203
Nonzamo Seniors' Club 101–102
Norway 114
Nussbaum, M. 30, 45, 91, 116

Obergefell v. Hodges 121
occupation 24–29
  dark side to 27
  as an element of social division of labour 65–66
  manifesto for ix–xi
  societal structures and 27–28

translations into other languages 25–26
understandings of 25–27, 114–115
'occupation as ends' 129, 130, 131, 137, 138, 139
Occupation-based Community Development (ObCD) framework 91–105, 204, 210, 211
critical race theory applied to domestic work 93–95
Mitchell's Plain Workgroup 95–97
Nonzamo Seniors' Club 101–102
participatory methods to facilitate change 98–102
phases 92–93
photovoice methods 98–102
politics of human occupation 95–98
therapists' self-critique 94–95
occupational
apartheid 28, 64, 68
deprivation 39, 68
fulfilment 129, 138, 139
justice 38, 39–40, 41–42, 68, 116–117, 130–131, 188–189
reconstruction framework 43, 107–108, 119–121
science 37–38, 95, 115, 116, 132
older people *see* Nonzamo Seniors' Club; Taieri Blokes Shed
OOFRAS (Occupational Opportunities for Refugees and Asylum Seekers) 40
O'Reilly, D. 10

participation
ladder of citizen 15, 85
in local community development 16
ObCD and facilitating 98–102
political 85–86
social inclusion and 14–15, 39
struggle for social inclusion and occupational 133–137
sustainable 138–139
participatory art
conceptual foundations overlapping with occupational therapy 111–114
'Pictures of Trash' 108–111, *109*, 113, 120
Participatory Occupational Justice Framework (POJF) 41–42
Pascual-Leone, A. 224
Pecket Learning Community 80–81, 84
Pereira, R.B. 98, 129, 130, 131, 137, 138, 139, 145
Peters, L. 43, 91, 92, 93, 95, 97, 101, 189, 204, 210, 211
photo-elicitation interviews 100
photography-based art projects 57–60
photovoice methods 98–102
Nonzamo Seniors' Club 101–102
'Pictures of Trash' 108–111, *109*, 113, 120
Pilgram, A. 15

planetary citizenship 76–77
play facilities 211
Play Strategy 41
political participation 85–86
politics of human occupation 95–98
Pollard, N. 28, 38, 41, 67, 68, 107, 116, 160, 201, 210
positive collective occupations 207–209
poverty 9, 11, 12, 16, 70
  in Africa 202
power
  critical theory and 94, 95, 116, 117, 118, 119
  Dewey's treatment of 118
problematic situations 118–119
public health
  'fifth wave' interventions 156–157, 158
  interventions to reduce FASD 184–185

radical social action 118–119
recognition
  Arendt's concept of 82
  Honneth's theory of 16–17, 132–133
  Rose's struggle for 133–137
  social inclusion as 145
Reilly, M. 37, 114–115
religion and social exclusion 4–5
Rice, D. 220
rights, occupational 39
  see also human rights
Rose's story 133–137
Royal Society for the Blind - Canberra Blind Society 218

Sakellariou, D. 38, 41, 116, 210
Saloojee, A. 130, 145
Scotland
  community-based approaches to social inclusion 41
  NHS mental health services 156, 157–158
  public health 156–157
  see also Tayberry Social Enterprise
Sen, A. 14, 17, 30, 41, 116, 131, 145
sensory
  storytelling 161–162
  workshops 217, 218, 219–220, 222–225
The Shed *see* Taieri Blokes Shed
The Situationalist International 113
situations, concept of 113
slang 48–49

slavery 6
Smart, P. 48, 81
social being, labour as central ontological category of 63–65
social enterprise 43, 156–166, 210
social healing to redress legacies of colonisation 185–186
social inclusion
  approaches to 16–19
  context 10–15
  in context of development 16
  dimensions 18
  history 3–10
  key theoretical framings 145
  northern model of 9
  as a process 15–16
social inclusion, occupation-based
  across micro, meso and macro levels 44–49
  in Africa 202–209
  challenges for practice 137–139
  in context 130–132
  historical overview 36–41
  Rose's story 133–137
  theory and approaches 41–44
social movements 84–85, 119, 120, 121
social occupational therapy 37, 87, 107
  occupational reconstruction and 119–121
  overlapping conceptual foundations with participatory art 111–114
social reproduction 62, 66, 68, 69
social transformation 107–128
  concept of occupation 114–115
  Deweyan practice and critical theories 117–119
  healing in context of 185–186
  occupational reconstructions and 119–121
  in occupational therapy's social turn 116–117
  overlapping conceptual foundations 111–114
  participatory art 108–111, *109*
South Africa
  critical race theory applied to domestic work 93–95
  deaths from non-communicable diseases 203
  education in 204
  Mitchell's Plain Workgroup 95–97
  Nonzamo Seniors' Club 101–102
  positive collective occupation in Limpopo 207
  xenophobic protesting 206–207
  see also foetal alcohol spectrum disorder (FASD)
spaces
  for inclusion 46

in which to practice citizenship 84–85
Spain 4–5
Steinert, H. 14–15
storytelling
critical 101–102
sensory 161–162
strike, Chicago railroad workers' 118–119
Sustainable Development Goals (SDGs) 13, 16
sustainable participation 138–139
Sztompka, P. 167–180

Taieri Blokes Shed 167–180, *179–180*
community contribution 175–176
constructive work and learning 170–172
governance 172–173
health and safety 172
origins 169
research methodology 169–170
social inclusion 173–175
Tayberry Social Enterprise 156–166
activities 161–162
case studies of 163–164
developing 160–163
drumming 160, 161
governance 162–163
performing arts 162
sensory storytelling 161–162
setting up 157–160
staffing 163
training canteen 162
Taylor, C. 16, 17
Taylorism 64
'Theater of the Oppressed' 114
Thibeault, R. 83, 121, 137, 138
Tiao, photograph and portrait of *109*, 110
Todmorden 107
Townsend, E.A. 28, 38, 39, 42, 95, 98, 116, 129, 130, 131, 139, 188
Toyotism 64
toys 211

"ubuntu" 206
Uganda 120, 208
unemployment
marginalisation through 133–137
support for moving out of *see* Tayberry Social Enterprise
United Kingdom

colonisation 5–6, 7
disabled people's rights 12
Mental Health, Social Inclusion and the Arts project 40
NHS mental health services 156, 157–158
occupational therapy case study 149–155
Pecket Learning Community 80–81, 84
reading and writing difficulties 48
see also Scotland
United Nations Convention on the Rights of Persons with Disabilities (CRPD) 12
United Nations Department of Social and Economic Affairs (UN DESA) 12, 15, 16, 18, 45
United States of America 25, 27, 111, 113
AIDS 121
Black Lives Matter protests 120
labour problems 118–119
LGBTQ community 121
Native Americans 5–6

Venkatapuram, S. 29, 30, 31, 138
virtual space 84–85
visual impairments *see* museums, including people with visual impairments in
vocational models of rehabilitation 157, 161
see also Tayberry Social Enterprise
volunteering 210–211

Wapner, Joseph 218
Waste Land 108
Whiteford, G.E. 28, 39, 40, 42, 95, 98, 107, 116, 121, 130, 131, 132, 134, 137, 138, 139, 145, 188, 202
Wilcock, A.A. 24, 26, 28, 31, 38, 39, 69, 84, 95, 116, 129, 130, 131, 132, 137, 181, 189, 201, 204
'Woman Ironing (Isis)' 110
World Federation of Occupational Therapists 68
World Health Organization (WHO) 11, 12, 16, 28, 29, 31, 39, 184, 185, 202, 203, 204, 207
World Summit for Social Development (WSSD) 1995 9, 15

Zimbabwe 207

www.ingramcontent.com/pod-product-compliance
Lightning Source LLC
Chambersburg PA
CBHW081431270326
41932CB00019B/3169
9781861776044